MICROBIOLOGY RECALL

RECALL SERIES EDITOR

LORNE H. BLACKBOURNE, MD FACS
Fellow, Trauma/Surgical Critical Care
Department of Surgery
University of Miami
Jackson Memorial Hospital
Miami, Florida

MICROBIOLOGY RECALL

EDITORS

ALFA OMAR DIALLO
Class of 2004
University of Virginia School of Medicine
Charlottesville, Virginia

VINAY CHANDRASEKHARA
Class of 2004
University of Virginia School of Medicine
Charlottesville, Virginia

ASSOCIATE EDITORS

MATTHEW O'CONNOR
Class of 2004
University of Virginia School of Medicine
Charlottesville, Virginia

ROURKE M. STAY
Class of 2004
University of Virginia School of Medicine
Charlottesville, Virginia

FACULTY REVIEWING EDITOR

JULIE D. TURNER, PhD
Department of Microbiology
University of Virginia School of Medicine
Charlottesville, Virginia

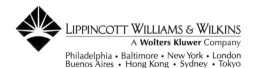

LIPPINCOTT WILLIAMS & WILKINS
A **Wolters Kluwer** Company
Philadelphia • Baltimore • New York • London
Buenos Aires • Hong Kong • Sydney • Tokyo

Editor: Neil Marquardt
Managing Editor: Emilie Linkins
Marketing Manager: Scott Lavine
Production Editor: Christina Remsberg
Compositor: TechBooks Inc.
Printer: RR Donnelly-Crawfordsville

Library of Congress Cataloging-in-Publication Data

CIP data has been requested from the Library of Congress and is available upon request.

Dedication

To my parents who instilled in me a passion for life and who gave me a personal standard to which I aspire.

Alfa Omar Diallo

To my parents and my sister whose endless love and spiritual guidance empowered me to follow my passion.

Vinay Chandrasekhara

Contents

SECTION IV
PARASITOLOGY

SECTION V
IMMUNOLOGY

SECTION VI
ORGAN SYSTEM

SECTION VII
APPENDICES

Contributing Authors

Madeline Adams, Medical Student, Class of 2004, University of Virginia School of Medicine

Sarah Bass, Medical Student, Class of 2004, University of Virginia School of Medicine

Julian Bick, Medical Student, Class of 2004, University of Virginia School of Medicine

R. Elaine Bucheimer, MD/PhD Candidate, University of Virginia School of Medicine

Paris Butler, Medical Student, Class of 2004, University School of Medicine

Rachel Clingenpeel, Medical Student, Class of 2004, University of Virginia School of Medicine

Stephen R. Collins, Medical/M. S. Student, Class of 2005, University of Virginia School of Medicine

Diana Diesen, Medical Student, Class of 2004, University of Virginia School of Medicine

Michelle Dunn, Medical Student, Class of 2004, University of Virginia School of Medicine

Lisa Edsall, Medical Student, Class of 2004, University of Virginia School of Medicine

Chloé Estrera, Medical Student, Class of 2004, University of Virginia School of Medicine

Dayna Finkenzeller, Medical Student, Class of 2004, University of Virginia School of Medicine

John H. Flint, Medical Student, Class of 2004, University of Virginia School of Medicine

Aaron M. Freilich, Medical Student, Class of 2004, University of Virginia School of Medicine

Leo M. Gazoni, MD, Resident, Department of Surgery, University of Virginia Health System

Ali Reza Gohari, Medical Student, Class of 2004, University of Virginia School of Medicine

Christopher P. Ho, Medical Student, Class of 2004, University of Virginia School of Medicine

Joseph A. Jackson, Medical Student, Class of 2004, University of Virginia School of Medicine

Owen N. Johnson III, Medical Student, Class of 2004, University of Virginia School of Medicine

Shawn Kapoor, Medical Student, Class of 2004, West Virginia School of Osteopathic Medicine

Sohah N. Iqbal, Resident, Department of Internal Medicine, New York-Presbyterian Hospital, Columbia University Medical Center

Adnan Malik, Medical Student, Class of 2004, University of Virginia School of Medicine

Farnaz Milani Gazoni, Medical Student, Class of 2004, University of Virginia School of Medicine

Randall T. Myers, Medical Student, Class of 2004, University of Virginia School of Medicine

Matt O'Connor, Medical Student, Class of 2004, University of Virginia School of Medicine

Justin Rackley, Medical Student, Class of 2004, University of Virginia School of Medicine

Mark Sawyer, Medical Student, Class of 2004, University of Virginia School of Medicine

Sebastian Schubl, Medical Student, Class of 2004, University of Virginia School of Medicine

Anne H. Smith, Medical Student, Class of 2004, University of Virginia School of Medicine

Amita Sudhir, Medical Student, Class of 2004, University of Virginia School of Medicine

Mukta Srivastava, Medical Student, Class of 2004, University of Virginia School of Medicine

Matthew P. Traynor, Medical Student, Class of 2004, University of Virginia School of Medicine

Patrick L. West, Medical Student, Class of 2004, University of Virginia School of Medicine

James M. Winger, Medical Student, Class of 2004, University of Virginia School of Medicine

Rebecca Youkey, Medical Student, Class of 2004, University of Virginia School of Medicine

Faculty Reviewers

Jay C. Brown, PhD, Professor of Microbiology, Department of Microbiology, University of Virginia School of Medicine

Kevin Hazen, PhD (ABMM), Professor of Pathology and Microbiology, Department of Medical Pathology, University of Virginia School of Medicine

Robert J. Kadner, PhD, Professor of Microbiology, Department of Microbiology, University of Virginia School of Medicine

Julie D. Turner, PhD, Assistant Professor of Microbiology, Department of Microbiology, University of Virginia School of Medicine

Manuscript Reviewers

Lippincott Williams and Wilkins acknowledges the following people who served as manuscript reviewers:

Matt Jackson, Department of Immunology and Microbiology, Wayne State University School of Medicine, Detroit, Michigan

Johann Farley, Medical College of Wisconsin, Racine Family Practice, All Saints Healthcare System, Racine, Wisconsin

Miguel del Mazo, Class of 2005, Emory University School of Medicine, Atlanta, Georgia

Leslie-Ann Williams, Class of 2006, Wayne State University School of Medicine, Detroit, Michigan

Figure Acknowledgments

Used by permission of University of Virginia: Figures 1-2, 1-3; 3-1; 4-2, 4-3; 5-1, 5-2, 5-3; 6-1; 7-1, 7-5; 9-1; 10-1; 11-2; 12-1, 12-2; 14-1; 15-1; 18-1; 22-2; 32-2; 33-7, 33-8, 33-9; 35-1, 35-2, 35-3, 35-5, 35-6; and Color Photo 10

Used by permission from Koneman EW, Allen SD, Janda WM, Schreckenberger PC, and Winn WC, Jr.: *Color Atlas and Textbook of Diagnostic Microbiology*, 5th edition. Philadelphia, Lippincott Williams & Wilkins, 1997. Figures 4-1, 6-2; 7-7; 11-1; 22-1; 23-2; 27-1; 30-4; 32-4; 33-2, 33-3, 33-5, and 33-7

Used by permission from Strohl WA, Rouse H, Fisher BD, *Lippincott's Illustrated Reviews: Microbiology* (Harvey RA, Champe PA, Series Editors). Philadelphia, Lippincott Williams & Wilkins, 2001. Figures: 7-3, 7-4, 7-6; 8-1; 10-2; 13-1; 15-2; 21-1, 21-2; 22-3; 33-4, 33-6

Used by permission from Rubin ER, Farber, JL, eds. *Pathology*, 3rd edition. Philadelphia, Lippincott Williams & Wilkins, 1999. Figure 28-1

Foreword

I hear and I forget.
I see and I believe.
I do and I understand.
—Confucius (551–479 B.C.)

Action uncovers understanding; an active process of study is endorsed by the editors of *Microbiology Recall* for medical students approaching USMLE Step I. If a student is actively engaged in replying, responding, and even retorting to a series of questions, then I believe that student will learn, digest material, and grow in his or her mastery of the subject. True mastery of the academic framework of knowledge laid in medical school will occur when it is questioned and contorted, separated and sifted, to the further edification of the student.

As I page through the content of this book, I am struck by the level of collaboration and clarity of communication attained by the student writers. This team—directed by Alfa Diallo and Vinay Chandrasekhara—approach their material from a vantage point unique to study guides: recent USMLE experience (Step I), current academic exposure to microbial etiologies, and relevant clinical encounters on the wards. The benefit of their career stage is clear: a high-yield approach to studying with rapid-fire queries stocked with pithy, positive feedback.

Microbiology Recall is a straightforward engagement with bacteria, viruses, fungi, and parasites. It is my hope that readers find themselves pulled into the discipline, actively questioning the causes of disease in the twenty-first century. Such action will uncover understanding, and understanding will drive us to new cures for old diseases.

Julie Davis Turner, PhD
Department of Microbiology
University of Virginia
Charlottesville, Virginia

Preface

This book was started during our third year of medical school, after having just completed our microbiology course and taken Step I of the USMLE. It was written with the primary goal of creating a student-to-student study aid that is high-yield, concise, and overseeable, and that can serve as a microbiology companion guide for class, exam preparation, and the wards.

The book is structured in such a way as to provide the reader with valuable bite-sized bits of information when only a few minutes are available, as well as the opportunity to fully grasp a given topic when there is more time.

We suggest that you use this guide as an adjunct to your class. Consider reading the Recall section you will cover in your notes or in class to "prestudy," and again after you have covered the material in your class. As test time nears, consider using the book to quiz classmates in small, power-review sessions. This book covers clinical pearls, so you may find the book useful as a quick review to brush up on infectious diseases, including their clinical presentation and management while on the wards.

To enhance your ability to pinpoint information, we have included the following icons in the text:

 refers to high-yield information that is commonly tested on Steps 1 and 2 of the USMLE.

 denotes "memory aids" that will help you learn the information faster.

 designates "clinical correlations" that are useful for the wards.

Microbiology is a fact-driven subject, for which repetition is the key to success. For this reason, try limiting yourself to a few study aids but know them well. When test time comes around, you'll remember, "Oh, it was that mnemonic on the bottom left of the page." By sticking to a few high-yield sources, "taking a sip of water out of the microbiology fire hydrant" will be easier.

Best of luck,
Alfa and Vinay

Section I

Bacteriology

1

Bacterial Structure, Growth, and Metabolism

GENERAL

What three shapes do most bacteria assume?

1. Cocci (spheres)
2. Bacilli (rods)
3. Spirochetes (spirals)

What are three configurations of cocci?

1. Staphylococci (clusters)
2. Streptococci (chains)
3. Diplococci (doublets) (see Fig. 1-1)

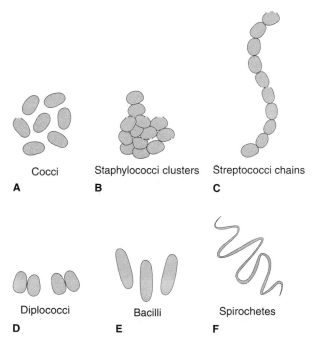

Cocci

A

Staphylococci clusters

B

Streptococci chains

C

Diplococci

D

Bacilli

E

Spirochetes

F

Figure 1-1. A-F. Appearance of bacteria and cocci.

What are pleomorphic bacteria?

Bacteria that do not have a defined shape

What is one example?

Mycoplasma, which lacks cell walls

What is the average size of a bacterium?	1 to 5 microns (μm) in diameter
How does this compare to viruses and eukaryotic cells?	100 times larger than a virus 10 times smaller than a eukaryotic cell

CELL ENVELOPE

What is the cell envelope?	The material external to and enclosing the cytoplasm
What are the two main functional layers of the cell envelope?	Cell membrane and cell wall
What is the cell membrane made of?	Phospholipid bilayer and proteins
What is the main component of the cell wall?	Peptidoglycan (murein), which forms a cross-linked mesh
What is the "peptido" portion of the peptidoglycan made of?	Short string of amino acids
What is the "glycan" portion of the peptidoglycan made of?	Alternating monosaccharides N-acetylglucosamine (NAG) and N-acetylmuramic acid (NAM) forming the "back bone" of the mesh
How is the peptidoglycan mesh formed?	Amino acids cross-link glycan backbones (NAG and NAM) at NAM subunits
What is the purpose of the peptidoglycan mesh?	Determines cell shape and size and provides stability against lysis
Which two bacterial genera do not contain peptidoglycan?	1. *Mycoplasma* 2. *Chlamydia*
What stain is used for microscopic identification of peptidoglycan in bacterial cell walls?	Gram stain
What two categories of bacteria are delineated by this stain?	1. Gram-positive, which appear purple (thick wall, retains dye) (see Fig. 1-2) 2. Gram-negative, which appear pink (thin wall, dye washes out) (see Fig. 1-3)

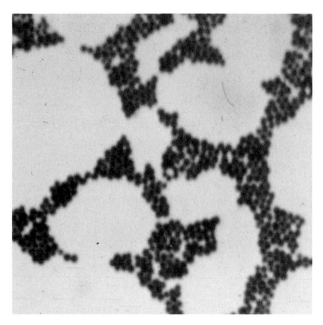

Figure 1-2. Gram-positive bacteria (see also Color Photo 1).

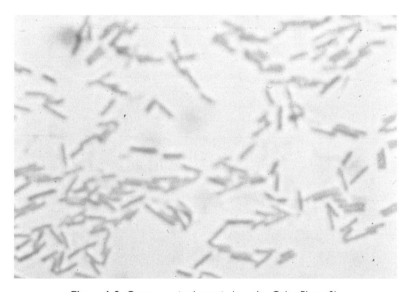

Figure 1-3. Gram-negative bacteria (see also Color Photo 2).

What are the five steps of a Gram stain reaction?

1. Heat fix specimen to slide, add crystal violet, let react for 1 minute, rinse slide
2. Add iodine, let react for 1 minute, rinse slide

3. Decolorize with acetone or alcohol, rinse with water
4. Add safranin counterstain rinse with water
5. Blot dry, and visualize under microscope (see Fig. 1-4)

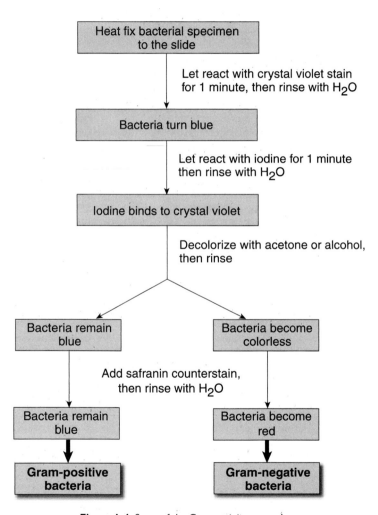

Figure 1-4. Steps of the Gram staining procedure.

What are two components of a Gram-positive cell wall?

Teichoic acid and a thick, multilayered peptidoglycan layer (see Fig. 1-5A)

What is teichoic acid?

Why is it significant?

Glycerol polymers that are bonded covalently to peptidoglycan and lipids
1. Involved in adherence of bacteria to host cells
2. Serves as a cell surface antigen
3. Promotes inflammatory response

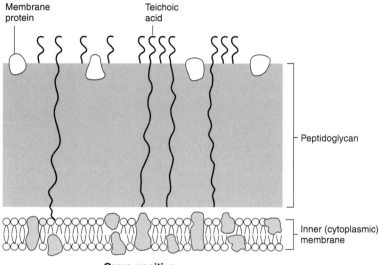

Gram-positive

A

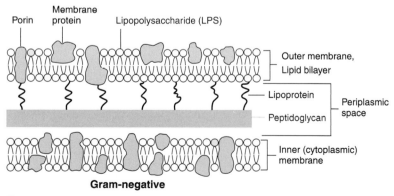

Gram-negative

B

Figure 1-5. A. Gram-positive bacteria have cell walls containing a thick peptidoglycan layer and teichoic acid. B. Gram-negative bacteria have cell walls with multiple layers, including an outer layer containing the LPS endotoxin and the periplasmic space containing enzymes that confer antibiotic resistance.

What are the five components of a gram-negative cell wall in order from external to internal layer?

1. Outer membrane
2. Lipoprotein
3. Thin peptidoglycan layer
4. Periplasmic space
5. Inner (cytoplasmic) membrane (see Fig. 1-5B)

What makes up the outer membrane?

Lipid bilayer with embedded lipopolysaccharides (LPS) and proteins

What is the antigenic portion of the lipopolysaccharide of the outer membrane?

O-polysaccharide

Why is it important?

Highly antigenic virulence factor used to identify species and strains

What is the toxic lipid portion of the lipopolysaccharide of the outer membrane?

Lipid A (endotoxin)

What makes this virulent to humans?

Activates complement and coagulation pathways and induces secretion of tumor necrosis factor (TNF) and interleukin-1 (IL-1)

What does lipoprotein do?

Links the peptidoglycan with the outer membrane

What is the periplasmic space?

Space between the inner and outer membranes

What is contained within the periplasmic space?

1. Peptidoglycan layer
2. Penicillin-binding proteins
3. Hydrolytic enzymes (including β lactamases)

What are three external components of the cell envelope?

1. Polysaccharide coating
2. Flagella
3. Pili

What is the adhesive, viscous polysaccharide coating external to the cell wall?

Capsule or glycocalyx

What is the coating called if it is tightly bound to the cell and organized?

Capsule

What is the coating called if it is loosely bound to the cell and amorphous?

Glycocalyx

What is the purpose of a capsule or glycocalyx?

1. Adherence to surfaces
2. Protection from antibodies and phagocytosis
3. Barrier against some antibiotics

What laboratory test is used to detect organisms with a capsule?

Quellung reaction

How is it performed?

Mix antiserum with capsular polysaccharides, resulting in swelling of the capsule

What are two kinds of appendages that project from the cell wall?

Flagella and pili

What are some characteristics of each?

Flagella are highly antigenic tubular structures that rotate to propel bacteria toward chemotactic stimuli
Pili promote attachment to other cells and are shorter than flagella

CYTOPLASM

What are the components of the cytoplasm?

Amorphous fluid with enzymes, ions, metabolites, ribosomes and a nucleoid

What is the bacterial nucleoid?

A concentration of single circular double-stranded deoxyribonucleic acid (DNA), ribonucleic acid (RNA), RNA polymerase, and other proteins without a nuclear membrane

What is the purpose of a ribosome?

Protein synthesis

What are the ribosomal subunits in bacteria?

30S and 50S subunits, which combine to form a 70S ribosome

Why are bacterial ribosomes important in antibiotic treatment?

Antibiotics may be specifically targeted for bacterial ribosomes, which are different from human ribosomes that combine to form 80S complexes, thereby impairing protein synthesis and causing death or stasis of bacteria without affecting human cells

What are plasmids?

Small, circular, double-stranded DNA molecules capable of self-replication frequently containing genes that convey antibiotic resistance or toxin production

How are plasmids different than transposons?

Plasmids are capable of self-replication

SPORES

What are spores?

Metabolically dormant, protected bodies highly resistant to heat, desiccation, and chemicals, and are capable of germinating and establishing colonies

Why are spores formed?

Adaptive mechanism to survive adverse environments such as excess heat, cold, or conditions lacking sufficient nutrients

What confers resistance to heat?

Thick keratin coat containing calcium dipicolinate and a low water content

When do spores germinate?

When they are exposed to appropriate nutrients and water

Which two gram-positive rods produce spores?

Bacillus and Clostridium

BACTERIAL GROWTH

How do bacteria reproduce?

Binary fission

What are the four stages of growth?

1. Lag phase
2. Log (Exponential) phase
3. Stationary phase
4. Death phase (see Fig. 1-6)

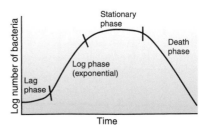

Figure 1-6. The four phases of bacterial growth.

Which phase corresponds with ...	
Cells adapting to a new environment?	Lag phase
Constant rate of cell doubling?	Log (Exponential) phase
Balance of bacterial growth and death?	Stationary phase
Accumulation of toxic metabolites or lack of nutrients?	Death phase
What are heterotrophs?	Bacteria requiring organic compounds for growth
Which element do all heterotrophs require for growth?	Organic carbon
What are autotrophs?	Bacteria capable of synthesizing organic compounds from carbon dioxide, eliminating a need for preformed organic compounds for growth
What are obligate intracellular bacteria?	Bacteria that must invade host cells in order to survive and replicate
Name four obligate intracellular bacteria	1. *Rickettsia* 2. *Chlamydia* 3. *Coxiella* 4. *Ehrlichia*
What are facultative intracellular bacteria?	Bacteria that can survive either inside or outside a cell
Name seven facultative intracellular bacteria	1. *Listeria monocytogenes* 2. *Salmonella typhi* 3. *Yersinia* 4. *Legionella* 5. *Brucella* 6. *Francisella tularensis* 7. *Mycobacterium*
What gas requirement can be used to categorize bacteria?	Dependence for oxygen

What are bacteria that can grow in the presence of oxygen called?

Aerobes

What are bacteria that require oxygen for growth called?

Obligate aerobes

Why do these organisms require oxygen?

Obligate aerobes must use oxygen as the terminal electron acceptor in energy production

What are bacteria that grow in the presence or absence of oxygen called?

Facultative anaerobes

What is their oxygen preference?

True facultative anaerobes prefer to use oxygen as the terminal electron acceptor but do not require it for survival

What are bacteria that require or tolerate oxygen at lower than atmospheric pressures called?

Microaerophilic

What are bacteria that prefer or require carbon dioxide at higher than atmospheric pressures called?

Capnophilic

What is an example?

Neisseria

What are bacteria that can grow without oxygen called?

Anaerobes

What are bacteria that grow only in the absence of oxygen called?

Obligate anaerobes

What enzymes are present in aerobes that are not present in anaerobes?

Either superoxide dismutase, catalase, peroxidase, or all three

What reaction does superoxide dismutase catalyze?

Conversion of free radical superoxide and hydrogen to hydrogen peroxide and oxygen

$$2O_2{}^* + 2H^+ \rightarrow H_2O_2 + O_2$$

What reaction does catalase catalyze?

Conversion of hydrogen peroxide to water and oxygen

$$2\ H_2O_2 \rightarrow 2H_2O + O_2$$

What reaction does peroxidase catalyze?

Conversion of hydrogen peroxide to water and a hydroxide compound

$$RH + H_2O_2 \rightarrow ROH + H_2O$$
(see Table 1-1)

Table 1-1.   Oxygen Requirements of Typical Bacteria

Oxygen Usage	Bacterial Examples
Obligate aerobes	*Pseudomonas* spp., *Mycobacterium tuberculosis, Mycoplasma* spp., *Nocardia, Bordetella pertussis, Francisella tularensis, Brucella* spp.
Obligate anaerobes (Moderate)	*Bacteroides fragilis, Clostridium perfringens, Fusobacterium nucleatum*
Obligate anaerobes (Strict)	*Clostridium haemolyticum, Clostridium tetani, Clostridium difficile, Clostridium novyi* type B *Treponema denticola: Prevotella-Porphyromonas*
Facultative anaerobes	*Escherichia coli, Enterococcus, Salmonella, Shigella, Staphylococcus aureus,* coagulation-negative *Staphylococcus* spp., *Yersinia, Haemophilus* spp., *Actinobacillus* spp., *Bacillus anthracis, Bacillus cereus, Corynebacterium* spp., *Listeria monocytogenes, Erysipelothrix*
Microaerophilic	*Campylobacter jejuni, Helicobacter pylori, Streptococcus pyogenes, Streptococcus pneumoniae*

Can be both facultative anaerobes AND strict anaerobes: *Actinomyces, propionibacterium, lactobacillus;* Treponemes were once thought to be strict anaerobes; however, recently they have been shown to use glucose oxidatively; Streptococci are often listed as "facultative anaerobes," however these organisms are Catalase-negative and often grow poorly in the presence of oxygen.

ENERGY PRODUCTION AND METABOLISM

What are the three categories of metabolism?

1. Aerobic respiration
2. Anaerobic respiration
3. Fermentation

What form of energy is produced?

Adenosine triphosphate (ATP)

How is energy produced by respiration?

Oxidative phosphorylation

Where does this take place?

Cell membrane, because prokaryotic bacterial cells lack mitochondria and other organelles

What compound serves as the final electron acceptor in electron chain transport in aerobic respiration?

Oxygen

What compound serves as the final electron acceptor in electron chain transport in anaerobic respiration?

Inorganic compounds, e.g., nitrate, sulfate, and carbon dioxide

What is fermentation?

Breakdown of a monosaccharide (glucose, galactose, and maltose) to pyruvic acid, which is usually converted to lactic acid or other organic end products

How is energy produced by fermentation?

Substrate-level phosphorylation

What compound serves as the final electron transporter in fermentation?

Organic compounds that are formed from the breakdown of monosaccharides

2

Bacterial Genetics

GENERAL

**What are four differences
between prokaryotes and
eukaryotes?**

1. Prokaryotes lack nuclei and
   membrane-bound organelles
2. Prokaryotes have a single chromosome
   while eukaryotes have multiple linear
   chromosomes
3. Prokaryotes have cell walls while most
   eukaryotes lack cell walls
4. Prokaryotes do not multiply by sexual
   reproduction, but many eukaryotes
   reproduce sexually

**Are bacteria prokaryotes or
eukaryotes?**

Prokaryotes

**What does the bacterial
genome consist of?**

1. Linear or circular double-stranded
   deoxyribonucleic acid (DNA)
   chromosomes
2. Plasmids
3. Bacteriophage (see Fig. 2-1)

What is a nucleoid?

Another term for bacterial chromosomal
DNA

**What does the chromosome
contain?**

All the essential genes for bacterial
survival

**What is the ploidy of
bacterial DNA?**
  What does this mean?

Haploid

Haploid cells contain one set of
chromosomes

**What is the average
genome size of bacterial
DNA?**
  **How does this compare
  to the average genome
  size of eukaryotes?**

0.876–8 million base pairs (Mbp)

Much smaller than eukaryotic DNA,
which is typically 500 times greater than
bacterial DNA

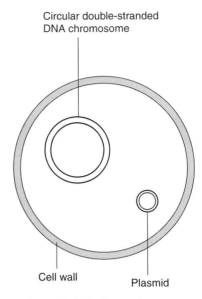

Figure 2-1. The bacterial genome.

Where is DNA located in bacteria?	Within the cytoplasm because bacteria lack membrane-bound nuclei
What is found in eukaryotic DNA but not in bacterial DNA?	Histones and nucleosomes
What are plasmids?	Small extrachromosomal segments of circular DNA
What do they contain?	May contain transposons and genes encoding for toxins, antibiotic resistance, and proteins that promote transfer of the plasmid to other cells
What are transposons?	Mobile DNA sequences that can move from plasmid to plasmid and/or from plasmids to chromosomal or bacteriophage DNA

DNA REPLICATION

What is the name for the special sequence of DNA that is required for replication in prokaryotic cells?	Replication origin, also known as "ori"

How many replication origins (ori) are present in bacterial DNA?	One
What is the name for the region of DNA that contain these sequences?	Replicons
What enzymes are important for adding DNA base pairs during replication?	DNA polymerases
In which direction do they work?	Bidirectionally, but always 5' → 3' (see Fig. 2-2)

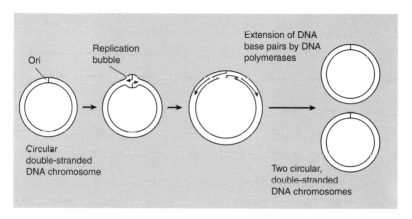

Figure 2-2. Bidirectional replication of circular DNA in bacteria.

How do plasmids replicate?	Independently of the main chromosome

GENE TRANSFER

What are three distinct mechanisms by which DNA is transferred between bacteria?	1. Conjugation 2. Transduction 3. Transformation
What is conjugation?	Process where bacteria transfer genetic material from one cell to another by means of cell-to-cell contact
What structure assists in conjugation between bacteria?	Sex pili

How?

They are hair-like projections that bind donor and recipient cells, bringing them closer together

What genetic material is transferred during conjugation?

Conjugative plasmids

What portion of the plasmid is transferred during conjugation?

Only one strand of the double-stranded plasmid is transferred to the recipient cell

The complementary plasmid strand is synthesized by the recipient cell (see Fig. 2-3)

What is the prototypic conjugative plasmid found in *Escherichia coli*?

F, or fertility, plasmid

What medically important genes are often contained within plasmids?

Antibiotic resistance genes and structural genes for the pilus protein

What is the name for bacteria in which the F plasmid becomes integrated into the bacterial chromosome?

Hfr (high frequency of chromosomal recombinants)

What is transduction?

Process where viruses transfer genetic material from one bacteria to another by means of a bacteriophage without any cell-to-cell contact

What is a bacteriophage?

Virus that replicates within bacterial cells

What is the composition of a bacteriophage?

Single or double-stranded nucleic acid (DNA or ribonucleic acid [RNA]) within a protective protein coat

What are five stages of bacteriophage replication?

1. Phage attachment (adsorption)
2. Injection of phage DNA (penetration)
3. Synthesis of phage DNA or proteins
4. Assembly of new phage particles
5. Lysis of cell and release of new phage progeny (see Fig. 2-4)

What are two types of phage?

Virulent and temperate

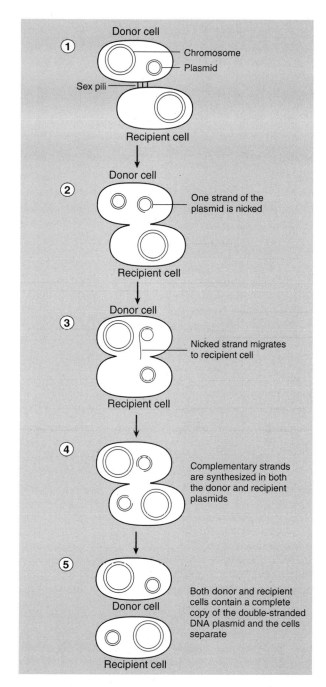

Figure 2-3. Conjugation involving the transfer of one strand of a plasmid from a donor to a recipient cell.

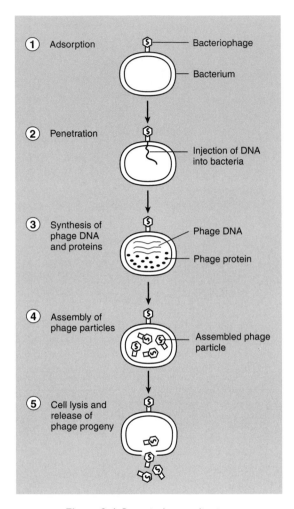

Figure 2-4. Bacteriophage replication.

What is the name of the virulent phage replication cycle?

Lytic cycle

What are the steps of this cycle?

1. Virulent phage infect cells
2. Replicate intracellularly
3. Lyse and kill host cells
4. Release new phage particles

What is the name of the temperate phage replication cycle?

Lysogenic cycle

What are the steps of this cycle?

1. Temperate phage infect cells
2. Phage genome integrates into the host chromosomal DNA
3. Remains silent and replicates as part of the host chromosome

What is the name for a phage that is integrated within the host chromosome?

Prophage

What prevents expression of the phage once it has been integrated within the host chromosome?

The phage encodes a repressor protein that prevents expression of other phage genes

What are two types of transduction?

1. Generalized transduction
2. Specialized transduction

What is generalized transduction?

Process where phage enzymes cleave bacterial DNA into fragments which are randomly packaged in a phage protein coat and released during cell lysis (see Fig. 2-5A)

What is specialized transduction?

Process where chromosomal bacterial genes closely upstream or downstream to the prophage insertion site are transferred because they are randomly excised and packaged into a phage protein coat and released during cell lysis (see Fig. 2-5B)

What type of phage is involved in specialized transduction?

Temperate phage

What is transformation?

Process where transfer of genes occurs by cellular uptake of naked DNA fragments

What is the term for the ability of a recipient cell to take up naked DNA?

Competency

How does naked DNA enter a cell?

It binds to the cell wall and is taken up intracellularly or passes through defects in the cell wall

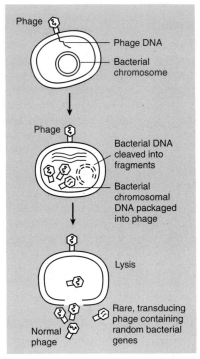

A

Figure 2-5. Transduction. A. Generalized transduction.

| How does it become integrated? | One strand of the naked DNA binds to a region of sequence homology on the recipient chromosome, replacing the original complementary strand, while the second strand of naked DNA is destroyed by cell nucleases (see Fig. 2-6) |

GENETIC MUTATIONS

What is a wild type organism?	A standard to which genetic mutants are compared
What is a mutant?	An organism that deviates from normal in some recognizable characteristic (phenotype)
What is a mutation?	A change in the base sequence of DNA (genotype)

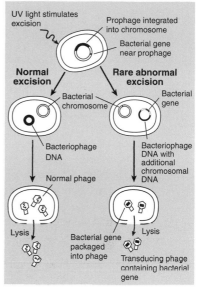

B

Figure 2-5. (*Continued*) B. Specialized transduction.

What is an unstable mutation?	A mutation which frequently changes back to its original state
How are nucleotides classified?	Purines: adenine (A), guanine (G) have two rings Pyrimidines: cytosine (C), thymine (T) have one ring Pyrimidines contain the letter "Y"
What is a point mutation? What are two types?	A mutation that only affects one base pair 1. Transition substitution 2. Transversion substitution
What is a transition substitution?	A point mutation where a purine is substituted for a purine or a pyrimidine is substituted for a pyrimidine
What is a transversion substitution?	A point mutation where a purine replaces a pyrimidine or vice-versa
What is . . . **An inversion mutation?**	A mutation where a string of base pairs are deleted and reinserted in the same position, but in the opposite direction

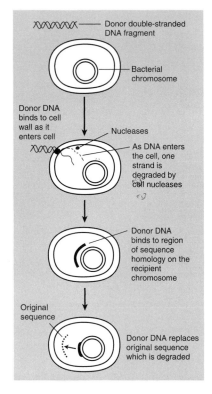

Figure 2-6. Transformation.

A silent mutation?	A mutation that alters base pairs, but not the specific amino acid they encode
A missense mutation?	A mutation that alters base pairs, resulting in the replacement one amino acid residue for another
A nonsense mutation?	A mutation resulting in a stop codon, prematurely terminating the elongation of a polypeptide chain
A frame-shift mutation?	A mutation that changes the reading frame of the genetic code, resulting in a misreading of all downstream nucleotides and altering the encoded amino acids of the polypeptide chain, often resulting in early stop codons (see Fig. 2-7)

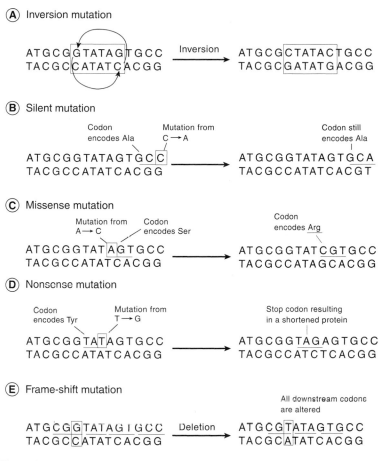

Figure 2-7. A. Inversion mutation; B. Silent mutation; C. Missense mutation; D. Nonsense mutation; E. Frame-shift mutation.

What common properties are used to categorize mutants?	Nutritional needs, temperature-sensitivity, capability to suppress mutations, and capability to regulate gene expression
What are seven classes of mutagenic agents?	1. Base analogs (e.g., 5-bromouracil) 2. Chemical modifiers (e.g., nitrous acid, hydroxylamine, alkylating agents) 3. Frame-shift mutagens (e.g., acridine) 4. Radiation (e.g., UV light, x-rays) 5. Mobile genetic elements (e.g., transposons)

6. Oxidizing agents (e.g., hydroxyl radicals, superoxide)
7. Intercalating agents (e.g., ethidium bromide, daunomycin)

What laboratory test can be used to detect mutagens? What is this test?

Ames test

A laboratory test that allows investigators to identify mutagens by performing the following steps:
1. Potential mutagens are added to strains of *Salmonella* that have been genetically modified to require histidine for growth
2. These bacteria are plated on medium lacking histidine
3. Bacteria that grow in the absence of histidine are presumed to have acquired a mutation allowing them to produce histidine

GENETIC REGULATION

How do bacteria demonstrate negative control for gene expression?

Bacteria encode repressor proteins (repressors) that bind to operator sites, preventing expression of downstream genes

What is an inducer?

A protein or molecule that binds to and inhibits the repressor, allowing expression of downstream genes

What is an activator?

A protein or molecule that binds to chromosomes, increasing gene expression

BACTERIAL PHYLOGENY

How are bacteria classified?

See Fig. 2-8

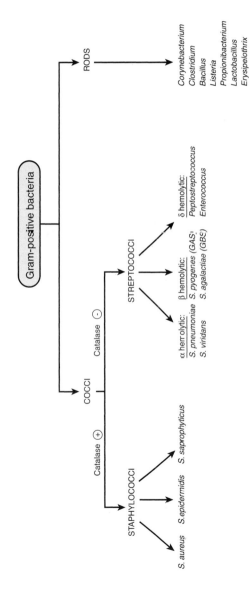

Figure 2-8. Bacterial phylogeny.

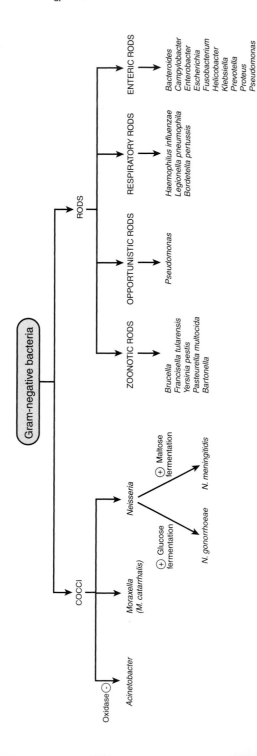

Figure 2-8. (*Continued*)

3

Gram-Positive Cocci: *Staphylococcus*

OVERVIEW

What are three medically important gram-positive cocci?	1. *Staphylococcus* 2. *Streptococcus* 3. *Enterococcus*
What test is positive in *Staphylococcus* and negative in *Streptococcus*?	Catalase test
What is the mechanism of catalase?	Converts hydrogen peroxide to water and oxygen: $2H_2O_2 \rightarrow 2\,H_2O + O_2$ Catalase inactivates toxic peroxide species, while superoxide dismutase inactivates toxic oxide radicals
What is the difference between staphylococci and streptococci on Gram stain?	Staphylococci appear as spherical cocci arranged in irregular grape-like clusters Streptococci appear as diplococcal pairs or chains rather than as clusters (see Fig. 3-1)
What are three pathogenic types of *Staphylococcus*?	1. *Staphylococcus aureus* 2. *Staphylococcus epidermidis* 3. *Staphylococcus saprophyticus*
Which staphylococci sometimes demonstrate hemolytic properties? **What type of hemolytic reaction do they demonstrate?**	*S. aureus* β-hemolytic or complete hemolysis characterized by red cell lysis resulting in a clear ring around the colony when cultured on blood agar

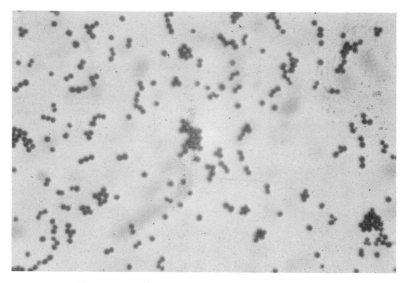

Figure 3-1. Staphylococci appearing as "Cluster of grapes"

What are two tests that can be used to distinguish between strains of Staphylococcus?	1. Coagulase Test – to determine if the enzyme is present 2. Mannitol Test – to determine if the organism is able to ferment mannitol
What is coagulase?	Bacterial enzyme which when released activate both prothrombin and the coagulation cascade
What results would you see with the coagulase test for the three pathogenic staphylococci?	(+) S. aureus (–) S. epidermidis (–) S. saprophyticus
What does a coagulase positive test look like?	"Clumping" on latex agglutination test
What results would you see with the mannitol test for the three pathogenic staphylococci?	(+) S. aureus (–) S. epidermidis (–) S. saprophyticus (see Table 3-1)
Which of the three pathogenic types of staphylococci. . .	

Table 3-1.   Staphylococci at a Glance

	Catalase	Coagulase	Mannitol Fermentation
S. aureus	+	+	+
S. epidermidis	+	−	−
S. saprophyticus	+	−	−

Are often found in normal flora?	*S. aureus* and *S. epidermidis*
Produces exotoxin?	Only *S. aureus*
Is most virulent?	*S. aureus*
Have capsules?	*S. aureus* and *S. epidermidis*
What defense mechanism do encapsulated bacteria utilize?	Demonstrate antiphagocytic properties
Do staphylococci contain endotoxin?	No, endotoxins are never produced by gram positive bacteria. Instead of endotoxins, *Staphylococcus aureus*, like all Gram positive bacteria, stimulate cytokine production by producing surface components including peptidoglycan, teichoic acids, and lipoprotein
What can make *Staphylococcus* potentially difficult to treat?	*Staphylococcus*, commonly produces β-lactamases and/or penicillin binding proteins which result in antibiotic resistance, e.g., methicillin-resistant *S. aureus* (MRSA) or vancomycin-resistant *S. aureus* (VRSA) (see Table 3-1)

STAPHYLOCOCCUS AUREUS

What is the origin of the word aureus?	Aureus comes from the Latin root for gold
What is the relevance of this?	*S. aureus* colonies appear golden on some media
Does *S. aureus* grow in the presence of air?	Yes, all staphylococci are facultative anaerobes

Where are you most likely to find S. aureus in a healthy, non-infected person?	Mucous membranes of anterior nares
What are three major mechanisms that S. aureus uses to cause disease in the host?	1. Direct tissue destruction 2. Exotoxin release 3. Promotes immunologic dysfunction
What S. aureus proteins contribute to pathogenicity?	Protein A, hemolysins, coagulase, leukocidins, penicillinase, superantigens and many enzymes
What does Protein A bind? **How does this contribute to pathogenecity?**	The heavy chain constant domain (Fc) of IgG antibodies Decreases the likelihood of immune system to "see" bacteria and therefore decrease opsonization and phagocytosis
What is the result of hemolysins and leukocidins?	Destruction of RBC and WBC, respectively
What is a specific hemolysin? **How does it work on a molecular level?**	Alpha toxin Polymerizes into tubes that pierce membranes resulting in osmotic lysis
What are the clinical implications of alpha toxin?	Causes marked necrosis of the skin and hemolysis
What is penicillinase?	Secreted form of β-lactamase
What is the mechanism of action?	Inactivates β-lactam antibiotics via the disruption of the β-lactam portion of the penicillin molecule
What are three proteins made by S. aureus that are specifically used to destroy tissue?	1. Hyaluronidase 2. Staphylokinase 3. Lipase
How does hyaluronidase work?	Breaks downs proteoglycans in connective tissue

How does staphylokinase work?	Lyses fibrin clots
How does lipase work?	Catabolism of fats and oils allowing for sebaceous gland colonization
What are superantigen exotoxins?	Exotoxins which interact the V_b domain of the T-cell receptor (TCR) and the major histocompatibility complex (MHC) class II molecules on the surface of antigen-presenting cells directly activating them regardless of antigen specificity
What are two effects of superantigens?	1. CD_4^+ T cell and antigen-presenting cell proliferation 2. Substantial increase in the release of CD_4^+ T cell cytokines, e.g., IL-1, IL-2, IFN-γ, and TNF
What are two pyrogenic superantigen exotoxins released by S. aureus?	1. Enterotoxin (Heat stable) 2. Toxic shock syndrome toxin (TSST) Exfoliatin is released by S. aureus but is *not* a super-antigen
What is the result of the release of exfoliatin exotoxin?	Results in scalded skin syndrome where the skin desquamates and sloughs off
What is the pathogenesis?	The toxin attacks the intercellular adhesive layer of the stratum granulosum with resulting desquamation of the epidermis, i.e., epidermolysis
Which patient population is usually affected?	Newborns with recently severed umbilical cords or children with skin infections
Will the skin of a child with scalded skin syndrome contain S. aureus?	No, just the exotoxin
What is the result of heat stable enterotoxin release?	Gastroenteritis leading to vomiting and diarrhea Enterotoxin, also a superantigen, is much more stable than S. aureus and may still cause gastroenteritis from cooked foods

What is the time course of the enterotoxin mediated gastroenteritis?

Rapid onset (1–6 hrs) of acute period of nausea and non-bloody, explosive vomitus from presence of pre-formed enterotoxin

What type of foods facilitates growth of S. aureus?

Foods such as custards, egg salad, cream pastry, mayonnaise, and potato salad

What causes Toxic shock syndrome (TSS)?

TSST
TSS can be caused by 1) TSST + S. aureus, 2) TSST + streptococci, or 3) circulating enterotoxin

What is the pathogenesis of TSST?

Superantigen induced IL-1, IL-2, IFN-γ, and TNF expression

What in the past has been associated with TSS?

1970's TSS epidemic from super absorbent tampons

What are six major symptoms of TSS?

1. Fever
2. Nausea and vomiting
3. Watery, non-bloody diarrhea
4. Erythematous rash similar to scarlet fever
5. Epidermolysis of palms and soles
6. Septic shock and organ damage

What determines the extent of symptoms?

Presence of the exotoxin rather than the presence of bacteria

What organ systems are directly affected by S. aureus?

Skin, heart, lungs, brain, bones and joints

What are five examples of skin infections caused by S. aureus?

1. Folliculitis
2. Abscess
3. Furuncles
4. Carbuncles
5. Wound infection
Impetigo (pyoderma) and cellulitis are skin manifestations primarily seen with Group A streptococci

What is folliculitis?

An inflammatory reaction in hair follicles

What is an abscess?

A collection of pus

What is a furuncle?

Abscess produced by an infected hair follicle deep in the subcutaneous tissue often forming around foreign bodies, e.g., splinters

What is a carbuncle?

A much larger, deeper, painful version of a furuncle in which lesions occasionally lead to bacteremia

What is a wound infection?

Infection at a site of skin trauma, often associated with surgical contamination

What is the most severe complication of *S. aureus* bacteremia on the heart?

Acute endocarditis

How do patients with *S. aureus* endocarditis present?

Sudden onset of fever, chills, myalgia and evidence of septic emboli

What are the ultimate results of acute endocarditis?

Valvular destruction and septic embolizations to brain, lung, and spleen, and classic stigmata of endocarditis, i.e., Janeway lesions, Roth's spots, Osler's nodes, splinter hemorrhages

What is the most common cause of acute endocarditis from *S. aureus*?

IV drug use

In IV drug users, which heart valves are likely to be affected by *S. aureus* endocarditis?

Right heart valves, usually tricuspid valve IV injections go into the vein and veins drain back to the right side of the heart

What effect does *S. aureus* have on the lungs?
Who is most likely to be affected?

Severe, necrotizing pneumonia

Middle aged adults living in the community following influenza viral infection

What is the clinical course of pneumonia?

Acute fever and chills with lobar consolidation of lung with potential cavitation secondary to destruction of the lung parenchyma

What are likely sequelae of cavitations?

Effusions and empyema

What effect does S. aureus have on the brain?

Meningitis, cerebritis, and brain abscess

How do patients with meningitis present?

High fever, nuchal rigidity, headache, change in mental status (obtundation), focal neurologic signs or coma

What effect does S. aureus have on the bones?
  Who is most likely to have it?

Acute and chronic osteomyelitis infection

Males less than 12

How do patients with osteomyelitis present?

Asymmetrical, swollen, warm tissue over bone; systemic fever and shakes secondary to bacteremia

What effect does S. aureus have on the joints?
  Is this a medical emergency?

Septic arthritis secondary to synovial membrane invasion
Yes, pus can rapidly cause irreparable cartilage damage

What is the most common overall cause of septic arthritis?

S. aureus

Who is most likely to be affected by S. aureus induced septic arthritis?

The young and the old, i.e., pediatric age group and adults over 50

What is the most common cause of septic arthritis in the middle age population?

N. gonorrhea

How do patients with S. aureus septic arthritis present?
  How would you diagnose it?

Acutely painful, swollen, red-hot joint

Yellowish fluid on arthrocentesis with >100,000 neutrophils along with positive Gram stain or culture

How would you treat it?

1. Drain the joint
2. Antimicrobial therapy

Why are most S. aureus types resistant to Penicillin G?	Presence of penicillinase-encoding plasmids and transposons, commonly found in community and hospital acquired strains
What is MRSA?	Methicillin-Resistant *Staphylococcus Aureus*, which carries β-lactam enzymes used for peptidoglycan synthesis that are insensitive to the antibiotic effects of methicillin
Where do these type of infections usually develop?	In hospitals or nursing homes where broad spectrum antibiotics are used
How is MRSA transmitted between patients?	Usually via hand contact of health care workers
How can this be prevented?	Frequent, proper hand washing
What is the gold standard treatment for severe MRSA infections?	Vancomycin, although resistance has developed

STAPHYLOCOCCUS EPIDERMIDIS

What is S. epidermidis?	A coagulase negative organism found as normal flora on the skin
Does S. epidermidis have a low or high virulence compared to S. aureus?	Low
Does S. epidermidis have an increased or decreased likelihood of drug resistance when compared to S. aureus?	More frequent than S. *aureus*
Why?	Innately more resistant
What population groups are frequently infected with S. epidermidis?	1. Patients with Foley catheters, IV lines or any indwelling lines 2. Patients with prosthetic devices or damaged heart valves 3. Immunocompromised patients
What gives S. epidermidis a predilection for prosthetic devices?	Formation of biofilms on implanted surfaces resulting in adherence of the polysaccharide capsule

**How do you determine if
S. epidermidis bacteremia
is of a blood-origin or from
contamination?**

Sterilely draw more than one blood
sample from two different sites
15 minutes apart

STAPHYLOCOCCUS SAPROPHYTICUS

What is S. saprophyticus?

A coagulase negative organism which
causes urinary tract infections and cystitis

**Where is S. saprophyticus
found?**

Normal flora of the vagina

**What test can be
performed to help
distinguish S. saprophyticus
from other staphylococci?**

Novobiocin (antibiotic) sensitivity

**What results would you see
with the novobiocin
sensitivity test for the three
pathogenic staphylococci?**

S. saprophyticus is (+), or resistant,
demonstrating growth
S. aureus and S. epidermidis are (−), or
sensitive, demonstrating no growth

**Who is most likely to be
infected?**

Young healthy sexually-active females

4

Gram-Positive Cocci: *Streptococcus* & *Enterococcus*

OVERVIEW

What type of organisms are *Streptococcus*?

Gram-positive, catalase-negative bacteria that assemble in chains (see Fig. 4-1)

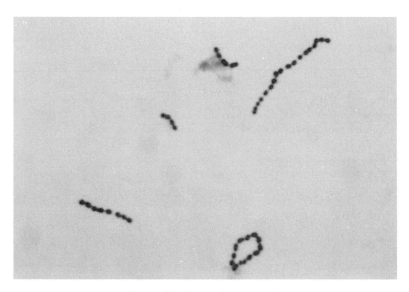

Figure 4-1. Chains of streptococci.

What is a simple way to distinguish between *Staphylococcus* and *Streptococcus*?

Streptococcus is a catalase-negative organism

Staphylococcus is a catalase-positive organism

What are the oxygen requirements for *Streptococcus*?

Streptococcus is a microaerophilic organism

What does this mean?	*Streptococcus* can grow in the presence of air, but prefers low oxygen tension
What lab conditions are used to grow *Streptococcus*?	Usually grown aerobically, in candle jars or 5% CO_2 incubators
What are three ways in which *Streptococcus* can be classified?	1. Hemolytic properties 2. Metabolic and growth properties 3. Serologic groups, i.e., Lancefield grouping system
What are the three types of hemolytic reactions?	α-, β-, and γ-hemolysis
What is α-hemolysis?	α-Hemolytic *Streptococcus* causes partial red blood cell lysis, resulting in a green ring around their colonies when cultured on blood agar
What are two α-hemolytic streptococci? **How can you distinguish the two?**	1. *Streptococcus pneumoniae* 2. *Viridans streptococcus* *S. pneumoniae* has a capsule (+ Quellung reaction) and shows sensitivity to Optochin *Viridans streptococcus* has no capsule and is Optochin resistant (see Fig. 4-2)
What is β-hemolysis?	β-Hemolytic *Streptococcus* causes complete red blood cell lysis, resulting in a clear ring around the colony when cultured on blood agar
What are two β-hemolytic streptococci? **How can you distinguish the two?**	1. *S. pyogenes* 2. *S. agalactiae* *S. pyogenes* is bacitracin sensitive *S. agalactiae* is bacitracin resistant
What is γ-hemolysis?	γ-Hemolytic *Streptococcus* causes no red blood cell lysis, resulting in no color change when cultured on blood agar
What are two γ-hemolytic streptococci?	1. *Enterococcus* (e.g., *E. faecalis*) 2. *Peptostreptococcus*

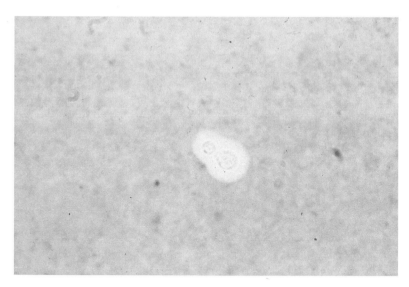

Figure 4-2. Positive Quellung reaction (see also Color Photo 3).

	Some *Enterococcus* can also demonstrate α- or β-hemolytic properties
How can you distinguish between the two?	*Enterococcus,* e.g., *E. faecalis,* can be grown in bile and 6.5% NaCl *Peptostreptococcus* is obligate anaerobic organism
What is the Lancefield grouping system?	Serologic classification system that primarily categorizes β-hemolytic *Streptococcus*
What is the basis of this grouping system?	C-carbohydrate polysaccharides that are found in cell walls of most *Streptococcus* and are classified in groups A through U
Which groups are of major medical importance?	Group A *Streptococcus* (GAS) corresponding to *S. pyogenes* Group B *Streptococcus* (GBS) corresponding to *S. agalactiae*
Which four streptococci are not classified under the Lancefield system?	1. *S. pneumoniae* 2. *Viridans streptococcus* 3. *S. mutans* 4. *Enterococcus* (see Table 4-1)

Table 4-1. Hemolytic Classification of Commonly Encountered Streptococci

α-Hemolytic	β-Hemolytic	γ-Hemolytic
S. pneumoniae	S. pyogenes (GAS)	Enterococcus[b]
S. viridans[a]	S. agalactiae (GBS)	Peptostreptococcus[b]

GAS = group A streptococci Lancefield classification; GBS = group B streptococci Lancefield classification.
[a] May also demonstrate γ-hemolytic properties.
[b] May also demonstrate α- or β-hemolytic properties.

α-HEMOLYTIC STREPTOCOCCUS

STREPTOCOCCUS PNEUMONIAE

What is S. pneumoniae?

Encapsulated, α-hemolytic, Optochin-sensitive streptococci

What are two major virulence factors of S. pneumoniae?

1. Capsule
2. Pneumolysin

What is the Quellung reaction?

When the bacterial capsule appears to swell when mixed with type-specific antisera

What type of Quellung reaction do S. pneumoniae display?

Positive Quellung reaction

What other organisms also give a positive Quellung reaction?

1. Neisseria meningitides
2. Haemophilus influenzae
3. Klebsiella

Who is at risk of S. pneumoniae infection?

1. Individuals who have had their spleens removed or who have a decrease in splenic function, e.g., secondary to Sickle cell disease
2. Individuals with decreased respiratory function or after anesthesia, e.g., infants, the elderly, alcoholics

Splenic function is critical in clearing encapsulated bacteria such as S. pneumonia

How many different serotypes of S. pneumoniae exist?

85 distinct serotypes

What are the serotypes based on?

The capsule

What is the function of the capsule that surrounds *S. pneumoniae*?

Confers antiphagocytic properties

What is pneumolysin?

How does this occur?

An important virulence factor that lyses phagocytes and is released when *S. pneumoniae* lyses itself

1. *S. pneumoniae* is engulfed by phagocytic cells
2. *S. pneumoniae* releases autolysins to lyse itself
3. Pneumolysin, which was intrabacterial, is now present inside the phagocyte and degrades the cell from the inside out

Think of this being a last ditch effort for *S. pneumoniae* to exert revenge on the phagocyte, i.e., "I'm going down but I'm taking you with me"

What clinical syndromes are associated with *S. pneumoniae*?

1. Pneumonia (most common cause)
2. Otitis media (most common cause)
3. Sinusitis
4. Meningitis
5. Sepsis

What commonly predisposes an individual to get pneumonia?

Previous viral infection and being immunocompromised

What key laboratory tests are useful when identifying *S. pneumoniae*?

1. Sputum or blood culture on blood agar
2. Optochin sensitivity

What is a characteristic finding in a patient with *S. pneumoniae*?

Rusty-colored sputum

Which antibiotics are useful against *S. pneumoniae* strains?

Penicillin G or a cephalosporin, although resistance is spreading rapidly

What treatment is indicated for resistant forms of *S. pneumoniae*?

Vancomycin, erythromycin, or clindamycin

What vaccines are available for *S. pneumoniae*?

1. Pneumovax: a polyvalent capsular polysaccharide vaccine that immunizes against 23 serotypes
2. Prevnar: a heptavalent conjugate vaccine which is made up of 7 pneumococcal antigens conjugated to a nontoxic diphtheria toxin

Which vaccine is used in infants?

The heptavalent conjugate vaccine (Prevnar) in children <2 years old "Pneumovax is used in 23-year-olds and Prevnar is used in 7-year-olds"

VIRIDANS STREPTOCOCCUS

What are *Viridans* streptococcus?

Unencapsulated, Optochin-resistant α-hemolytic streptococcus

Where are they normally found?

Oral flora

What is the predominant species?

Streptococcus mutans

What are two clinical concerns regarding *S. mutans*? Based on this, what would be appropriate prophylactic management?

1. Subacute bacterial endocarditis
2. Dental caries
Certain vulnerable patients, e.g., those with artificial heart valves or valve abnormalities, may be treated with penicillin before undergoing dental procedures

β-HEMOLYTIC STREPTOCOCCUS

STREPTOCOCCUS PYOGENES (GAS)

What is *S. pyogenes*?

Encapsulated, bacitracin sensitive, β-hemolytic *streptococcus*, also known as Group A *Streptococcus* (GAS)
Remember that the two most clinically relevant groups of β-hemolytic *streptococcus* are Lancefield groups A and B
S. pyogenes is the most virulent member of the group A β-hemolytic *streptococcus* (GAS) (see Fig. 4-3)

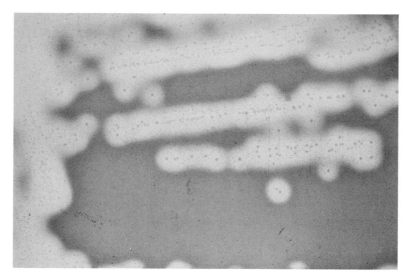

Figure 4-3. β-Hemolytic streptococci (see also Color Photo 4).

What is the structure of S. pyogenes?

Gram-positive, nonmotile cocci that can appear as long chains, pairs, clusters, or individual cocci

What are the two postinfectious immunological sequelae that are associated with S. pyogenes?

1. Acute rheumatic fever
2. Acute glomerulonephritis

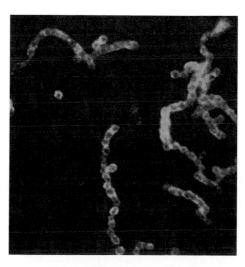

Figure 4-4. Chains of S. Pyogenes.

What is the most common means of S. pyogenes transmission?

Aerosolized respiratory droplets

What is another means of transmission?

Direct spread can occur, e.g., by invading intact skin

What is unique about the capsule of group A S. pyogenes?

Composed of hyaluronic acid

What is the significance of the capsule?

The body does not recognize it as foreign because hyaluronic acid mimics the outer layer of human connective tissue

What are nine virulence factors associated with S. pyogenes?

1. M proteins and teichoic acids
2. C-carbohydrate
3. Protein F
4. Streptococcal pyrogenic exotoxins (SPEs)
5. Streptolysin O and S
6. Streptokinase
7. Streptodornases
8. C5a Peptidase
9. Hyaluronidase

Which four virulence factors are components of the cell wall?

1. M proteins
2. Teichoic acid
3. C-carbohydrate
4. Protein F

What confers antiphagocytic properties of S. pyogenes?

1. Fibrillar M proteins with highly variable N-terminus regions
2. Adherence to some epithelial cells

What is the significance of the high variability?

Variability gives the bacteria new "camouflage," limiting the host's use of antibodies that would opsonize the bacteria

What is the function of protein F?

Attachment of S. pyogenes to host tissues, e.g., to pharyngeal epithelium

What is SPE A?

A superantigenic exotoxin corresponding to classic erythrotoxin

How is SPE A expressed?

Carried by bacteriophages that lysogenize S. pyogenes

What is the pathogenesis of SPE A?	Superantigen-mediated response that increases T-cell/antigen-presenting cell mitogenicity and cytokine expression, i.e., interleukin (IL)-1, IL-2, interferon (IFN)-γ, and tumor necrosis factor (TNF)
What are two clinical manifestations associated with SPE A?	1. Rash of scarlet fever 2. Toxic shock-like syndrome
What is SPE B?	A superantigenic exotoxin corresponding to cysteine protease
How is SPE B expressed?	Chromosomally encoded cysteine protease that is variably expressed
What is a clinical manifestation of elevated levels of SPE B?	Necrotizing fasciitis
What is streptolysin O?	An antigenic, oxygen-labile hemolysin that can lyse mammalian cells, releasing enzymes that damage tissue
What are antibodies against streptolysin O useful for?	Documenting recent group A *Streptococcus* infection
What is streptolysin S?	An oxygen stable, but nonimmunogenic hemolysin that lyses leukocytes, platelets, and red cells
How is this useful for diagnosis?	Responsible for the clear ring observed around β-hemolytic streptococci colonies on blood agar
What is streptokinase?	Catalyses the conversion of plasminogen to plasmin resulting in lysis of clots and facilitating rapid spread of group A *Streptococcus* Streptokinase is not, in the biochemical sense, a kinase
What are streptodornases?	Bacterial deoxyribonuclease (DNAses) made by *S. pyogenes* that degrade viscous deoxyribonucleic acid (DNA) in tissue, further facilitating spread of infection
What is the role of C5a peptidase?	Inactivates C5a that is interfering with complement-mediated recruitment of white blood cells

What is hyaluronidase?

Hydrolyzes hyaluronic acid in the ground substance of connective tissue, further aiding spread of infection

What are eight clinical syndromes caused by S. pyogenes?

1. Cellulitis (a major cause)
2. Acute pharyngitis/epiglotitis
3. Impetigo
4. Erysipelas
5. Puerperal sepsis
6. Necrotizing fasciitis
7. Acute rheumatic fever
8. Acute glomerulonephritis

What is cellulitis?

Rapidly spreading inflammation of the skin and subcutaneous tissue

What is pharyngitis?

Redness and edema of the throat and tonsils frequently covered with yellow-white exudates

What is the treatment for acute pharyngitis?

Penicillin G or a macrolide if the patient is allergic to penicillin

What is impetigo?

Common superficial infection usually on the face of children with small vesicles turning into pustules and eventually spread into a thick yellowish crust

What is the treatment for impetigo?

Topical mupirocin or a systemic first-generation cephalosporin

What is erysipelas?

An advancing erythematous cellulitis with a defined border, usually on the face or lower limbs

What is puerperal sepsis?

A postpartum infection of the uterine endometrium that presents as a purulent vaginal discharge with systemic signs of infection

What is necrotizing fasciitis?

A rapidly spreading systemic infection caused by S. pyogenes, which is also known as "flesh-eating bacteria"

What is acute rheumatic fever?

An autoimmune disease appearing 3 weeks after streptococcal pharyngitis leading to fever, rash, arthritis and pancarditis

4 Gram-Positive Cocci: Streptococcus & Enterococcus 49

What is the pathogenesis?	A cross-reaction between streptococcal antigens and host tissues associated with specific M proteins
What is acute glomerulonephritis?	A postinfectious sequelae appearing 10 days after streptococcal pharyngitis or 3 weeks after cutaneous *S. pyogenes* infection
What is the pathogenesis?	Believed to be caused by antigen–antibody complexes being deposited in the basement membrane of the glomerulus

STREPTOCOCCUS AGALACTIAE (GBS)

What is S. agalactiae?	Unencapsulated, bacitracin resistant, β-hemolytic streptococci, also known as Group B *Streptococcus* (GBS)
Where is S. agalactiae found?	Vagina, urethra, and gastrointestinal (GI) tract
How is S. agalactiae spread?	1. Sexually transmitted 2. During childbirth (parturition)
What are the clinical syndromes caused by S. agalactiae?	1. Neonatal sepsis and meningitis (leading cause) 2. Endometritis 3. Pneumonia 4. Lower-extremity infections in diabetics
Which antibiotics are useful against S. agalactiae?	Penicillin and ampicillin
What measures should be taken to prevent S. agalactiae transmission from a mother to her child during prolonged labor?	A prophylactic course of penicillin or ampicillin should be administered during prolonged labor, fever, or prior evidence of GBS colonization/amnionitis

γ-HEMOLYTIC STREPTOCOCCUS

ENTEROCOCCUS

What are enterococci?	γ-Hemolytic group D streptococcus Some *Enterococcus* can also demonstrate α- or β-hemolytic properties

USMLE

What are the two clinically important species of enterococci?

1. *E. faecalis*
2. *E. faecium*

Why is *Enterococcus* a prominent cause of nosocomial infections?

Resistance to multiple antibiotics

Where is *Enterococcus* found?

Normal part of the fecal flora

How is *Enterococcus* identified in the laboratory?

1. Group D Lancefield grouping
2. Can survive in bile salts and 6.5% NaCl
3. Yields a positive pyrrolidonyl arylamidase (PYR) test

What property do *Enterococcus* and *Streptococcus* bovis share?

Group D Lancefield classification

How is *S. bovis* differentiated from *Enterococcus*?

Enterococcus yields a positive PYR test
S. bovis does not yield a positive PYR test

What are two clinical manifestations of *Enterococcus*?

1. Urinary tract infection (UTI)
2. Subacute endocarditis

Are these infections easily treated?

No; enterococci infections are often resistant and survive on infected surfaces for a long time

PEPTOSTREPTOCOCCUS

What is *Peptostreptococcus*?

γ-Hemolytic anaerobic streptococci that are relatively avirulent

Why is *Peptostreptococcus* not part of the Lancefield system?

Peptostreptococcus lacks the C-carbohydrate cell wall antigen and thus is not part of Lancefield system

What distinguishes peptostreptococci from other streptococci?

Peptostreptococci, unlike other streptococci, are obligate anaerobes

What clinical manifestations are associated with *Peptostreptococcus*?

Infections in soft tissues, pneumonia and genitourinary infections

5

Gram-Positive Rods: *Clostridia, Corynebacteria, Listeria, & Bacillus*

OVERVIEW

What are seven gram-positive rods?

1. *Clostridia*
2. *Corynebacteria*
3. *Listeria*
4. *Bacillus* (see Fig. 5-1)
5. *Propionibacterium*
6. *Lactobacillus*
7. *Erysipelothrix*

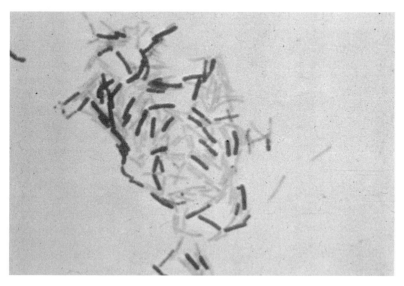

Figure 5-1. Gram-positive rods, *Bacillus cereus* (see also Color Photo 5).

CLOSTRIDIA

What is the morphology of Clostridia?	Gram-positive rods
What are the oxygen requirements of Clostridia?	Obligate anaerobes
What are four important species of Clostridium?	1. *C. perfringens* 2. *C. botulinum* 3. *C. difficile* 4. *C. tetani*
Which of these Clostridia form spores?	All *Clostridia* form spores
Which of these Clostridia are motile?	All *Clostridia* except *C. perfringens*
Where is Clostridia commonly found?	Human intestines, aquatic areas, soil, and sewage
Why is Clostridia difficult to kill?	They form endospores that are resistant to many disinfectants and to short periods of boiling
What process is effective in killing Clostridia?	Autoclaving at 121°C (250°F), under pressure, for 15 minutes

CLOSTRIDIUM PERFRINGENS

Where can C. perfringens be found in humans?	Normal flora of the lower gastrointestinal (GI) tract and vagina
Where are C. perfringens spores commonly found?	Soil
What is the rate of growth for C. perfringens?	Fast; population can double every 10 minutes
What are three pathogenic substances secreted by C. perfringens?	1. Exotoxins 2. Enterotoxins 3. Degradative enzymes
How are C. perfringens strains grouped?	By the activity of their exotoxins

What are the different groups?

Groups A to E

What is the most common strain in human infections?

Type A strains

What are two major toxins elaborated by *C. perfringens*?

1. Alpha toxin
2. Enterotoxin

What is alpha toxin?

A lecithinase (phospholipase C3)

What makes alpha toxin pathogenic?

Lyses endothelial cells, erythrocytes, leukocytes, and platelets

Where does enterotoxin act?

Terminal small intestine

What makes enterotoxin pathogenic?

Binds epithelial cell receptors and interferes with ion transport, eventually causing loss of intracellular proteins and fluids

What are some of the degradative enzymes produced by *C. perfringens*?

Deoxyribonucleases (DNAses), hyaluronidases, proteases, and collagenases

What makes DNAses pathogenic?

Degrades viscous deoxyribonucleic acid (DNA) in necrotizing tissue, promoting the spread of infection

What makes hyaluronidase pathogenic?

Disturbs the extracellular matrix of proteins/ground substance, promoting the spread of the infection

What are five conditions commonly associated with *C. perfringens*?

1. Myonecrosis (gas gangrene)
2. Cellulitis
3. Food poisoning
4. Necrotizing enteritis
5. Endometritis

What is myonecrosis?

Bacterial invasion of healthy muscle tissue producing crepitations secondary to subcutaneous gas formation

What are two common predisposing factors for myonecrosis?

Open wounds and fractures

Do other organisms normally infect sites of *C. perfringens* infections?
Yes, other anaerobes and facultative bacteria are commonly present

What is seen in smears of tissue and exudates of affected tissue?
Large, gram-positive rods, cellular debris, often other bacteria, rarely spores, and no neutrophils

What is the characteristic finding on *C. perfringens* colonies in blood agar?
Double zone of hemolysis

What produces the gas in myonecrosis?
Fermentation of carbohydrates

What is the prognosis of untreated clostridial myonecrosis?
Death within a couple of days from gangrene

What is the cause of death in myonecrosis?
Shock and multi-organ failure secondary to intravascular dissemination of exotoxins

What is key to prevention and treatment of myonecrosis?
Cleaning and débridement of the wound

Which antibiotic is commonly used to treat myonecrosis?
Penicillin

What else can be helpful in disrupting the progression of myonecrosis?
Hyperbaric oxygen chambers

What is clostridial cellulitis?
What is the treatment?
An acute inflammatory disorder of the skin without myonecrosis
Incision of the skin in front of the infectious leading edge

What are the most common vehicles for *C. perfringens* food poisoning?
Poultry, fish, beef, and pork

What causes *C. perfringens* food poisoning?
Heat-labile toxin

What are the common symptoms?
Nausea, abdominal cramps, and diarrhea without fever or diarrhea with fever

How soon after eating food contaminated with *C. perfringens* does one become symptomatic?

8–18 hours after ingestion because bacteria has to grow and produce the toxin

What is the treatment for *C. perfringens* food poisoning?

Supportive care because the disease is self-limiting

What is necrotizing enteritis?

An uncommon acute ulcerative process in the small intestine resulting in separation of the mucosal and submucosal layers forming large denuded areas

What is necrotizing enteritis also known as?

Enteritis necroticans or pigbel

What is the mortality rate?

50%

What is endometritis?

Infection of the uterine endometrium frequently caused by anaerobic organisms

What predisposes an individual to clostridial endometritis?

Inadequately sterilized instruments or incomplete abortion

What is the clinical progression of untreated clostridial endometritis?

Gangrene of uterine tissue, toxemia, and eventual bacteremia

CLOSTRIDIUM BOTULINUM

Where are *C. botulinum* spores classically found?

Soil

What do the spores usually contaminate?

Foods, including honey, vegetables, and meats

When does *C. botulinum* become a problem for humans?

When contaminated foods are canned and vacuum packed without adequate sterilization, leading to germination and toxin production

What causes botulism?

A neurotoxin called botulinum toxin

What are the most common toxin types?

A, B, and E

What is the pathogenesis of botulinum toxin?	A zinc metalloprotease that blocks the release of acetylcholine (ACh) at peripheral cholinergic synapses by cleaving specific SNARE (soluble N-ethylmaleimide-sensitive factor attachment protein receptor) proteins, e.g., synaptobrevins
What is the resultant type of paralysis?	Flaccid paralysis
How does the toxin reach the peripheral cholinergic synapses?	Hematogenous spread secondary to intestinal absorption
When are symptoms first observed after toxin ingestion?	12–36 hours
What are three clinical manifestations of C. botulinum?	1. Infant botulism 2. Classic botulism 3. Wound botulism
What is the most common form of botulism in the United States?	Infant botulism (floppy baby syndrome)
What is the classic source of C. botulinum spores causing this disease?	Honey
What are the common symptoms?	Feeding difficulties, lethargy, and decreased muscle tone
What are common symptoms of classic botulism? **What is the mortality rate?**	Double vision (diplopia), difficulty swallowing (dysphagia), and other cranial nerve dysfunctions 15%
What is the most common cause of death?	Respiratory failure
What is wound botulism?	Botulism occurring as a result of absorption of toxin from an infected wound
How is botulism commonly treated?	Trivalent antitoxin against the three common toxin types, i.e., A, B, and E

How can botulinum toxin be used therapeutically?	In small doses, botulinum toxin can be used to relieve strabismus, to decrease poststroke spasticity, or to reduce wrinkles

CLOSTRIDIUM DIFFICILE

What percentage of the population carries *C. difficile* in their GI tract?	~3%
What is the disease most commonly associated with *C. difficile*?	Pseudomembranous colitis
What is the classic finding?	A pseudomembrane
What is it composed of?	The pseudomembrane is composed of mucus, inflammatory cells, fibrin, and cellular debris
What is the classic presentation?	Nonbloody diarrhea after broad-spectrum antibiotic treatment, e.g., clindamycin or β-lactam antibiotics
Why does it occur after broad spectrum antibiotic treatment?	Suppression of normal flora by antibiotics allows proliferation of *C. difficile*
Are neutrophils found in the diarrhea?	Approximately 50% of the time
How is *C. difficile* transmitted?	Fecal–oral route or by contact with spores found on bedding and toilets
What are the exotoxins produced by pathogenic strains called?	Exotoxins A and B
Which toxin is an enterotoxin?	Toxin A
Which toxin is a cytotoxin?	Toxin B
Which toxin is predominantly responsible for pseudomembrane formation?	Toxin B

What laboratory test is used to diagnose *C. difficile*?	Enzyme-linked immunoabsorbent assay (ELISA) test for exotoxins A and B
How is pseudomembranous colitis generally treated?	Supportive care, discontinuation of offending drug, and starting of new antibiotics
Which antibiotics are most commonly used?	Metronidazole or vancomycin
Why are these two antibiotics used?	These antibiotics suppress *C. difficile* and allow normal flora to reestablish themselves

CLOSTRIDIUM TETANI

What is the characteristic histologic morphology of *C. tetani*?	Tennis-racket-shaped rod (see Fig. 5-2)
Are smears and cultures generally effective in diagnosis?	No

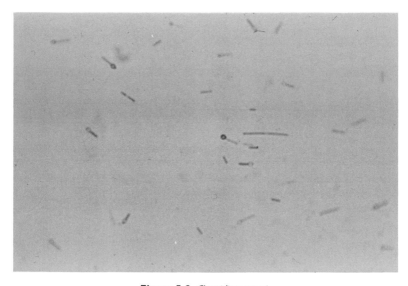

Figure 5-2. *Clostridium tetani.*

What is a common portal of entry for *C. tetani*?	Wound contact (e.g., puncture lesions) with infected soil

What is the incubation period for *C. tetani* toxin production?	4 days to several weeks
What is another term for tetanus toxin?	Tetanospasmin
What is the structure of the toxin?	A light fragment (A) bonded to a heavy fragment (B) by a disulfide bond
What role does the light fragment (A) play?	Acts as a protease and blocks release of inhibitory neurotransmitter glycine and gamma-aminobutyric acid (GABA)
What role does the heavy fragment (B) play?	Controls binding to neurons and aids in the cellular penetration of light fragment A
How is tetanus toxin transported...	
Systemically?	Hematogenously
Neuronally?	Retrograde neuronal transport
How does tetanus typically present?	Spastic paralysis at site of infection
What symptom is pathognomonic for tetanus?	Lock jaw (trismus)
What is the characteristic grimace in affected people called?	Risus sardonicus
What is the most common cause of death?	Respiratory failure
What is crucial in effective diagnosis and treatment?	Clinical suspicion because treatment is empirical
What is used in the pharmacologic treatment of tetanus?	Antitoxin
What else is used in treating tetanus?	1. Sedatives and muscle relaxants to prevent spasms 2. Penicillin and common wound care

Why is tetanus rare today in developed countries?

Childhood immunization against the tetanus exotoxin and booster shots have decreased incidence

What is given for tetanus immunizations?

Tetanus toxoid

What is it?

Formalin inactivated, but antigenic, tetanus toxin

What other vaccines are usually given with this vaccine during childhood immunizations?

Diphtheria toxin and pertussis antigens (diphtheria, tetanus toxoids and acellular pertussis [DTaP])

What is the recommended immunization schedule?

1. 2, 4, 6, and 18 months
2. Booster upon school entry
3. Boosters every 10 years afterward

Why is tetanus seen more often in the elderly?

Failure to followup on booster shots

CORYNEBACTERIA

What are the two non-spore forming gram-positive rods?

1. *Corynebacterium diphtheriae*
2. *Listeria monocytogenes*

What are their oxygen requirements?

Facultative anaerobic

What is the morphology of *C. diphtheriae*?

Small, pleomorphic, unencapsulated gram-positive rods

What disease is *C. diphtheriae* commonly known for?

Diphtheria

How are collections of *C. diphtheriae* commonly described?

Chinese characters/letters (see Fig. 5-3)

How is *C. diphtheriae* usually spread?

Respiratory droplets

How else can one become infected with *C. diphtheriae*?

Puncture wound or cut

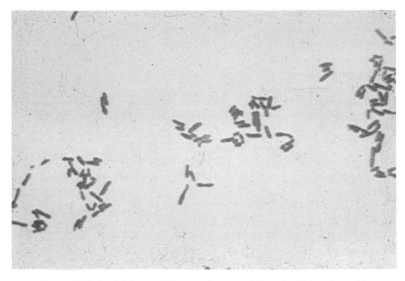

Figure 5-3. C. diphtheriae "Chinese characters." (see also Color photo 6.)

What is the pathogenesis of diphtheria?	Absorption of an exotoxin composed of an A and a B fragment
How does this diphtheria toxin affect the cell?	Inhibits eukaryotic protein synthesis
What is the role of fragment A?	Adenosine diphosphate (ADP) ribosylation of elongation factor-2 (EF-2) resulting in EF-2 inactivation and blockage of the translocation of polypeptidyl-transfer ribonucleic acid (tRNA)
What is the role of fragment B?	Binding to cell and delivery of fragment A
Where is the toxin encoding DNA found?	In a bacteriophage
Which strains of bacteriophages can produce C. diphtheriae capable of active infection?	Lysogenic strains
Why can lysogenic strains do this?	Lysogeny allows bacteriophage integration into the bacterial genome and toxin (protein) expression

Where does *C. diphtheriae* usually infect humans?

Throat and nasopharynx

What is a classic clinical manifestation of *C. diphtheriae* infection? What is this?

Pseudomembrane pharyngitis

An adherent, thick and gray exudative pseudomembrane forming in the throat or nasopharynx with lymphadenopathy

What are two rare clinical manifestations of diphtheria?

1. Myocarditis
2. Neuritis of cranial nerves

How does the host neutralize the toxin?

Antibody formation

How is clinical *C. diphtheriae* diagnosed?

Although no quick and reliable lab tests exist, cultures may yield gram-positive rods with blue and red (metachromatic) granules

How is *C. diphtheriae* definitively diagnosed?

Isolation of *C. diphtheriae* via potassium tellurite containing Tinsdale agar and demonstration of toxin production via precipitin reaction

How is diphtheria treated?

Empiric treatment, i.e., immediate administration of horse serum antitoxin and antibiotics

Which antibiotics can be used?

Penicillin G and erythromycin

How is the disease prevented?

DTaP vaccine

What are diphtheroids?

Corynebacterium species similar to *C. diphtheriae*

What patient population gets affected by diphtheroids?

Immunosuppressed

Which antibiotic is used to treat diphtheroids?

Vancomycin

LISTERIA MONOCYTOGENES

What is the morphology of *Listeria*?	Intracellular, small, gram-positive rods
What type of hemolytic reaction do the rods show?	Narrow zone of β-hemolysis
What feature helps distinguish *Listeria* **from** *Streptococcus*?	*Listeria* are catalase positive; *Streptococcus* are catalase negative
What morphologic features do *Listeria* **and** *Corynebacterium* **share?**	Nonspore-forming gram-positive rods
What nonmorphologic feature distinguishes *Listeria* **from** *Corynebacterium*?	*Listeria* exhibit a tumbling motion and motility at room temperature
What is the important pathogenic species of *Listeria*?	*Listeria monocytogenes*
What populations are most commonly infected by *Listeria*?	1. Pregnant women 2. Fetuses of infected mothers 3. Immunocompromised individuals
How do most people become infected?	Via food, e.g., contaminated meat, dairy products, or vegetables
Does transmission from mother to child occur across the placenta or during the delivery?	Transmission can occur in both situations
How does *Listeria* **enter cells?**	Via phagocytosis
How does *Listeria* **penetrate the phagocytic vacuole to enter the cytoplasm?**	Production of listeriolysin O toxin
Can *Listeria* **move from cell to cell?**	Yes

How does it move from cell to cell?	Forms a "battering ram" by "hijacking" host cell actin to provide a portal of entry from one cell to another
What type of enzymes aid in this passage across the cell membrane?	Phospholipases
What are three clinical manifestations of Listeria infections (Listeriosis)?	1. Meningitis 2. Sepsis 3. Gastroenteritis outbreaks
What are two uncommon clinical manifestations of *Listeria*?	1. Endocarditis 2. Lymphadenitis
How do infected mothers present?	Flu-like illness or asymptomatically
What is characteristic of gastroenteritis secondary to listeriosis?	Watery diarrhea, fever, and headache
How is the diagnosis of *Listeria* infection usually made?	Gram stain and culture
What are the antibiotics commonly prescribed to treat *Listeria* infections?	Ampicillin and gentamicin (especially in newborns) *or* Trimethoprim-sulfamethoxazole *and* Supportive care

BACILLUS

What is the morphology of *Bacillus*?	Blunt-ended gram-positive rods
What are their oxygen requirements?	Obligate or facultative aerobes
Does *Bacillus* form endospores?	Yes
What are the two more commonly known pathogenic species?	1. *Bacillus anthracis* 2. *Bacillus cereus*

BACILLUS ANTHRACIS

What do *B. anthracis* affect more commonly, humans or animals?	Animals
Which animals are commonly affected?	Herbivores, e.g., sheep
How are humans exposed to *B. anthracis*?	Inhalation of spores, ingestion of contaminated food, and contact with contaminated animal products
What are common entry sites?	Skin, mucous membranes and respiratory tract
When exposed, what is the contaminating agent?	Endospores
Are *B. anthracis* spores easily killed?	No, the spores are both heat resistant and difficult to eradicate via chemical or physical means
What are three virulence factors of *B. anthracis*?	1. Antiphagocytic capsule (D-glutamate polymers) 2. Edema factor (exotoxin) 3. Lethal toxin (exotoxin)
What is edema factor?	A calmodulin-dependent adenylate cyclase, increasing cyclic adenosine monophosphate (cAMP) resulting in severe edema
What is lethal toxin?	A protease responsible for cleaving the kinase that activates the mitogen-activated protein kinase (MAPK) signal transduction pathway, inhibiting cell growth, increasing the production of tumor necrosis factor (TNF) and causing cell death
What are two clinical manifestations of *B. anthracis*?	1. Cutaneous anthrax 2. Pulmonary anthrax
What is the most common form of anthrax seen in humans?	Cutaneous anthrax
What are the five stages of cutaneous anthrax?	1. Papule 2. Black, painless "malignant" pustule

3. Invasion of regional lymph nodes
4. Invasion of bloodstream
5. Sepsis

What is the overall morta-lity of cutaneous anthrax?

20%

What antibiotics are commonly used for the treatment of anthrax?

Penicillin, tetracyclines, and ciprofloxacin

What is another term for pulmonary anthrax?

Woolsorter disease

USMLE

What is the cause of pulmonary anthrax?

Inhalation of *B. anthracis* spores

What findings are characteristic of pulmonary anthrax?

Mediastinal widening and sometimes hemorrhagic lymphadenitis

What is the overall mortality of untreated pulmonary anthrax?

Almost 100%

BACILLUS CEREUS

How is *B. cereus* morphologically different from *B. anthracis*?

They are unencapsulated and motile

What is *B. cereus* classically associated with?

Food poisoning, especially from reheated fried rice

What is the route of entry for disease causing *B. cereus* spores?

The gastrointestinal tract

What are the two toxins produced by *B. cereus*?

1. Heat-labile toxin
2. Heat-stable toxin

Can each toxin produce different types of food poisoning?

Yes

How is the heat-labile toxin similar to cholera toxin?

Both result in ADP ribosylation of a G-protein that stimulates the production of cAMP via adenylate cyclase

What is the presentation of disease caused by the heat-labile toxin?

Watery, nonbloody diarrhea, nausea, and abdominal pain 18 hours after ingestion lasting 12–24 hours

What is the presentation of disease caused by the heat-stable toxin?

Acute onset of nausea and vomiting with some diarrhea 4 hours after ingestion

How do you treat food poisoning caused by *B. cereus*?

Supportive care

MISCELLANEOUS GRAM-POSITIVE RODS

Which anaerobic bacteria is associated with acne?

Propionibacterium acnes

Which gram-positive rod is normal flora for mucous membranes and produces lactic acid?

Lactobacillus

Which gram-positive rod is associated with skin infections found most often in those who deal with animal meat, i.e., butchers?

Erysipelothrix rhusiopathiae

6

Gram-Negative Cocci: Neisseria, Moraxella, & Acinetobacter

NEISSERIA

What is *Neisseria*?

Facultative, anaerobic, gram-negative *Diplococcus*

What is the classic morphology of *Neisseria* on light microscopy?

"Kidney bean"-shaped diplococci (see Fig. 6-1)

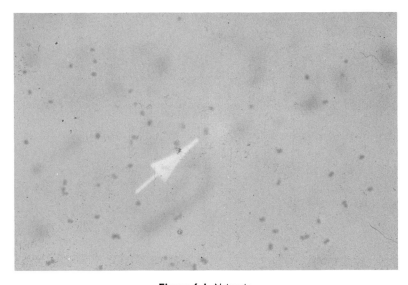

Figure 6-1. *Neisseria.*

Which environment provides optimal growth for *Neisseria*?

High CO_2 concentration

What are two important enzymes that *Neisseria* possess?

1. Cytochrome C oxidase
2. Catalase

What is the function of each?

Cytochrome C oxidase is an enzyme that is part of electron transport and nitrate metabolism that can accept electrons from other substrates

Catalase is an enzyme that inactivates toxic oxygen species by converting hydrogen peroxide to water and oxygen

What selective media is used for culturing *Neisseria*?

Thayer-Martin VCN

What is the composition of this media?

Chocolate agar with *v*ancomycin, *c*olistin (polymyxin), and *n*ystatin (VCN)

What makes this media selective?

Vancomycin kills the gram-positive organisms; colistin (polymyxin) kills all gram-negative organisms except *Neisseria*; nystatin eliminates fungi

What are two *Neisseria* species that cause disease in humans?

1. *N. meningitidis*
2. *N. gonorrhoeae*

How are they metabolically differentiated?

N. meningitidis can metabolize maltose and glucose; *N. gonorrhoeae* can only metabolize glucose

How are they structurally differentiated?

N. meningitidis is encapsulated and will have a positive Quellung reaction; *N. gonorrhoeae* is unencapsulated and will have a negative Quellung reaction

NEISSERIA MENINGITIDIS

What is *N. meningitidis*?

Encapsulated facultative, anaerobic, gram-negative diplococcus capable of fermenting maltose and glucose

What is another name for *N. meningitidis*?

Meningococcus

What are the virulence factors of meningococcus?

1. Antiphagocytic polysaccharide capsule
2. Lipooligosaccharide (LOS) endotoxin
3. Immunoglobulin (Ig) A1 protease
4. Pili-facilitating adherence

5. Transferrin-binding proteins A and B, i.e., proteins that extract iron from human transferrin

What are two ways of classifying *N. meningitidis*?

1. Serotype
2. Serogroup

What is the basis for serotype differentiation?

Outer membrane proteins and LOSs

How many serotypes exist?

>20

What is the basis for serogroup differentiation?

Polysaccharide capsule

How many serogroups exist?

>13

Which serogroups are infectious?

Serogroups A, B, C, W, and Y

Which serogroup is the predominant cause of meningococcal disease in the United States?

Serogroup B

Which virulence factor is responsible for the petechial rash of meningococcal infections?

LOS

What is the only natural host for *N. meningitidis*?

Humans

What is the mode of transmission for *N. meningitidis*?

Inhalation of aerosolized respiratory droplets

What are two populations at increased risk for meningococcal infections?

1. Infants (6 months–2 years)
2. Individuals living in close quarters such as schools, prisons, and military barracks

Why do infants younger than 6 months of age have a smaller risk of meningococcal infection?

Maternal antibodies (IgG) confer protection

What are three predisposing risk factors for meningococcal disease?	1. Recent upper respiratory tract infection 2. Active or passive smoking 3. Deficiencies in the late complement components, e.g., deficiency of C5b-C9 membrane attack complex (MAC)
How does *N. meningitidis* most commonly affect humans?	Asymptomatic nasopharyngeal colonization
How does *N. meningitidis* adversely affect humans?	1. Meningitis 2. Meningococcemia 3. Waterhouse-Friderichsen syndrome (fulminant meningococcemia)
What is a classic sign of these infections?	Petechial rash progressing to purpura
What is the most common form of meningococcal disease?	Meningitis
What is meningitis?	Inflammation of the protective tissues covering the brain
What are five symptoms of meningitis?	1. Nuchal rigidity 2. Severe headache—"worst headache of my life" 3. Altered mental status 4. Photophobia 5. Nonspecific symptoms including fever, vomiting, irritability, and lethargy
What is meningococcemia?	Presence of *N. meningitidis* in the blood
What is the classic skin finding seen with meningococcemia?	Petechial rash
What are the symptoms of meningococcemia?	1. Spiking fevers 2. Chills 3. Arthralgias 4. Myalgias

What is the drug of choice for treating meningococcemia in the adult?	Ceftriaxone or cefotaxime
What is Waterhouse-Friderichsen syndrome?	Bilateral hemorrhage of the adrenal glands leading to adrenal insufficiency causing hypotension, tachycardia, disseminated intravascular coagulation (DIC), coma, and death
What is used for N. meningitidis prophylaxis?	Rifampin
When is prophylaxis indicated?	For individuals who are close-contacts of patients infected with *N. meningitidis*
Is there a vaccine available for N. meningitidis?	Yes
Who should get it?	College students living in dormitories, military recruits, and travelers visiting endemic areas
What serogroups does this vaccine protect against?	Serogroups A, C, W, and Y Unfortunately serogroup B is not effectively covered by this vaccine because it has a capsule containing polysialic acid, which does not elicit an adequate immune response

NEISSERIA GONORRHOEAE

What is N. gonorrhoeae?	Unencapsulated, facultative, anaerobic gram-negative diplococcus capable of fermenting glucose
How is N. gonorrhoeae spread?	1. Sexually transmitted 2. During parturition with an infected mother
What is another name for N. gonorrhoeae?	Gonococcus
What are the virulence factors of gonococcus?	1. Pili 2. IgA1 protease 3. Outer membrane proteins (OMPI and OMPII)

What are three functions of pili?	1. Adherence to host cells 2. Prevention of phagocytosis from macrophages and neutrophils 3. Highly variable antigens protecting against antibodies
What two mechanisms allow gonococcus to avoid the host's immune system? **What is gene conversion?**	1. Gene conversion 2. Phase variation Process by which *N. gonorrhoeae* produces pilin molecules with different antigens by recombining pilin genes
What is phase variation?	Reversible lack of pilin expression
How does this occur?	When a pilin gene is moved
What is the clinical significance of gene conversion and phase variation?	1. Inability to create an effective vaccine because of highly variable bacterial antigens 2. Reinfection may occur after first infection because initial infection does not confer immunity to gonococci with different antigens
What are common symptoms of gonococcal infection in males?	Dysuria and purulent discharge from urethra
What are complications of gonococcal disease in males?	1. Epididymitis 2. Prostatitis 3. Urethral strictures 4. Gonococcal bacteremia 5. Septic arthritis
What are common symptoms of gonococcal infection in females?	Dysuria, purulent vaginal discharge, and pain with sexual intercourse (dyspareunia) Gonorrhea is more frequently asymptomatic in women than in men
What are complications of gonococcal disease in females?	1. Pelvic inflammatory disease (PID) 2. Septic arthritis 3. Endometriosis 4. Gonococcal bacteremia 5. Infertility 6. Increased rate of ectopic pregnancy

Who is most likely to contract gonococcal septic arthritis?

Sexually active individuals

Why is gonococcal bacteremia less frequent than meningococcal bacteremia?

Unlike encapsulated meningococci, unencapsulated gonococci have a limited ability to multiply in the bloodstream

What are complications of gonococcal bacteremia?

1. Pericarditis
2. Endocarditis
3. Meningitis

What are less common sites of *N. gonorrhoeae* infection in sexually active individuals?

Anorectal area and throat

How is *N. gonorrhoeae* diagnosed?

Gram stain and culture of infected fluid or discharge
Culture of infected fluid or discharge is the gold standard for diagnosis because Gram stain is often negative

What do you look for on Gram stain?

Gram-negative diplococci within polymorphonuclear neutrophils (PMNs)

What are two rapid tests for detection of gonorrhea?

1. Enzyme-linked immunoabsorbent assay (ELISA) for detection of gonococcal antigens
2. Deoxyribonucleic acid (DNA) probe assay for detection of gonococcal ribosomal genes

What is the drug of choice for the treatment of gonococcal infections?

Ceftriaxone

Why is doxycycline often added to the treatment regimen for gonorrhea?

Patients with gonorrhea are also often coinfected with *Chlamydia trachomatis*

What clinical manifestation occurs with *N. gonorrhoeae* infection during parturition?

Ophthalmia neonatorum

What other organism causes this disease?

C. trachomatis

What type of damage results from this disease?

Damage to the cornea may cause blindness

How is this disease prevented?

Newborn prophylaxis with erythromycin eye drops

How is this disease treated?

Systemically with ceftriaxone

MORAXELLA

What is *Moraxella*?

Nonmotile, aerobic, gram-negative coccus usually found in pairs that resemble *Neisseria*

Is *Moraxella* oxidase positive or negative?

Oxidase positive

Does *Moraxella* ferment glucose?

No, it does not ferment any carbohydrates

Which species of *Moraxella* is the most important human pathogen?

M. catarrhalis (see Fig. 6-2)

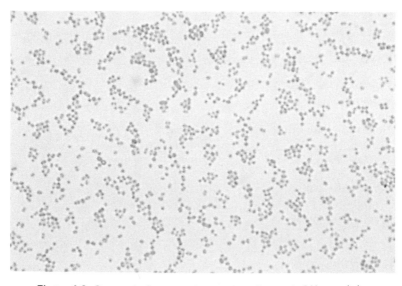

Figure 6-2. Gram stain demonstrating gram-negative cocci of *M. catarrhalis*.

What infections does it cause?	1. Otitis media 2. Sinusitis 3. Bronchitis 4. Pneumonia
How is it treated?	Because most strains are resistant to penicillins, trimethoprim-sulfamethoxazole is often used
Which species of Moraxella is a common cause of blepharitis (infection of the eyelid)?	*M. nonliquefaciens*
What is another common cause of blepharitis?	*Staphylococcus aureus*

ACINETOBACTER

What is *Acinetobacter*?	Encapsulated, nonmotile, obligately aerobic coccobacillus that resembles *Neisseria*
Is *Acinetobacter* oxidase positive or negative?	Oxidase negative
Does *Acinetobacter* ferment glucose?	No, it does not ferment any carbohydrates
Where is *Acinetobacter* found?	Widely distributed in soil and water, but also part of normal skin flora
Which species of *Acinetobacter* usually causes human infection?	*A. calcoaceticus*
What infections does it cause?	1. Sepsis 2. Pneumonia 3. Urinary tract infection
Which two patient populations are at higher risk for infection?	1. Immunocompromised patients 2. Hospitalized patients with indwelling catheters or who are using respiratory ventilation

7

Gram-Negative Rods: Enteric Pathogens

OVERVIEW

What are enteric bacteria?	Gram-negative bacteria that are associated with gastrointestinal flora or disease
What are six families of enteric bacteria?	1. Enterobacteriaceae 2. Vibrionaceae 3. Pseudomonadaceae 4. Bacteroidaceae 5. Campylobacteraceae 6. Helicobacteraceae
What are eight genera that are part of the Enterobacteriaceae family?	1. *Escherichia* 2. *Salmonella* 3. *Shigella* 4. *Klebsiella* 5. *Proteus* 6. *Enterobacter* 7. *Serratia* 8. *Yersinia*
What are the oxygen requirements of most gram-negative rods?	Facultative anaerobes
What are three exceptions?	*Pseudomonas* and *Bacteroides* are obligate anaerobes *Campylobacter* is microaerophilic
What are three common metabolic characteristics of most gram-negative rods?	1. Ferment glucose to produce acid and gas 2. Reduce nitrates to nitrites 3. Oxidase negative
What is the one exception?	*Pseudomonas* does not ferment glucose and is oxidase positive

What biochemical properties can be used to differentiate enteric bacteria?

1. Ability to ferment lactose
2. Ability to produce urease
3. Ability to produce hydrogen sulfide (H_2S)

Which three pathogenic enteric bacteria ferment lactose?

1. *Escherichia*
2. *Enterobacter*
3. *Klebsiella*

EEK! A mouse eats cheese (lactose)

Which three intestinal pathogens cannot ferment lactose?

1. *Shigella*
2. *Salmonella*
3. *Pseudomonas*

Which five enteric bacteria produce urease?

1. *Helicobacter*
2. *Klebsiella*
3. *Proteus*
4. *Providencia*
5. *Morganella*

What is the function of urease?

Metabolizes urea to form carbon dioxide, ammonia, and water, producing a habitable alkaline environment

What differential media can be used to isolate enteric bacteria from gram-positive bacteria?

Eosin-methylene blue (EMB) agar, MacConkey agar, and Hektoen enteric (HE) agar

What characteristic do these agar select for?

Gram-negative bacteria

How does EMB inhibit growth of gram-positive bacteria?

Aniline dyes

How does MacConkey agar inhibit growth of gram-positive bacteria?

Bile salts and crystal violet

How does Hektoen enteric agar inhibit growth of gram-positive bacteria?

Bile salts

What characteristic do these agars screen for?

Lactose-fermenting versus lactose-nonfermenting bacteria

How do lactose-fermenting bacteria appear on EMB?

Metallic-green colonies

How do lactose-fermenting bacteria appear on MacConkey agar?	Pink (see Fig. 7-1)

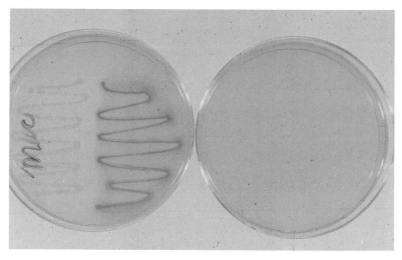

Figure 7-1. Lactose-fermenting bacteria on MacConkey agar. (see also Color Photo 7.)

How do lactose-fermenting bacteria appear on Hektoen enteric agar?	Yellow or orange
How do nonlactose-fermenting bacteria appear on EMB?	Translucent
How do nonlactose-fermenting bacteria appear on MacConkey agar?	Translucent
How do nonlactose-fermenting bacteria appear on Hektoen enteric agar?	Blue-green
What other media selects against gram-positive organisms?	*Salmonella-Shigella* agar
Which four surface antigens are used to differentiate among enteric bacteria?	O antigen, H antigen, K antigen, and pili

What is the O antigen?

Heat-stable cell wall antigen located on the most external surface of lipopolysaccharide (LPS)

Remember "O" for outer

What part of the O antigen confers unique characteristics to different O antigens?

Sugars, e.g., the O157 subtype, which is differentiated by its sugar moiety

What is the H antigen?

Antigen located on the flagella

Only those bacteria with "flag-hella" will have an H antigen

What is the K antigen?

Antigen associated with the capsule or fimbriae

Remember "K" for "kapsule"

What are pili?

Antigenic fimbriae responsible for attachment and colonization of an organism (see Fig. 7-2)

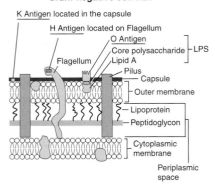

Figure 7-2. Pili and the O, H, and K antigens.

What three characteristics make enteric bacteria pathogenic?

1. Enterotoxins
2. Endotoxins
3. Capsule

How are enterotoxins pathogenic?

They cause transduction of fluid into the ileum

How are endotoxins different from enterotoxins?

Enterotoxins are released from bacteria

Endotoxins are found in the LPS complex of the bacterial outer membrane

What endotoxin do almost all gram-negative rods contain?	LPS
What is a common component in most endotoxins?	Toxic lipid A
Why are endotoxins pathogenic?	1. Stimulate release of tumor necrosis factor (TNF), interleukin-1 (IL-1), and (IL-6) leading to hypotension 2. Stimulate release of IL-1 and IL-6 leading to fever 3. Hemorrhage in the intestine, adrenal glands, heart, and kidneys
How is the capsule pathogenic?	It suppresses phagocytosis
Where do gram-negative rods usually cause disease?	Intraintestinal, extraintestinal, or both, depending on genera
Which gram-negative rods cause disease primarily inside the enteric tract?	*Shigella, Vibrio,* and *Helicobacter*
Which gram-negative rods cause disease outside of the enteric tract?	*Klebsiella, Enterobacter, Serratia, Proteus, Providencia, Morganella, Pseudomonas,* and *Bacteroides*
Which gram-negative rods cause disease both inside and outside of the enteric tract?	*Escherichia, Salmonella, Yersinia,* and *Campylobacter*

ESCHERICHIA COLI

What is E. coli?	Lactose-fermenting, oxidase-negative, gram-negative enteric rod
Where is E. coli found?	Part of the normal flora of the human gut
What are three metabolic characteristics of E. coli?	1. Facultative anaerobes 2. Ferment glucose and lactose 3. Reduce nitrates to nitrites
How is E. coli transmitted?	Fecal–oral and food-borne transmission

What enables *E. coli* to adhere to the epithelium of the gastrointestinal (GI) tract?	Pili or fimbriae
How are *E. coli* strains typed?	O, H, and K antigens
What is the most common clinical manifestation of *E. coli* infection?	Diarrhea

What extraintestinal diseases does *E. coli* commonly cause?

1. Urinary tract infections
2. Cystitis
3. Pyelonephritis
4. Sepsis
5. Neonatal meningitis
6. Hemolytic uremic syndrome
7. Endotoxic shock
8. Pneumonia

How is *E. coli* infection diagnosed?	Culture, biochemical tests, and serological tests
Which antibiotics are commonly used to treat *E. coli* infection?	Ampicillin, cefotaxime, ciprofloxacin (Cipro), and trimethoprim-sulfamethoxazole (Bactrim)

What are five common pathogenic species of *E. coli*?

1. Enterotoxigenic *E. coli* (ETEC)
2. Enteropathogenic *E. coli* (EPEC)
3. Enterohemorrhagic *E. coli* (EHEC)
4. Enteroinvasive *E. coli* (EIEC)
5. Enteroadherent *E. coli* (EAEC)

Which strains cause bloody diarrhea?	EHEC and EIEC

ENTEROTOXIGENIC E. COLI

What does ETEC commonly cause?	Traveler's diarrhea
What are two enterotoxins released by ETEC?	1. Heat-labile toxin (LT) 2. Heat-stable toxin (ST)
How many subunits does heat-labile toxin have?	2 subunits: A and B

What is the pathogenesis of heat-labile toxin?

Subunit A: activates adenylate cyclase, increases cyclic adenosine monophosphate (cAMP), increases secretion of water and chloride ions, and inhibits sodium reabsorption leading to electrolyte imbalance, hypermotility, and diarrhea (similar to cholera toxin) Subunit B: binds G_{M1} ganglioside at the brush border of the small intestine, facilitating entry of Subunit A Heat-labile toxin is essentially the same as the cholera toxin produced by *Vibrio cholerae*

What is the pathogenesis of heat-stable toxin?

Activates guanylate cyclase in epithelial cells of the small intestine, increasing cyclic guanosine monophosphate (cGMP) and causing fluid secretion

How does ETEC cause disease?

Attaches to the small intestinal epithelium via pili and produces enterotoxins that cause hypersecretion of chloride ions and block absorption of sodium, resulting in massive amounts of water in the lumen of the gut

ENTEROPATHOGENIC *E. COLI*

What does EPEC commonly cause?

Watery diarrhea in infants

When does EPEC infection usually take place?

During parturition (birth) or in utero

How does EPEC cause disease?

Bacteria in the gastrointestinal tract attach to mucosal cells in the small intestine and destroy microvilli with attaching and effacing lesions, also resulting in an inflammatory response

ENTEROHEMORRHAGIC *E. COLI*

What is the primary reservoir for EHEC?

Cattle

How does this relate to outbreaks of EHEC?

Eating undercooked beef

What does EHEC commonly cause?	Hemorrhagic colitis and bloody diarrhea
How does EHEC cause disease?	Attaches to and destroys mucosal cells with attaching and effacing lesions and also produces verotoxin, a Shiga-like toxin that enters the bloodstream causing endothelial damage and platelet aggregation, resulting in thrombus formation
Does EHEC invade the bloodstream?	No, only the Shiga-like toxin and LPS enter the blood
What life-threatening condition is associated with EHEC?	Hemolytic uremic syndrome (HUS)
What strain of EHEC has resulted in recent outbreaks and hemolytic uremic syndrome?	*E. coli* O157:H7
What sugar is not fermented by this strain that is fermented by other strains of *E. coli*?	Sorbitol

ENTEROINVASIVE *E. COLI*

What disease does EIEC cause?	Dysentery (bloody diarrhea and fever) similar to shigellosis

ENTEROADHERENT *E. COLI*

What disease does EAEC cause?	Traveler's diarrhea and persistent diarrhea in children

SALMONELLA

What is *Salmonella*?	Nonlactose-fermenting, oxidase-negative, gram-negative rods with flagella located over the entire surface of the bacteria (see Fig. 7-3)
How many different species of *Salmonella* exist?	One, *S. enterica*

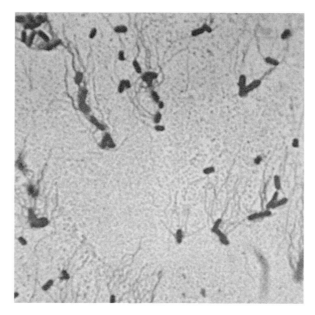

Figure 7-3. *Salmonella* with multiple flagella. (see also Color Photo 8.)

How many different serotypes of *S. enterica* exist?	More than 1,500
Which serotype is an exclusively human pathogen?	*S. typhi*
Where are the other serotypes found?	Animals (reptiles, birds, mammals, pet turtles) and foods (eggs and poultry)
How is salmonella transmitted?	Ingestion of bacteria, usually from food
What natural host defense inhibits *Salmonella* infection?	Stomach acid Decreased stomach acid increases the risk of *Salmonella* infection
What populations are particularly susceptible to *Salmonella* infection?	1. Elderly 2. Young children 3. Patients who have had a gastrectomy 4. Those who chronically take antacids

What hematological disease classically predisposes children to *Salmonella* infection, including osteomyelitis?

Sickle cell anemia

Where is *S. typhi* usually found in chronically infected individuals?

Gall bladder

Where are most other strains usually found?

Bone marrow

What are two metabolic characteristics of *Salmonella*?

1. Produces acid and gas during the fermentation of glucose
2. Produces hydrogen sulfide from sulfur-containing compounds

What are three virulence factors of *Salmonella*?

1. LPS
2. Vi capsular antigen (found in *S. typhi*)
3. RCK (resists complement killing)

What is the capsular antigen similar to?

K antigen of *E. coli*

What are the different diseases caused by *Salmonella*?

1. Gastroenteritis (*S. enteritidis* and *S. typhimurium*)
2. Enteric and typhoid fever (*S. typhi*)
3. Sustained bacteremia, which occurs when the bacteria seed atherosclerotic plaques

What are the symptoms of gastroenteritis caused by *Salmonella*?

Nausea, vomiting, nonbloody diarrhea, fever, and cramping caused by *S. enteritidis* serotype within 48 hours of consumption of contaminated food or water

How long do these symptoms last?

Usually resolve within 72 hours

What is the treatment for gastroenteritis?

No antibiotic treatment is needed, only symptomatic treatment with rehydration
Antibiotics may actually prolong the course of the disease

How does *S. typhi* cause enteric fever?

1. Bacteria enters the gastrointestinal system

2. Bacteria invade small intestinal epithelial cells
3. Bacteria pass to the submucosa
4. Phagocytosed by macrophages
5. Survive in the macrophages and are transported to the reticular endothelial system
6. *Salmonella* can then reenter the gut via the liver and bile

What are the symptoms of enteric fever?

Life-threatening systemic illness with fever, abdominal pain, and a truncal maculopapular rash caused by *S. typhi* serotype

What is the incubation period for *Salmonella* enteric fever?

1–3 weeks

What are the complications of enteric fever?

Intestinal hemorrhage, focal infections, and endocarditis

What agar is used to isolate *Salmonella*?

MacConkey agar

What is the treatment for *Salmonella*?

1. Enterocolitis—resolves without treatment; antibiotics may prolong excretion
2. Enteric fever—using either ceftriaxone or ciprofloxacin substantially decreases mortality from 15% to 1%

Is there a vaccine available for *Salmonella*?

Yes, but only for S. typhi serotype, which offers 50% to 80% protection

SHIGELLA

What is *Shigella*?

Nonmotile, nonlactose-fermenting, oxidase-negative, gram-negative enteric rods

What is the reservoir for *Shigella*?

Humans only, there is no other animal reservoir

How is *Shigella* transmitted?

Fecal–oral and food-borne transmission
Four F's: fingers, flies, food, feces

Is the infectious dose low or high for Shigella?	Very low
What does this mean?	Even a low number of organisms (~200) can cause disease if ingested
How many different serotypes of Shigella exist?	40 serotypes are organized into 4 species based on the polysaccharide O antigen
What serogroup is the most common in the United States?	S. sonnei
What toxin is associated with Shigella?	Shiga toxin, which is only produced by S. dysenteriae serotype 1
What is it?	An exotoxin with cytotoxic properties
How does Shigella cause disease?	Invades and destroys the mucosa of the large intestine, but does not cause bacteremia
What disease does Shigella commonly cause?	Dysentery
What are the symptoms of this disease?	Bloody diarrhea, mucus, and painful abdominal cramping; seizures in children
How long do symptoms last?	Untreated dysentery resolves in 1 week
What selective agar can be used to identify Shigella?	Hektoen agar
What is this?	Agar that can differentiate on the basis of lactose fermentation and hydrogen sulfide production and which contains bromthymol blue pH indicator and bile salts for inhibition of gram-positive organisms
What is the treatment for Shigella dysentery?	Ciprofloxacin or azithromycin can reduce the duration of the illness, but concerns about resistance and increased frequency of hemolytic uremic syndrome have made treatment controversial

CAMPYLOBACTER

What is *Campylobacter*?   Curved, comma, or S-shaped organisms
with a single polar flagellum (see Fig. 7-4)

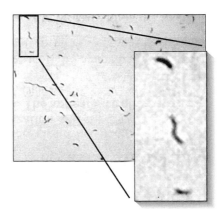

Figure 7-4. Micrograph demonstrating
"S"-shaped *C. jejuni.*

What are the oxygen   Microaerophilic, i.e., they require 5%
requirements for   oxygen, not atmospheric oxygen (21%)
Campylobacter?

What are the reservoirs of   Mammals and birds
Campylobacter?

How is *Campylobacter*   1. Fecal–oral transmission
transmitted to humans?   2. Direct contact (especially poultry)
3. Contaminated water

Who is typically susceptible   Children
to *Campylobacter* infection?

What species of   *C. jejuni*
Campylobacter is a major
human pathogen?

What is the pathogenesis of   Following oral ingestion, *C. jejuni* colo-
C. jejuni?   nizes intestinal mucosa and invades intestinal epithelium, with resultant ulceration and bleeding of mucosal surface
Rarely, *C. jejuni* may enter the bloodstream, disseminating to multiple
organs, particularly in the
immunocompromised

**What diseases does
C. jejuni cause?**

Acute enteritis, traveler's diarrhea,
pseudoappendicitis, and bacteremia

**What is the incubation
period for acute enteritis?**

1–7 days

**What are three
complications of C. jejuni
infection?**

1. Guillain-Barré syndrome
2. Septic abortion
3. Reactive arthritis

**How is Campylobacter
infection diagnosed?**

Growth on selective media in
microaerophilic conditions

**What is the treatment for
C. jejuni?**

Symptomatic treatment with fluid and
electrolyte replacement
Treat with ciprofloxacin for persistent
infection or bloody diarrhea

**Which strain of Campy-
lobacter causes vascular
and central nervous system
(CNS) infection?**

C. fetus

**What is the treatment for
C. fetus?**

Symptomatic treatment with fluid and
electrolyte replacement
Treat with ampicillin or third-generation
cephalosporin for persistent symptoms
or bloody diarrhea

VIBRIO

What is Vibrio?

Rapidly motile short, curved,
oxidase-positive, gram-negative rods with
a single polar flagellum (see Fig. 7-5)

**What are the oxygen
requirements of Vibrio?**

Facultative anaerobes

**What are the natural
hosts?**

Marine shellfish and plankton

**How are the different
Vibrio strains classified?**

Based on their O antigens

**Which strains are
pathogenic?**

1. V. cholerae O1 strains
2. V. cholerae non-O1 strains
3. V. parahaemolyticus
4. V. vulnificus

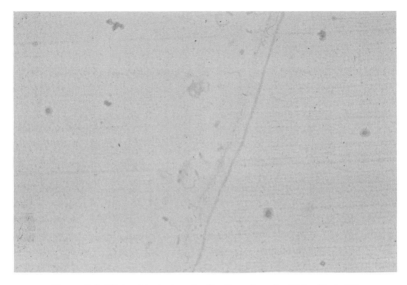

Figure 7-5. *Vibrio* with single polar flagellum. (see also Color Photo 9.)

How is *V. parahaemolyticus* infection differentiated from *V. cholera* infection?	*V. parahaemolyticus* grows in 8% NaCl solution, but *V. cholera* does not
How are the biotypes of *V. cholerae* 01 differentiated?	By differences in biochemical reactions
What are the two biotypes of *V. cholerae* 01?	El Tor and Classic
How do they differ?	El Tor produces hemolysins, has higher carriage rates, and can survive in water longer
How are *V. cholerae* transmitted?	By contaminated food and water
How do *V. cholerae* cause disease?	After ingestion, bacteria attach to the small intestine, but do not invade the mucosa, where they produce cholera toxin
How does cholera toxin cause disease?	Causes outpouring of water and chloride ions into the lumen of the intestine

How many subunits does cholera toxin have?

2: A (active) and B (binding)

What is the function of the A subunit?

A1 adenosine diphosphate (ADP) ribosylates Gs protein, activating adenylate cyclase, which increases cAMP yielding increased chloride ion and water flow to the lumen
A2 facilitates penetration of cell membranes

What is the function of the B subunit?

Binds to G_{M1} ganglioside receptor of epithelial cells

How is the diarrhea classically characterized in cholera?

"Rice water" stools

What is the cause of death from cholera?

Severe dehydration

What condition predisposes individuals to infection with Vibrio?

Reduced stomach acid, e.g., from gastrectomy or antacid use

How is V. cholerae identified?

Growth on standard media such as blood and MacConkey agars
Thiosulfate-citrate-bile salts-sucrose (TCBS) enhances isolation

What is the treatment for cholera?

Replacement of fluids and electrolytes can reduce death rates from 50% to less than 1%
Tetracycline can shorten symptoms

What food is associated with V. parahaemolyticus infection?

Inadequately cooked seafood

What are the clinical manifestations of V. parahaemolyticus infection?

Watery diarrhea, nausea, vomiting, abdominal cramps, and fever

What is the treatment for V. parahaemolyticus?

Symptomatic treatment only because antibiotics do not alter the course of infection

What are the clinical manifestations of *V. vulnificus* infection?	1. Soft-tissue infections (cellulitis) 2. Septicemia in the immunocompromised and in those with chronic liver disease

YERSINIA

What is *Yersinia*?	Small, encapsulated, gram-negative rods
What three species of *Yersinia* cause disease in humans?	1. *Y. enterocolitica* 2. *Y. pseudotuberculosis* 3. *Y. pestis*
What species causes disease of the gastrointestinal tract?	*Y. enterocolitica*, Y. pseudotuberculosis
What disease does *Y. pestis* cause?	Bubonic and pneumonic plague
What are the characteristics of *Y. enterocolitica* and *Yersinia pseudotuberculosis*?	1. They can grow at 4°C (39.2°F), 27°C (80.6°F) (room temperature), or 37°C (98.6°F) 2. Motile at 25°C (77°F) but not at 37°C (98.6°F) 3. Lactose negative
How are *Y. enterocolitica* and *Yersinia pseudotuberculosis* transmitted?	By ingestion of contaminated food
Which virulence factors are associated with *Yersinia*?	V and W antigens
How do *Y. enterocolitica* and *Yersinia pseudotuberculosis* cause disease?	They cause ulcerative lesions in terminal ileum and necrosis in Peyer patches with enlargement of mesenteric lymph nodes
What disease is caused by *Y. enterocolitica* and *Yersinia pseudotuberculosis*?	Enterocolitis
What are the symptoms of this disease?	Fever, abdominal pain, and diarrhea, which may mimic appendicitis

What are two complications of *Yersinia* infection?	1. Reactive polyarthritis 2. Erythema nodosum
How is *Yersinia* infection diagnosed?	Growth on MacConkey or cefsulodin-irgasan-novobiocin (CIN) agar
What is the treatment for *Y. enterocolitica* and *Yersinia* pseudotuberculosis infection?	Antibiotics are of questionable value if infection is limited to the gastrointestinal tract Ciprofloxacin or trimethoprim-sulfamethoxazole for systemic infection

HELICOBACTER

What is *Helicobacter*?	Curved or spiral organisms with multiple polar flagella (see Fig. 7-6)

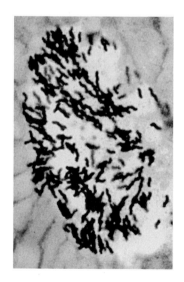

Figure 7-6. *Helicobacter* with multiple polar flagella.

What are the oxygen requirements of *H. pylori*?	Microaerophilic
What enzyme does *Helicobacter* produce? **What is the function of urease?**	Urease Metabolizes urea to form carbon dioxide, ammonia, and water, producing a local habitable alkaline environment in the normally acidic stomach

What is unusual about where some *Helicobacter* colonize humans?	They can only colonize the stomach, where most bacteria cannot
Where does *Helicobacter* live in the stomach?	In the mucus layers adjacent to the mucosa
How is *Helicobacter* transmitted?	Person to person
How long will a person be infected with *Helicobacter*?	If not treated, the infection can be life-long
How does *Helicobacter* cause disease?	Does not invade the epithelium, but causes chronic inflammation of the mucosa by releasing cytotoxins; the ammonia may also cause injury and potentiate the effects of the cytotoxin
What characterizes initial and chronic *Helicobacter* infection?	Initial infection is characterized by acute gastritis, occasionally with diarrhea Chronic infection is characterized by gastritis (usually asymptomatic) and can lead to gastric and duodenal ulcers, gastric carcinoma and gastric B-cell lymphoma
Are most infections symptomatic?	No, most are asymptomatic
What noninvasive tests can diagnose *Helicobacter* infection?	Enzyme-linked immunoabsorbent assay (ELISA) for serum antibodies to *H. pylori*; breath tests for urease
What invasive test can be used to diagnose *Helicobacter* infection?	Biopsy via endoscopy
What is the treatment of *H. pylori*?	Combination therapy, such as metronidazole, tetracycline, and bismuth or metronidazole, clarithromycin, and a proton pump inhibitor

ENTEROBACTER

What is *Enterobacter*?	Lactose-fermenting, motile, gram-negative rods

Who is usually susceptible to *Enterobacter* infection?

Hospitalized patients, in association with antibiotic treatment, catheters, or invasive procedures

What are the clinical manifestations of *Enterobacter* infection?

Pneumonia and urinary tract infections

KLEBSIELLA

What is *Klebsiella*?

Lactose-fermenting, nonmotile, gram-negative rods

What is the distinguishing characteristic of *Klebsiella*?

Has a large capsule, giving colonies a mucoid appearance

What infections can *Klebsiella* cause?

Necrotizing lobar pneumonia, urinary tract infections, and bacteremia

Which individuals are most susceptible to *Klebsiella* pneumonia?

Alcoholics, diabetics, patients with chronic obstructive pulmonary disease (COPD)

What does the sputum of a patient with *Klebsiella* pneumonia look like?

Currant-jelly appearance

SERRATIA

What is *Serratia*?

Motile, slow lactose-fermenting, gram-negative rods

What species of *Serratia* most commonly infects humans?

S. marcescens

What diseases does *Serratia* most commonly cause?

Pneumonia and urinary tract infections, mainly in the immunocompromised

How does *Serratia* appear in culture?

Some strains produce a red pigment

PROTEUS

What is a common clinical manifestation of *Proteus* infection?

Urinary tract infection

What additional complications are seen with *Proteus* infection in the immunocompromised?	Pneumonia, wound infection, and septicemia
What enzyme do *Proteus* species produce?	Urease
What is a significant complication of *Proteus* infection and increased urine pH?	Struvite stone formation containing magnesium, ammonium hydroxide, and phosphate
How does *Proteus* appear on agar plates?	Swarming bacteria (see Fig. 7-7)

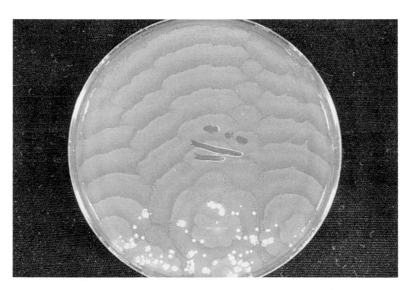

Figure 7-7. Swarming *Proteus*. (See also Color Photo 10.)

BACTEROIDES

What is *Bacteroides*?	Slender, gram-negative rods or coccobacillus
What are the oxygen requirements of *Bacteroides*?	Obligate anaerobes

Where is *Bacteroides* normally found?

It is the predominant organism of the human colon

Which *Bacteroides* species is a major human pathogen?

B. fragilis

What is the main virulence factor of *B. fragilis*?

Polysaccharide capsule

Why is the polysaccharide capsule the main virulence factor?

It conveys resistance to phagocytosis and can trigger abscess formation
The capsule contains little or no endotoxin

How does *B. fragilis* infection occur?

A break in the mucosal surface (usually secondary to local trauma) allows bacteria to enter the blood stream

What are three infections that *B. fragilis* causes?

1. Sepsis
2. Peritonitis
3. Abscess formation
These infections usually occur below the diaphragm

How does the presences of facultative anaerobes contribute to the pathogenesis of *B. fragilis*?

Facultative anaerobes (e.g., *E. coli*) utilize oxygen, thereby producing an environment with a reduced oxygen concentration which allows *B. fragilis* to grow

How are *B. fragilis* infections diagnosed?

1. Culture of infected site
2. Gas chromatography
3. Biochemical tests

How is *B. fragilis* cultured?

Growth in anaerobic conditions on blood agar plates containing kanamycin and vancomycin to inhibit growth of unwanted organisms

What does gas chromatography detect?

Short-chain fatty acids that are produced by *B. fragilis*

What is the treatment for *B. fragilis* infection?

Metronidazole

PREVOTELLA

What is *Prevotella*?	Slender, gram-negative rods
What are the oxygen requirements of *Prevotella*?	Obligate anaerobes
Where is *Prevotella* normally found?	Normal flora of the mouth and upper gastrointestinal and respiratory tracts
Which species of *Prevotella* is the most common human pathogen?	*P. melaninogenica*
How does *P. melaninogenica* infection occur?	A break in the mucosal surface (usually secondary to local trauma) allows bacteria to enter the bloodstream
What are two infections that *P. melaninogenica* causes?	1. Sepsis 2. Abscess formation These infections usually occur above the diaphragm
How are *P. melaninogenica* infections diagnosed?	1. Culture of infected site 2. Gas chromatography 3. Biochemical tests
How does *P. melaninogenica* appear on blood agar?	Forms black colonies
What is the treatment for *P. melaninogenica* infections?	Metronidazole

PORPHYROMONAS

What is *Porphyromonas*?	Anaerobic, gram-negative rods
What are two species of *Porphyromonas* that can cause disease in humans? **What diseases can they cause?**	1. *P. gingivalis* 2. *P. endodontalis* Periodontal disease, including gingivitis and dental abscess

8

Gram-Negative Rods: Respiratory Pathogens

OVERVIEW

What are three gram-negative rods associated with respiratory tract infections?

1. *Haemophilus influenzae*
2. *Legionella pneumophila*
3. *Bordetella pertussis*

What virulence factor do these organisms have in common?

Lipopolysaccharide (LPS), which is common to all gram-negative bacteria

What are their oxygen requirements?

Facultative anaerobes

HAEMOPHILUS

What is the structure of *Haemophilus*?
Why can they be difficult to visualize on Gram stain?

Pleomorphic: from coccobacillus to long slender rods
The organisms are small

What are two pathogenic species of *Haemophilus*?

1. *H. influenzae*
2. *H. ducreyi*

HAEMOPHILUS INFLUENZAE

How are serotypes of *H. influenzae* distinguished?

By their capsular polysaccharide (see Fig. 8-1)

How many different serotypes exist?

6
There is another type which is denoted "nontypeable" because it is unencapsulated

What is the natural host of *H. influenzae*?

Humans are the only natural host

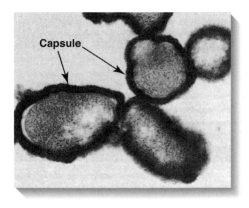

Figure 8-1. *Haemophilus influenzae* (electron micrograph) showing thick capsules.

Where is *H. influenzae* commonly found?

Normal flora of the upper respiratory tract

How is *H. influenzae* transmitted?

Respiratory droplets

What virulence factors enable *H. influenzae* to attach to respiratory mucosa?

Immunoglobulin (Ig) A protease and several types of adhesins

What are two general types of infections caused by *H. influenzae*?

1. Localized infections of the respiratory tract secondary to contiguous spread of bacteria (e.g., pneumonia)
2. Disseminated disease secondary to bacteremia (e.g., meningitis)

What part of *H. influenzae* enables it to cause disseminated disease?

The capsule

Do unencapsulated *H. influenzae* cause meningitis?

No; unencapsulated bacteria cannot survive in the bloodstream or cause disseminated disease

Which serotype of *H. influenzae* is associated with severe infections?

Type b

Why is type b associated with severe infections?

The capsule is composed of polyribose phosphate, facilitating tissue invasion

What are four major infections caused by *H. influenzae* in children?

1. Sinusitis
2. Otitis media
3. Meningitis
4. Epiglottitis

"SOME" is an acronym for the infections caused by *H. influenzae* in children

What makes epiglottitis a life-threatening disease?

The swollen epiglottis may obstruct the airway

What major adult infection is caused by *H. influenzae*?

Pneumonia

What population has an increased risk of infection?

Patients with chronic obstructive pulmonary disease (COPD) who cannot effectively clear the organism

What are other clinical manifestations of *H. influenzae*?

1. Septic arthritis
2. Purulent conjunctivitis
3. Brazilian purpuric fever

How is *H. influenzae* definitively diagnosed in the lab?

Culture on chocolate agar

Which two factors are required for growth of *H. influenzae* on laboratory media?

Factor V (NAD) and factor X (heme)

How can meningitis be diagnosed?

Cerebrospinal fluid (CSF) Gram stain, latex agglutination, immunoelectrophoresis, and radioimmune assay of CSF

How are upper respiratory tract infections treated?

Antibiotics, including trimethoprim-sulfamethoxazole

How are disseminated infections treated?

Third-generation cephalosporins such as ceftriaxone or cefotaxime

Why use third-generation cephalosporins?

Many of the type b organisms produce β-lactamase, which destroys penicillin and ampicillin

What percent of *H. influenzae* type b isolates produce β-lactamase, thus requiring treatment with a cephalosporin?

20–30%

What is the mortality rate for untreated *H. influenzae* meningitis?	~90%
How are *H. influenzae* infections prevented?	Administration of childhood conjugated vaccine
What are the components of the conjugated *H. influenzae* vaccine? **Why is it conjugated to diphtheria toxoid?**	Type b capsular polysaccharide conjugated to diphtheria toxoid or another carrier protein The toxoid is antigenic, increasing the immunogenic response to the vaccine
At what age is it administered?	2–15 months
How effective is the conjugated *H. influenzae* vaccine?	It has reduced the incidence of meningitis in immunized children by 90%
How has this affected the prevalence of *H. influenzae* meningitis?	Until introduction of the vaccine in the early 1990s, *H. influenzae* was the number one cause of meningitis in children
Which drug is used for prophylactically for close contacts of *H. influenzae*-infected patients? **Why is this drug used?**	Rifampin Rifampin is secreted in saliva and therefore reduces respiratory carriage of organisms

HAEMOPHILUS DUCREYI

How is *H. ducreyi* transmitted?	Sexually
What does *H. ducreyi* cause?	Chancroid on the genitals and inguinal lymphadenopathy (buboes)
How are *H. ducreyi* lesions distinguished from those of *Treponema pallidum* syphilitic lesions?	*H. ducreyi* chancres are very painful and tend to have ragged edges, whereas *T. pallidum* chancres are shallow, indurated, painless ulcers

LEGIONELLA

What is the structure of Legionella?

Unencapsulated slender rods that may appear coccobacillary

How many different species of Legionella exist?

34

Which species is responsible for 90% of human disease caused by Legionella?

Legionella pneumophila

What is the primary reservoir of Legionella?

Environmental water sources that contain stagnant water such as air conditioners

How is Legionella transmitted?

Inhalation of aerosolized organisms

Why is Legionella occasionally transmitted by swimming in pools?

It is chlorine tolerant

What type of immune response prevents Legionella infection?
How?

Innate immunity

Alveolar macrophages phagocytose bacteria, normally killing the organism

What allows Legionella to be pathogenic?

Failure of fusion between the phagosome and lysosome allows bacteria to multiply within the protected environment of the phagosome until it ruptures, releasing bacteria

What two infections are caused by Legionella?

1. Legionnaires' disease
2. Pontiac fever

What is Legionnaires' disease?

An atypical pneumonia with a lobar distribution

What percentage of patients exposed to Legionella develop Legionnaires' disease?

1–5%

Which populations are most susceptible to *Legionella* infection?	Elderly, smokers, alcoholics, and immune-suppressed individuals
What type of sputum is seen in *Legionella* pneumonia?	Scant and nonpurulent
What does Gram stain of sputum from a person with *Legionella* pneumonia demonstrate?	Neutrophils without bacteria
What nonrespiratory clinical findings accompany *Legionella* infection?	Confusion, fever, malaise, myalgias, anorexia, diarrhea, proteinuria, and hematuria, death
What metabolic abnormality is commonly associated with *Legionella* pneumonia?	Hyponatremia (low sodium)
What is the fatality rate for Legionnaires' disease?	5–30%
What percentage of cases of community-acquired pneumonia does *Legionella* cause?	1–5%
What is Pontiac fever?	An influenza-like illness
How is *Legionella* diagnosed? **Which method is the gold standard for diagnosis?**	1. Culture 2. Serology Culture
What are the culture requirements for *Legionella*?	Special medium containing buffered charcoal yeast extract with iron and L-cysteine
How is *Legionella* diagnosed by serology?	Antibody titers or urine antigen detection
What role does Gram stain have in the diagnosis of *Legionella*?	A minor one because *Legionella* stains poorly with Gram stain

What is the treatment for Legionella?	Legionnaires' disease is treated with erythromycin or azithromycin and supportive therapy; Pontiac fever is treated symptomatically

BORDETELLA

What is the structure of Bordetella?	Small, encapsulated coccobacillus that grows singly or in pairs
How are serotypes of Bordetella distinguished?	Cell-surface molecules called agglutinogens
What is the most common human pathogen of Bordetella?	B. pertussis
What disease does it cause?	Whooping cough
How is B. pertussis transmitted?	Respiratory droplets B. pertussis is highly contagious
What population is most susceptible to B. pertussis infection?	Infants and children
How does B. pertussis interact with the respiratory epithelium?	Attaches to cilia without invading the tissue, producing toxins and virulence factors that eventually cause cilia to die
What is the major toxin produced by B. pertussis?	Pertussis toxin
What is the structure of pertussis toxin?	Two subunits, including an enzymatically active A subunit and a B subunit that bind host cells
What is the function of the A subunit?	Stimulates adenylate cyclase resulting in increase camp by adenosine diphosphate (ADP) ribosylating (and therefore inactivating) G_i, the inhibitory subunit of the G protein
What makes pertussis toxin pathogenic?	1. Lymphocytosis 2. Increased histamine sensitivity 3. Insulin secretion secondary to pancreatic β-islet cell activation resulting in hypoglycemia

What are five other virulence factors produced by *B. pertussis*?	1. Filamentous hemagglutinin 2. Adenylate cyclase toxin 3. Dermonecrotic toxin 4. Tracheal toxin (peptidoglycan) 5. Agglutinogens
What is the mechanism of . . .	
Filamentous hemagglutinin?	Allows bacteria to attach to ciliated epithelial cells
Adenylate cyclase toxin?	Taken up by leukocytes, causing excessive accumulation of intracellular cyclic adenosine monophosphate (cAMP), resulting in decreased chemotaxis and phagocytosis of bacteria
Dermonecrotic toxin?	Vasoconstriction and ischemic necrosis
Tracheal cytotoxin?	Inhibits cilia movement and regeneration of damaged cells
Agglutinogens?	Facilitates attachment of bacteria to host cells
What part of the respiratory tract does *B. pertussis* infect?	Tracheobronchioles
What is the incubation period for pertussis?	1–3 weeks
What are the three stages of whooping cough?	1. Catarrhal phase 2. Paroxysmal phase 3. Convalescent phase
What are the symptoms of the catarrhal phase?	Nonspecific symptoms, including copious rhinorrhea, conjunctival infection, malaise, fever, and nonproductive cough
What are the symptoms of the paroxysmal phase?	Paroxysmal, productive hacking cough which often ends with an inspiratory "whoop" and may last up to 4 weeks
What are the symptoms of the convalescent phase?	Less-frequent and less-severe coughing episodes with gradual resolution after 1–3 months

How is *B. pertussis* infection diagnosed?
How is this confirmed?

Clinical suspicion with marked lymphocytosis
Culture of *B. pertussis* from nasopharynx of symptomatic patient or direct fluorescent antibody test
Blood cultures will always be negative

What type of medium is required for growth of *B. pertussis*?

Selective agar medium containing blood and charcoal supplemented with antibiotics to inhibit growth of other normal flora of the nasopharynx

What is the treatment for *B. pertussis*?

Erythromycin and supportive therapy

What two vaccines are available for *B. pertussis*?

1. Acellular vaccine containing proteins from inactivated pertussis toxin
2. Killed whole cells

Which one is approved for use in the United States?

Acellular vaccine usually given with diphtheria and tetanus toxoids (diphtheria, tetanus toxoids, and acellular pertussis [DTaP]) in 3 doses beginning at 2 months of age

9

Gram-Negative Rods: Opportunistic Pathogens

PSEUDOMONAS

What is *Pseudomonas*?

Oxidase-positive, pigment-producing, encapsulated rods with polar flagella

What are the oxygen requirements of *Pseudomonas*?

Obligate aerobe

What is a specific metabolic characteristic of *Pseudomonas*?

Unable to ferment carbohydrates, including glucose

Where is *Pseudomonas* found?

Soil, plants, and water (including humidifiers, ventilators, and tap water)

What is the main pathogen of the *Pseudomonas* family?
How is it transmitted?

P. aeruginosa

Water aerosols, aspiration, or fecal contamination

What parts of the body does it colonize?

Skin, upper respiratory tract, and colon

Which group of patients is at increased risk for *P. aeruginosa* infection?
What are two high-risk groups?

Hospitalized patients
P. aeruginosa is a major cause of nosocomial infection
1. Cystic fibrosis patients
2. Burn patients

Why are patients with cystic fibrosis at increased risk for infection?

The cilia of patients with cystic fibrosis are unable to effectively clear the organism from the respiratory tract

What are four virulence factors of *P. aeruginosa*?	1. Pili (type 4) 2. Glycocalyx 3. Toxins 4. Extracellular products
How do they contribute to pathogenesis?	Pili mediate attachment to the host's cells; the capsule is antiphagocytic
What toxins and extracellular products are produced by *P. aeruginosa*?	1. Extracellular pigments 2. Endotoxin 3. Exotoxins A and S 4. Extracellular proteases (e.g., elastase and alkaline protease) 5. Cytotoxin 6. Hemolysins
What pigments does *P. aeruginosa* produce?	Usually green (pyoverdin) and blue (pyocyanin) pigments, but may also produce red and black pigments (see Fig. 9-1)

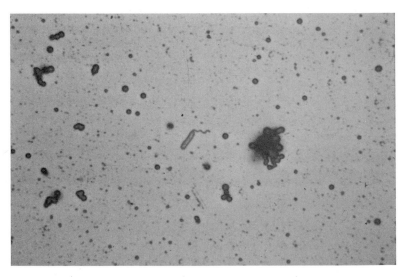

Figure 9-1. Pigments produced by *P. aeruginosa* (see also Color Photo 12).

What part of the endotoxin contributes to pathogenesis?	Lipid A moiety
What is the action of exotoxin A?	Adenosine diphosphate (ADP) ribosylates and inactivates elongation factor (EF-2), thereby

inhibiting mammalian protein synthesis
Diphtheria toxin produced by
Corynebacterium diphtheriae acts by this
mechanism

**What is the action of
exotoxin S?**

ADP ribosylates specific guanosine
triphosphate (GTP)-binding proteins

**What are four common
infections caused by
P. aeruginosa?**

1. Urinary tract infections
2. Wound infections
3. Pneumonia
4. Sepsis

**What is the mortality rate
for *P. aeruginosa* sepsis?**

50%

**What are three
less-common infections
caused by *P. aeruginosa*?**

1. Malignant otitis externa
2. Folliculitis
3. Corneal infections

**How is *P. aeruginosa*
infection diagnosed?**

Growth on blood or MacConkey agar and
biochemical tests

**What is noticeable about
P. aeruginosa growth on
culture?**

Fruity aroma

**How is *P. aeruginosa*
treated?**

Two bactericidal antibiotics are given
simultaneously to prevent resistance

**What classes of antibiotics
can be used for treatment?**

Aminoglycosides, antipseudomonal
β-lactams, and quinolones

**What other species of
Pseudomonas cause human
infection?**

1. *Burkholderia mallei*
2. *Burkholderia cepacia*
3. *P. pseudomallei*

**How does *B. mallei* differ
from other species of
Pseudomonas?**

It is nonmotile

**What infection does
B. mallei cause?**

Glanders, which is more common in
horses, donkeys, and mules

**What are the clinical
manifestations of *B. mallei*?**

Depending on the route of infection, it
can cause

1. Acute, localized suppurative infection of the eye, nose or lips
2. Acute pulmonary infection
3. Acute septicemic infection that is usually fatal
4. Chronic suppurative infection with multiple subcutaneous or intramuscular abscesses

What disease does *P. pseudomallei* cause?

Melioidosis

What are the clinical manifestations of *P. pseudomallei*?

Symptoms are similar to *B. mallei* infection

10

Gram-Negative Rods: Zoonotic Pathogens

What are five zoonotic gram-negative organisms?	1. *Brucella* 2. *Francisella tularensis* 3. *Yersinia pestis* 4. *Pasteurella multocida* 5. *Bartonella* sp.

BRUCELLA

What type of organism is *Brucella*?	Aerobic, facultative intracellular, unencapsulated coccobacillus found alone or in pairs
Which animals are reservoirs for *Brucella*?	Goats, sheep, cattle, pigs, and dogs
How is *Brucella* transmitted to humans?	Ingestion of contaminated, unpasteurized milk products or through cuts and skin abrasions
Which cells does *Brucella* typically infect?	Macrophages of the reticuloendothelial system
What is the incubation period for Brucella? **What is the major virulence factor?**	Several weeks; but can range from 5 days to months Lipopolysaccharide (LPS)
What is the host response to *Brucella* infection?	Granulomatous, with focal abscess formation
What are the clinical manifestations of *Brucella* infection?	1. Undulating fever (repeatedly rises then falls) 2. Flu-like symptoms including myalgias, anorexia, gastrointestinal (GI) symptoms, and headache
What is the name for this constellation of symptoms?	Brucellosis

How is *Brucella* infection diagnosed?

Serologic titers for antibody greater than 1:160

Specimen cultures taking up to 1 month for growth

How is *Brucella* treated?

Doxycycline and gentamycin for 6 weeks

FRANCISELLA TULARENSIS

What type of organism is *F. tularensis*?

Obligately aerobic, facultative intracellular, pleomorphic coccobacillus with lipid-rich capsules

What animals are reservoirs for *F. tularensis*?

Wild animals, including rabbits, deer, and rodents

How is *F. tularensis* transmitted to humans?
How does it present clinically?

By vectors such as ticks, lice, and mice, or by contact with animal hide

1. Ulcer at site of infection
2. Lymphadenopathy at multiple sites
3. Flu-like symptoms including fever, chills, headache, malaise, and anorexia

What is the name for this constellation of symptoms?

Tularemia

What is another name for this disease?

Rabbit or deerfly fever

What other disease presents with similar symptoms and must therefore be considered in the differential diagnosis?

Lyme disease; however, it presents with a rash and not an ulcer

What are less-common symptoms of *F. tularensis* infection?

1. Conjunctivitis
2. Pneumonia
3. Pharyngitis

How is *F. tularensis* infection diagnosed?

History of possible exposure confirmed with serologic studies including enzyme-linked immunoabsorbent assay (ELISA); rarely cultured from blood

What is an important ingredient of an _F. tularensis_ growth medium?	Cysteine to provide a sulfhydryl source
What is the treatment for _F. tularensis_?	Streptomycin or gentamycin

YERSINIA PESTIS

What is the structure of _Y. pestis_?	Encapsulated small rods or coccobacillus
Which animals are reservoirs for _Y. pestis_?	Prairie dogs, rats, and squirrels
Which is the predominant reservoir in the United States?	Prairie dogs
How is _Y. pestis_ transmitted to humans?	By fleas, respiratory droplets, or ingestion of contaminated human tissue
Does Y. pestis replicate in humans?	No, humans are dead-end hosts
What does this mean?	Dead-end hosts accidentally become infected and do not participate in the life cycle of the pathogen
What is the incubation period for _Y. pestis_?	2–8 days
How does the virulence of _Y. pestis_ compare to other organisms?	It is highly virulent; 1 to 10 organisms are sufficient to elicit disease
What are five major virulence factors of _Y. pestis_?	1. F-1 envelope antigen confers antiphagocytic properties 2. Endotoxin 3. Exotoxin 4. V antigen 5. W antigen
What are three clinical manifestations of _Y. pestis_?	1. Bubonic plague 2. Pneumonic plague 3. Meningitic plague
What are the symptoms of bubonic plague?	1. Buboes 2. Fever

3. Chills
4. Headache
5. Myalgias
6. Weakness

What are buboes?   Swollen, painful, sometimes weepy lymph nodes typically found in the groin, axilla, and neck (see Fig. 10-1)

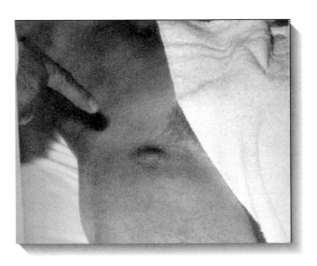

Figure 10-1. Bubo characteristic of *Y. pestis* infection.

What are the clinical manifestations of pneumonic plague?   Purulent pneumonia

What are the endotoxin-related symptoms of plague?
1. Disseminated intravascular coagulation (DIC)
2. Septic shock
3. Cutaneous hemorrhages
4. Hypotension

What is a complication of disseminated infection?   Plague meningitis

How is *Y. pestis* diagnosed?   Clinical presentation, Gram stain, and culture on MacConkey or blood agar

How does *Y. pestis* appear on Gram stain?   Rods or coccobacilli with bipolar staining

What does this mean?   Staining on either end of the organism with a central clear area (see Fig. 10-2)

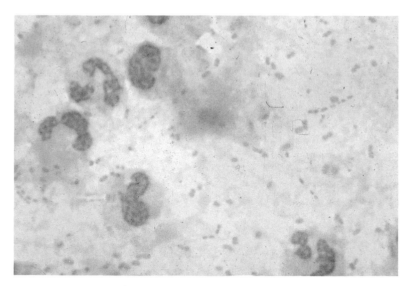

Figure 10-2. Bipolar staining seen with *Y. pestis* (see also Color Photo 13).

What is the treatment for *Y. pestis*?	Streptomycin is best, but gentamycin and tetracycline are alternatives
What is the treatment for plague meningitis?	Chloramphenicol, because of good central nervous system (CNS) penetration
What is the mortality rate of untreated bubonic plague?	50%
What is the mortality rate of untreated pneumonic plague?	Almost always fatal
What type of vaccine is available for *Y. pestis*?	Killed vaccine for those at high risk

PASTEURELLA MULTOCIDA

What is the structure of *P. multocida*?	Encapsulated coccobacillus or rods
What are the oxygen requirements of *P. multocida*?	Facultative anaerobe

Which animals are reservoirs for *P. multocida*?

Mammals and birds

How is *P. multocida* transmitted to humans?

Animal bites, cat scratches, and, rarely, by nasopharyngeal colonization

What are the clinical manifestations of *P. multocida* infection?

Wound infection or cellulitis near the site of inoculation with lymphadenitis, fever, local osteomyelitis, or arthritis

What is the concern associated with suturing animal bites?

Sutures provide a substrate for growth of *P. multocida*, which is common in animal bites

What is the gold standard for diagnosis of *P. multocida* infection?

Culture on blood agar

How does *P. multocida* appear on Gram stain?

Coccobacilli or rods with bipolar staining

How is *P. multocida* infection treated?

Penicillin along with wound cleaning/débridement for soft-tissue infections or surgical drainage for deeper infections

BARTONELLA

What type of organism is *Bartonella*?

Facultative, intracellular, slightly curved rods

What are three species of *Bartonella* that cause disease in humans?

1. *B. henselae*
2. *B. quintana*
3. *B. bacilliformis*

What disease does *B. henselae* cause?

Catscratch disease and bacillary angiomatosis

How does catscratch disease present?

Abscesses at site of cat scratch or bite followed by fever and lymphadenopathy

What is bacillary angiomatosis?

Disease of small blood vessels of skin and internal organs usually seen in immunocompromised persons

What disease does *B. quintana* cause?

Trench fever

How does this present clinically?	Mild, relapsing fever with maculopapular rash
What is the reservoir for B. quintana?	Humans
How is B. quintana transmitted?	Human body louse
What disease does B. bacilliformis cause?	Oroya fever
How does this present clinically?	Infectious anemia
Why?	The bacteria destroys red blood cells and damages the liver and spleen
How is B. bacilliformis transmitted?	Sandfly
Where does B. bacilliformis infection commonly occur?	South America
What antibiotics are used to treat Bartonella infections?	Azithromycin or rifampin plus doxycycline

11   Obligate Intracellular Bacteria: *Chlamydia, Rickettsia, Coxiella, & Ehrlichia*

OVERVIEW

How can you remember these four obligate intracellular bacteria?	"Reclaim the Step 1": *Rickettsia Ehrlichia Coxiella Chlamydia*

CHLAMYDIA

What are chlamydiae?	Obligate intracellular parasites (see Fig. 11-1)

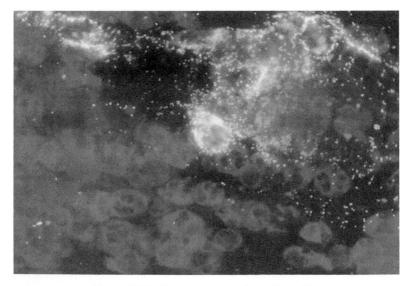

Figure 11-1. *Chlamydia* (see also Color Photo 14).

Why are they intracellular organisms?	Because they depend on the host cell for energy, e.g., adenosine triphosphate (ATP) and nicotinic acid dehydrogenase (NAD^+), and other conditions
What kind of cells do chlamydiae demonstrate tropism for?	Epithelial cells of mucous membranes or lungs
What are three reasons why chlamydiae are not classified as viruses?	1. Contain both ribonucleic acid (RNA) and deoxyribonucleic acid (DNA) 2. Synthesize proteins 3. Sensitivity to antibiotics
What are three species of *Chlamydia*?	1. *C. trachomatis* 2. *C. psittaci* 3. *C. pneumoniae*
What diseases are associated with the different *C. trachomatis* serotypes?	1. Nongonococcal urethritis and inclusion conjunctivitis of the newborn (D–K) 2. Trachoma (A–C) 3. Lymphogranuloma venereum (L_{1-3})
What disease is associated with *C. psittaci*?	Psittacosis, i.e., pneumonia
How many *C. psittaci* serotypes exist?	Many
What disease is associated with *C. pneumoniae*?	Community-acquired acute respiratory disease and possibly atherosclerosis
How many *C. pneumoniae* serotypes exist?	One
Do chlamydiae have a rigid cell wall?	Yes
How does the Chlamydiae cell wall differ from that of gram-negative bacteria?	Chlamydiae lack peptidoglycan
What toxins or virulence factors are responsible for chlamydiae pathogenesis?	None; Chlamydiae do not produce toxins or virulence factors

What are the two morphological forms of chlamydiae that are involved in the replicative cycle?	1. Elementary body 2. Reticulate body
What is the elementary body?	An extracellular, infectious small, spore-like particle which is metabolically inert Elementary body is extracellular
How does it enter the cell?	Through endocytosis into susceptible host cells
How does the elementary body escape cell-mediated destruction?	By inhibiting phagosome–lysosome fusion
What is the reticulate body?	A large, active, replicative, intracellular particle Reticulate body is replicative
How do the reticulate bodies replicate within the cell?	Binary fission
What are inclusion bodies?	Sites of reticulate body replication that appear within cells that can be stained and visualized microscopically
Why is Gram stain a poor choice in detecting chlamydiae?	Chlamydiae exist intracellularly and stain poorly on Gram stain
What are two methods for laboratory diagnosis of chlamydiae?	1. Giemsa stain 2. Immunofluorescence
What histologic finding is associated with *Chlamydia* infection?	Cytoplasmic inclusion bodies
What is used to grow chlamydiae in cell cultures? Why?	Cycloheximide Cycloheximide inhibits eukaryotic metabolism enhancing growth of *Chlamydia*

For which *Chlamydia* species is serology testing not useful?	*C. trachomatis*
Why is it not useful for *C. trachomatis*?	*C. trachomatis* infection is so frequent that many people already have antibodies against it
What two drug groups are effective for treating chlamydiae?	1. Tetracyclines (e.g., doxycycline) 2. Macrolides (e.g., erythromycin and azithromycin)
What vaccine is available for chlamydial disease?	None
What sexually transmitted infection is often found in patients with *Chlamydia*?	Gonococcus

CHLAMYDIA TRACHOMATIS

What four diseases are associated with *C. trachomatis*?	1. Nongonococcal urethritis 2. Inclusion conjunctivitis 3. Lymphogranuloma venereum 4. Trachoma

Nongonococcal urethritis

Which *C. trachomatis* serotypes cause nongonococcal urethritis?	D to K
What is the prevalence of nongonococcal urethritis?	The most common sexually transmitted infection
What are three causes of nongonococcal urethritis?	1. *C. trachomatis* 2. *Mycoplasma* 3. *Ureaplasma urealyticum*
What are four possible infection patterns in men with *C. trachomatis*?	1. Nongonococcal urethritis 2. Epididymitises 3. Prostatitis 4. Proctitis
What are three possible infection patterns in women with *C. trachomatis*?	1. Cervicitis 2. Salpingitis 3. Pelvic inflammatory disease (PID)

What are two symptoms of nongonococcal urethritis?	Dysuria with thick, mucoid discharge from the urethra of males or from the cervical os in females
What percentage of neonates born to C. trachomatis-infected mothers will contract the disease?	50%
What are three sequelae of a neonate born to C. trachomatis-infected mothers?	1. Mucopurulent eye infections, i.e., neonatal inclusion conjunctivitis 7–12 days after delivery 2. Chlamydial pneumonitis 2–12 weeks after birth 3. Reiter's syndrome, i.e., urethritis, arthritis, and uveitis
What is the treatment of choice for C. trachomatis infection?	Azithromycin

Inclusion Conjunctivitis

What is inclusion conjunctivitis?	An acute, purulent infection of conjunctiva around the eye that is named for the inclusions seen in infected conjunctival epithelial cells
How can one prevent the development of inclusion conjunctivitis in the newborn?	Erythromycin eye drops are prophylactically given to all newborns in the United States
How does C. trachomatis spread to the newborn?	Passage through birth canal, i.e., parturition

Lymphogranuloma Venereum

Which C. trachomatis serotypes cause lymphogranuloma venereum?	L_{1-3}
What is lymphogranuloma venereum?	A sexually transmitted infection characterized by transient papules on genitalia with inguinal/perirectal lymphadenopathy

Where is lymphogranuloma venereum endemic?	South America, Asia, and Africa
What is the treatment of choice for lymphogranuloma venereum?	Doxycycline

Trachoma

Which *C. trachomatis* serotypes cause trachoma?	A to C
What is trachoma?	Chronic conjunctivitis
What is the epidemiologic importance of trachoma?	The leading cause of preventable blindness worldwide
When does trachoma induced blindness develop?	10–15 years postexposure
What is the pathophysiology of trachoma-induced blindness?	1. Inflammation 2. Scar traction 3. Inversion of eyelid 4. Corneal scarring caused by eyelash friction against the cornea 5. Secondary bacterial infection 6. Blindness
What is the prophylactic treatment for trachoma?	Topical tetracycline
How are the inclusions in *C. trachomatis*-infected epithelial cells visualized?	Stained with iodine
Are the majority of genital tract infections caused by chlamydiae symptomatic?	No; especially in women, most infections are asymptomatic, undiagnosed, and untreated

CHLAMYDIA PNEUMONIAE

What disease is associated with *C. pneumoniae*?	Community-acquired acute respiratory infection, frequently asymptomatic
How many *C. pneumoniae* serotypes exist?	One

What organism is susceptible to *C. pneumoniae*?	Only humans
How is *C. pneumoniae* transmitted?	Inhalation of aerosols
Are the majority of *C. pneumoniae* infections symptomatic?	No, most infections are asymptomatic
What evidence indicates that *C. pneumoniae* is commonly acquired?	Approximately 50% of adults have developed antibodies to *C. pneumoniae*
Does *C. pneumoniae* cause invasive, disseminated infection?	Rarely
What is the treatment of choice for *C. psittaci* and *C. pneumoniae*?	Doxycycline

CHLAMYDIA PSITTACI

What disease is associated with *C. psittaci*?	Psittacosis, also known as ornithosis, which are types of pneumonia
How many *C. psittaci* serotypes exist?	Many
What organisms does *C. psittaci* infect?	Birds and mammals, including pets and domesticated animals
How does *C. psittaci* spread to humans?	Inhalation of organisms in dry bird feces
What are three symptoms of psittacosis?	Acute onset of fever, hacking dry cough, and flu-like symptoms

RICKETTSIA

What are rickettsiae?	Obligate intracellular parasites that divide by binary fission within host cells
What are three reasons rickettsiae are not considered viruses?	1. Contain both DNA and RNA 2. Synthesize own proteins 3. Susceptible to antibiotics

What molecule does rickettsiae require for growth?	ATP
What lipopolysaccharides do *Rickettsia* and *Proteus* share?	OX-2, OX-19, and OX-K
What is the implication of this?	Agglutination in the Weil-Felix test
What are three rickettsial diseases?	1. Rocky Mountain Spotted Fever (RMSF) 2. Typhus 3. Lyme disease
What is the classic triad of symptoms from rickettsial infection?	1. Headache 2. Fever 3. Rash
How does the rash in typhus spread?	Outward from the trunk to the extremities

How does the rash in RMSF spread?	Inward from the extremities to the trunk

What type of cells do rickettsiae have tropism for?	Endothelial cells that line blood vessels
What does this cause?	Vasculitis resulting in a rash with small, petechial hemorrhages
What is the treatment for most rickettsial infections?	Doxycycline, tetracycline, or chloramphenicol
How are rickettsiae transmitted?	Arthropod vector
What disease and most common vectors are associated with . . .	
R. rickettsii?	RMSF: tick
R. typhi?	Endemic typhus: flea
R. prowazekii?	Epidemic typhus: human body louse

What serological tests are used to diagnose rickettsial disease?	1. Enzyme-linked immunoabsorbent assay (ELISA) 2. Indirect immunofluorescence 3. Weil-Felix test
What does the Weil-Felix reaction detect?	Antirickettsial antibodies

Is the Weil-Felix reaction positive in . . .

RMSF?	Yes
Typhus?	Yes
How are rickettsiae cultured?	Inoculated into chick embryo yolk sac or cell culture

ROCKY MOUNTAIN SPOTTED FEVER

What is the causative organism in RMSF?	*R. rickettsii*
Is there human-to-human RMSF transmission?	No
Why?	*R. rickettsii* must complete its life cycle in the tick (vector)
How is RMSF transmitted? **What are two examples?**	Arthropod vector 1. Wood tick (*Dermacentor andersoni*) 2. Dog tick (*Dermacentor variabilis*)
What number of rickettsial diseases are caused by RMSF in the United States?	95% or ~ 1,000 cases per year
What time of year do most cases of RMSF occur?	Spring and early summer, i.e., when ticks are most active
Where in the United States is RMSF usually found?	East coast, e.g., Appalachian and Ozark mountains Not in the Rocky Mountains
What are three symptoms of RMSF?	1. Rash 2. Headache 3. Fever

How does the RMSF rash appear?

Migrates from the palms and soles to the wrists, ankles, and trunk

What are two other infectious causes of a rash on the palms and soles?

1. Syphilis caused by *Treponema pallidum*
2. Hand-foot-and-mouth disease caused by coxsackievirus, a *Picornaviridae*

What are six complications of RMSF?

Edema, delirium, disseminated intravascular coagulation (DIC), shock, coma, and death

What is the treatment for RMSF?

Doxycycline, tetracycline, or chloramphenicol

What is the prognosis for someone with RMSF? How does this affect treatment?

Potentially fatal if untreated, total cure if diagnosed and treated promptly
Treat empirically without delay

What are two preventative measures against acquiring RMSF?

1. Reduce exposure to arthropod vector with protective clothing and insect repellants
2. Frequent examination of skin for ticks

What kind of vaccine is used to protect against RMSF?

None, there is no vaccine against RMSF

TYPHUS

What is the difference between typhus and typhoid fever?

Typhus is a rickettsial disease with an arthropod vector
Typhoid fever is an enteric fever accompanied by bacteremia caused by *Salmonella enterica* (serotype typhi)

What are the causative organisms of typhus?

R. typhi or *R. prowazekii*

How is typhus transmitted?

Arthropod vector, i.e., human skin louse

What is the reservoir for *R. typhi* or *R. prowazekii*?

Only humans, there are no animal reservoirs

What are four symptoms of typhus?

1. Centrifugal maculopapular rash, i.e., spreads outward from trunk

2. Sudden onset chills
3. Fever
4. Headache

What are six complications of typhus?	1. Bacterial pneumonia 2. Severe meningoencephalitis 3. Delirium 4. Shock 5. Coma 6. Death
What sequence of events leads to typhus?	1. Human body louse bites a bacteremic individual and ingests the bacteria 2. Bacteria multiplies in louse gut epithelium 3. Excreted in feces of the louse during act of biting the next person 4. Autoinoculated by the person while scratching the bite
What is the treatment for typhus?	Doxycycline, tetracycline, or chloramphenicol
What is Brill-Zinsser disease?	A milder, recurrent form of epidemic typhus that occurs 10–40 years after initial infection
What kind of vaccine is used to protect against typhus?	Formalin-killed *R. prowazekii*
Who gets the vaccine?	Restricted for military use

COXIELLA

What are *Coxiella*?	Intracellular parasites
What are the clinical manifestations of *C. burnetii*?	Q fever
How is the disease transmitted?	Inhalation of aerosols
Is Weil-Felix reaction positive for Q fever?	No

Why is Q fever different from other rickettsial diseases?

No rash, no vector, negative Weil-Felix

What is the main organ involved with Q fever?

Lungs

What are three symptoms of Q fever?

1. Fever
2. Severe headache
3. Cough

What are the two most common comorbidities in Q fever?

1. Pneumonia
2. Hepatitis

What is the treatment for Q fever?

Doxycycline or tetracycline

What is the prognosis for someone with Q fever?

Good prognosis; recovery is expected even in the absence of antibiotics

What are three high-risk groups for contracting Q fever?

1. Veterinarians
2. Shepherds
3. Laboratory personnel
Very virulent if not grown in culture carefully

EHRLICHIA

What are *Ehrlichia*?
What cells do they show tropism for?

Obligate intracellular parasites
Leukocytes

What organelle do they infect?

Cytoplasmic vacuoles

What is the characteristic finding?

Inclusions called morulae

What are two types of pathogenic *Ehrlichia*?

1. Human monocytic ehrlichiosis (HME)
2. Human granulocytic ehrlichiosis (HGE)

What tick is the vector?

1. The Lone Star tick (HME)
2. Deer and dog ticks (HGE)

What time of year do most cases of *Ehrlichia* occur?

Spring and early summer, i.e., when ticks are most active

How is *Ehrlichia* infection diagnosed?

1. Serology
2. Polymerase chain reaction (PCR)

How is *Ehrlichia* infection treated?

Doxycycline

12

Mycobacteria

OVERVIEW

What are mycobacteria?

What are their oxygen requirements?

Acid-fast, long, slender, nonmotile, nonspore-forming, filamentous rods
Obligate aerobes

What test distinguishes mycobacteria from the majority of other bacteria?
Why is this test used?

Ziehl-Neelsen stain

Because *Mycobacterium* spp. contain a complex lipid coat, they are difficult to stain with Gram stain
Furthermore, once stained, *Mycobacterium* retain the dye and do not decolorize easily, even with acid, hence they are "acid fast"

How do they appear?

As red rods growing in a cord-like fashion (see Fig. 12-1)

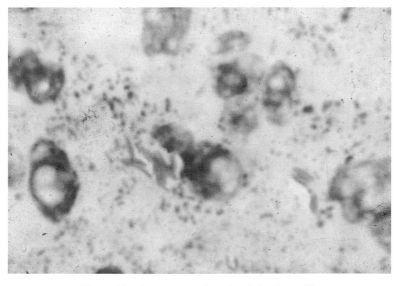

Figure 12-1. Mycobacteria (see also Color Photo 15).

What property accounts for this appearance?	High (60%) lipid content of mycobacterial cell walls
What is the name of these branched, long-chain fatty acids?	Mycolic acids
What are two major *Mycobacterium* species that cause disease in humans?	1. *M. tuberculosis* 2. *M. leprae*
What are four other species of *Mycobacterium*?	1. *M. avium-intracellulare* (MAC) 2. *M. bovis* 3. *M. kansasii* 4. *M. scrofulaceum* MAC is common in human immunodeficiency virus (HIV) patients

MYCOBACTERIA

MYCOBACTERIUM TUBERCULOSIS

What type of organism is *M. tuberculosis*?	Strictly aerobic, acid-fast, intracellular, filamentous rod
Which cells do *M. tuberculosis* show tropism for?	Macrophages, i.e., cells of the reticuloendothelial system
What are two mechanisms employed by *M. tuberculosis* to evade host cell defenses?	1. Pathogen resides within intracellular vesicles called phagosomes 2. Encodes proteins that prevent fusion of phagosomes with lysosomes
What form of immunity is important in fending off *M. tuberculosis*?	Cellular immunity
Why is it important?	Because *M. tuberculosis* is an intracellular organism
Is there an antibody response to *M. tuberculosis*?	Yes
Is the antibody response protective?	No
Why isn't it protective?	Because *M. tuberculosis* are intracellular pathogens that are protected from antibody activity

| What are five complex lipids and factors that contribute to the hardiness and virulence M. tuberculosis? | 1. Mycolic acids, which enable acid-fastness
2. Wax D, which enhances immunogenicity
3. Phosphatides, which result in caseous necrosis
4. Cord factor, which correlates with virulence
5. Arabinogalactan, which is a cell wall component
M. tuberculosis produces neither exotoxins nor endotoxins |

| How long must M. tuberculosis be cultured for growth to occur? | 6–8 weeks on solid media because it is an extremely slow-growing organism There is a new, faster liquid media in which growth occurs in 2–4 weeks |

| What is the special culture medium for M. tuberculosis? | Lowenstein-Jensen agar |

| How is M. tuberculosis transmitted? | Respiratory aerosol |

| Why is person-to-person transmission common with M. tuberculosis? | It can persist in the environment for prolonged periods, partly because the organism is resistant to desiccation |

| What is the reservoir for M. tuberculosis? | Only humans |

| What percentage of the world's population is infected with M. tuberculosis? | 33% |

| What is the overall percentage of developing reactivation disease after M. tuberculosis infection? | 10% |

| When is the risk for reactivation the greatest? | In the first 2 years after primary infection |

What is the overall percentage of developing reactivation disease after *M. tuberculosis* infection in patients with acquired immune deficiency syndrome (AIDS)?	33–50%
How does the yearly percentage correlate to developing reactivation disease?	Increases 10% annually
What are the possible clinical manifestations of tuberculosis?	1. Primary disease or initial host infection 2. Secondary disease or reactivation tuberculosis 3. Granuloma formation 4. Granuloma rupture with dissemination
What is the primary infection?	An infection, usually asymptomatic, often confined to the lungs and occurring after the first exposure to *M. tuberculosis*
Where is the site of primary tuberculosis infection?	Usually the lower lobes of the lung
What is the reactivation tuberculosis?	A secondary infection resulting from reactivation of dormant *M. tuberculosis* that persisted in inactive primary lesions
What causes reactivation?	Age, malnutrition, or other causes of decreased cell-mediated immunity
Where is the site of secondary tuberculosis infection?	Usually the upper lobes of the lung
Why does it occur there?	Prefers higher oxygen tension found there
What is a granuloma?	A central area of multinucleated giant cells, i.e., macrophages, that eventually necrose and fibrose, surrounded by a rim of epithelioid cells (see Fig. 12-2)
What is another name for granuloma?	Tubercle
Why does the body form granulomas?	To attempt to sequester the infectious process

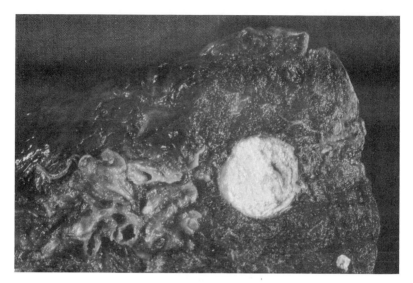

Figure 12-2. Granuloma secondary to M. tuberculosis.

What type of necrosis is seen inside a granuloma? What is this?	Caseous necrosis

A combination of liquefaction and coagulation necrosis resembling cottage cheese |
| **What is a fibrosed granuloma called?** | A Ghon complex, visualized as a solitary nodule on chest x-ray |
| **What are the clinical manifestations of a ruptured granuloma? Why does a ruptured granuloma cause these diseases?** | 1. Localized pulmonary involvement, e.g., chronic pneumonitis
2. Disseminated systemic involvement Spread of infectious, caseous material |
| **What is miliary tuberculosis?** | Disseminated tuberculosis in which multiple organs are seeded with small *M. tuberculosis* tubercles that resemble millet seeds |
| **What are four extrapulmonary manifestations of miliary tuberculosis?** | 1. Osteomyelitis
2. Meningitis
3. Intestinal infection
4. Erythema nodosum |

What virus predisposes individuals to reactivating tuberculosis?

HIV

When are these patients most susceptible?

When their CD4 count drops below 500

Why are these patients susceptible to developing tuberculosis?

Defective cell-mediated immunity

What test is used to screen for exposure to M. tuberculosis?

Purified protein derivative (PPD) test

Does a positive PPD test indicate active disease?

No; PPD tests detect *prior infection or exposure* to M. *tuberculosis, not active disease*

What are examples of a positive PPD test not caused by active disease?

History of vaccination, as well as for patients born in certain other countries

What is measured when evaluating a PPD test?

Diameter of *induration*, or skin elevation, at the injection site

What should not be measured?

Diameter of erythema

What type of reaction is responsible for induration?

Delayed (type IV) hypersensitivity

Under what conditions can a PPD test be positive?

1. Exposure to M. *tuberculosis*
2. Atypical mycobacteria present

What criteria are used for determining a positive PPD?

1. >15 mm of induration is considered positive in those without risk factors
2. >10 mm is positive for those with risk factors, e.g., homeless persons, immigrants from high-risk countries, or health care workers
3. >5 mm is positive in those with defective cell-mediated immunity, e.g., AIDS patients, or close contacts of those with active tuberculosis (TB)

Under what conditions can a PPD test be negative?

1. No previous exposure to M. *tuberculosis*
2. Exposure within 4–6 weeks of PPD test, i.e., it takes this amount of time to be able to amount an immune response

3. Anergy, i.e., defective cell-mediated immunity, e.g., in AIDS patients

How can a negative PPD be distinguished from anergy?

By placing a common allergen on the other arm when administering a PPD

What are the most common symptoms of tuberculosis?

Fatigue, night sweats, weight loss, cough, and hemoptysis
90% of *M. tuberculosis* infections are asymptomatic

What three laboratory tests are used to diagnose *M. tuberculosis* infection?

1. Acid-fast staining of sputum
2. Polymerase chain reaction (PCR) amplification of *M. tuberculosis* ribonucleic acid (RNA)/ deoxyribonucleic acid (DNA)
3. DNA probes

What are two major obstacles in the treatment of *M. tuberculosis*?

1. Emergence of multiple-drug-resistant strains of *M. tuberculosis*
2. Need for long therapy, which decreases compliance and selects for resistant strains

What are five drugs used to treat *M. tuberculosis* infection?

1. Rifampin
2. Isoniazid (INH) and vitamin B_6
3. Pyrazinamide
4. Ethambutol
"Be RIPE"

What is the time course for *M. tuberculosis* treatment?

6–9 months, depending on the drug regimen and local resistance rates to the drugs used
Note: Treatment time course is in constant flux

How long does it take for an infected patient to be rendered noninfectious with treatment?

2–3 weeks

What drug regimen is used for active *M. tuberculosis* prophylaxis?
  Who gets prophylaxis?

INH for 6–9 months with supplemental vitamin B_6

1. Asymptomatic persons with a positive PPD
2. Children exposed to patients with active TB

3. Patients with a positive PPD who will become immunosuppressed, e.g., HIV patients

What is one complication of INH prophylaxis?

Hepatitis

   Who is at increased risk for this complication?

1. Persons >35 year of age
2. Persons with a history of alcohol abuse

Is there a vaccine for *M. tuberculosis*?

Yes, the BCG (Bacille Calmette-Guérin) vaccine

   Is it given in the United States?

No

What type of vaccine is it?

Live-attenuated vaccine containing *M. bovis*

Should it be given to the immunocompromised?

No, because it is a live vaccine

ATYPICAL MYCOBACTERIA

What do atypical mycobacteria cause?

Tuberculosis, usually with disseminated rather than pulmonary manifestations

What are four atypical mycobacteria?

1. *M. avium-intracellulare* (MAC)
2. *M. kansasii*
3. *M. scrofulaceum*
4. *M. bovis*

Do these bacteria cause a positive PPD?

Yes, but not always

Which atypical mycobacterial opportunistic infection classically affects AIDS patients?

M. avium-intracellulare (MAC)

   What CD4 counts are usually associated with this?

CD4 <50

What is a common complication in the immunocompromised?

Disseminated, or miliary, disease

What disease is associated with MAC infection in the non-AIDS population?	Chronic obstructive pulmonary disease (COPD), e.g., emphysema or chronic bronchitis
What disease is *M. scrofulaceum* associated with?	Scrofula
What physical finding is seen in this disease?	Cervical lymphadenitis
What patient population is this disease commonly seen in?	Children
What is the etiology?	Either *M. tuberculosis* or *M. scrofulaceum*
What is the source of *M. bovis*?	Unpasteurized milk
What makes this *Mycobacterium* useful?	Attenuated strains of *M. bovis* are used to make a vaccine against tuberculosis
What is this called?	Bacille Calmette-Guérin (BCG) vaccine
Where is it used?	Internationally, but not in the United States

MYCOBACTERIUM LEPRAE

What are *M. leprae*?	Obligate, intracellular, acid-fast bacilli indistinguishable from other mycobacteria
What is an animal reservoir for *M. leprae*?	Armadillos
What temperatures does *M. leprae* prefer?	Cool temperatures (30°C [86°F])
What areas of the body does *M. leprae* infect?	Superficial areas that are "cooler," e.g., skin, superficial nerves
What are two clinical manifestations of *M. leprae*?	1. Tuberculoid leprosy 2. Lepromatous leprosy
How is *M. leprae* transmitted?	Prolonged contact with patients infected with lepromatous leprosy

What is the eponym for leprosy?

Hansen disease

What are the major differences between the two forms of leprosy?

Tuberculoid leprosy:
1. Cell-mediated immune response
2. Granuloma formation
3. Containment
Lepromatous leprosy:
1. Humoral response
2. No granuloma formation
3. Dissemination

Clinically, what is the significance of these differences?

Tuberculoid leprosy has few lesions and little tissue destruction
Lepromatous leprosy has many lesions with extensive destruction of bone and overlying soft tissues, resulting in the typical "leonine facies"

Which form of leprosy has a worse prognosis?

Lepromatous leprosy

What is a feared complication of lepromatous leprosy?

Erythema nodosum leprosum

What is the treatment?

Thalidomide

In which form of leprosy is the lepromin skin test positive?

The tuberculoid form

Can M. leprae be grown in culture?

No

How is M. leprae diagnosed?

Acid-fast stain of infected tissue samples

What is the treatment for leprosy?

Dapsone, rifampin, and clofazimine for approximately 2 years

What are two complications of this prolonged course of treatment?

1. Hemolysis
2. Methemoglobinemia

13

Mycoplasma

What are *Mycoplasma*?

Pleomorphically shaped organisms having a cholesterol bilaminar cell membrane and no peptidoglycan cell wall

What are four *Mycoplasma* species?

1. *M. pneumoniae*
2. *Ureaplasma urealyticum*
3. *M. hominis*
4. *M. incognitus*

What is unique about *Mycoplasma*?

Only bacteria to contain cholesterol in its cell membrane

Does *Mycoplasma* have cell walls?

No

What do some *Mycoplasma* colonies look like?

They have a "fried egg" appearance (see Fig. 13-1)

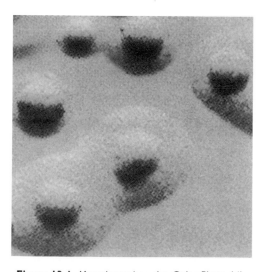

Figure 13-1. *Mycoplasma* (see also Color Photo 16).

MYCOPLASMA PNEUMONIAE

What disease does *M. pneumoniae* cause in humans?

Atypical pneumonia

What is another name for this disease?

"Walking pneumonia"

What medium is used to culture *M. pneumoniae*?

Eaton agar

How many serotypes of *M. pneumoniae* exist?

1

How is *Mycoplasma* transferred between humans?

By respiratory aerosols

Which age group is commonly affected?

Young adults living in close quarters
Think "army recruits in barracks at boot camp" or college students in dorms

How does an atypical pneumonia present clinically?

Gradual onset of headache, malaise, and a nonproductive cough

How does this differ from the presentation of pneumococcal pneumonia?

Patients with atypical pneumonia do not usually have severe symptoms, unlike the abrupt onset of pneumococcal pneumonia

What are five causes of atypical pneumonias?

1. *M. pneumoniae*
2. *Legionella* (*L. pneumophilia*)
3. *Chlamydia* (*C. trachomatis*)
4. *Viral pneumonias*
5. Q fever (*Coxiella bumetii*)

What unique antibodies are associated with *M. pneumoniae* infection?
What are they?

Cold agglutinins; these are produced in approximately 60% of infected patients
Immunoglobulin (IgM class antibodies directed against red blood cell (RBC) antigens

What is the effect of temperature with these antibodies?

No physiologic effect, but agglutination with RBCs at 0°C (32°F) to 4°C (39.2°F), but not at 37°C (98.6°F)

What is the diagnostic value of these antibodies?

Minimal because their presence is nonsensitive and nonspecific

How is *M. pneumoniae* infection diagnosed?

By serology, i.e., detection of specific antibodies to *M. pneumoniae* is diagnostic

What is the treatment for *M. pneumoniae*?

Erythromycin or tetracycline; however, the disease will resolve spontaneously in most individuals with supportive treatment

Why are penicillins and cephalosporins ineffective against *M. pneumoniae*?

Penicillins and cephalosporins destroy the integrity of cell walls, which is ineffective against *Mycoplasma* because they lack cell walls

Which is worse, the patient's clinical presentation or the appearance of the chest x-ray?

The chest x ray looks worse
The degree of pulmonary infiltrates is striking compared to the relatively mild clinical symptoms and x-ray findings usually remain several weeks after symptom resolution

Is reinfection possible?

Yes, and it is common

What is the severity of symptoms of *M. pneumoniae* in reinfection?

Reinfection results in worse symptoms than those seen on the first exposure

OTHER MYCOPLASMA

Besides *M. pneumoniae*, what two *Mycoplasma* species infect humans?

1. *U. urealyticum*
2. *M. hominis*

Where do these bacteria reside?

The human genitourinary tract

What disease does *U. urealyticum* cause?

Nongonococcal urethritis

What does *U. urealyticum* secrete?

Urease

What organism, implicated with ulcers, also secretes this?

Helicobacter pylori

What disease does *M. hominis* cause?

Postpartum fever

14   Actinomycetes: Actinomyces israelii & Nocardia asteroides

OVERVIEW

What are *Actinomycetes*? Gram-positive bacteria with branching filaments resembling fungal hyphae (see Fig. 14-1)

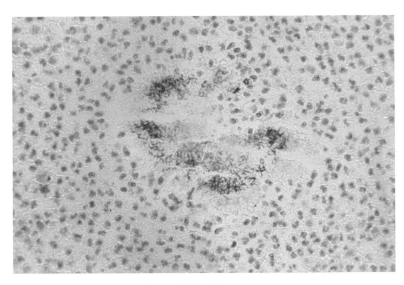

Figure 14-1. *Actinomycetes.*

What are two medically important *Actinomycetes*?	1. *A. israelii* (anaerobic) 2. *Nocardia asteroids* (aerobic)
Is person-to-person transmission of *Actinomyces* or *Nocardia* possible?	No

ACTINOMYCES ISRAELII

Where do *A. israelii* reside?	Normal flora of oral cavity
What are the oxygen requirements of *A. israelii*?	Obligate anaerobic
How does *A. israelii* appear microscopically?	Sulfur granules surrounded by neutrophils
Do sulfur granules contain sulfur?	No, their yellowish appearance only resembles sulfur

How can one be infected with *A. israelii*?

1. Trauma to the face or mouth
2. Victim of a human bite
3. Poor dental hygiene

What are three clinical manifestations of *A. israelii*?

1. Pus containing sulfur granules
2. Nontender abscesses, typically in the head and cervical region
3. Drainage through sinus tracts

How is *Actinomyces* treated?	Penicillin

NOCARDIA ASTEROIDES

Where is *Nocardia* found?	In the soil
How is *Nocardia* usually contracted?	Inhalation of aerosolized particles
What are the oxygen requirements of *Nocardia*?	Obligate aerobic
What property does *Nocardia* share with *Mycobacterium tuberculosis*?	Both are acid-fast
Which of these stains more weakly?	*Nocardia* stains more weakly with acid-fast reagents than *M. tuberculosis*

What are two clinical manifestations of *Nocardia*?

1. Pneumonia
2. Abscess formation in various organs following pneumonia

How is *Nocardia* infection treated?	Trimethoprim-sulfamethoxazole

15 Spirochetes

OVERVIEW

What are spirochetes?

Long, slender, motile, flexible, and undulating gram-negative bacteria that have a characteristic helical shape (see Fig. 15-1)

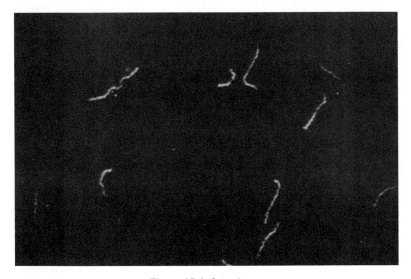

Figure 15-1. Spirochetes.

What are three elements of spirochete structure?

1. Cell wall
2. Axial filaments
3. Protoplasmic cylinder

What are axial filaments?

Thin endoflagella located between the cell wall and outer sheath

What is the purpose of axial filaments?

Axial filaments cause the cell to rotate, enabling tissue invasion in a corkscrew manner

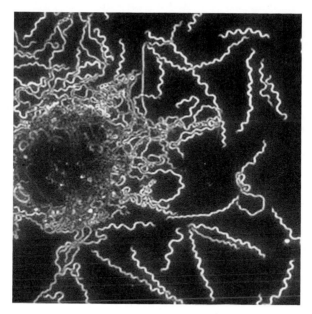

Figure 15-2. Spirochetes under dark-field microscopy (see also Color Photo 17).

What are four ways in which spirochetes are identified?

1. Dark-field microscopy (see Fig. 15-2)
2. Immunofluorescent stain
3. Enzyme-linked immunoabsorbent assay (ELISA)
4. Western blot

Which method is most sensitive?

Western blot

What are three genera of spirochetes that are important human pathogens?

1. *Treponema*
2. *Borrelia*
3. *Leptospira interrogans*

What are distinguishing morphological characteristics of each?

Treponema are tightly wound spirals

Borrelia are large loosely wound irregular coils

Leptospira are tight spirals with hooked ends

What are their oxygen requirements?

Microaerophilic

TREPONEMA

Which *Treponema* species is a major human pathogen?

Treponema pallidum

What disease does it cause?	Syphilis
How is it transmitted?	Sexually or transplacentally
How are the stages of syphilis categorized?	Primary, secondary, and tertiary stages

What are the clinical manifestations of primary syphilis?

1. Chancre, shallow, indurated, painless ulcers at the site of contact 3–6 weeks postexposure that heal spontaneously
2. Asymptomatic period (3–24 weeks) with hematogenous/lymphatic spread throughout body

What are the clinical manifestations of secondary syphilis?

1. Maculopapular rash on palms and soles
2. Condyloma latum
3. Systemic involvement
4. Heals over 6 weeks, then may enter latent phase

What is condyloma latum?

A moist, erythematous papule in anogenital areas pathognomonic of syphilis
Condyloma latum is caused by *T. pallidum*
Condyloma acuminatum is caused by human papillo- mavirus

What are four clinical manifestations of secondary systemic involvement?

1. Chorioretinitis
2. Hepatitis
3. Nephritis
4. Meningitis
This is why syphilis is called the "great mimic"

What are the clinical manifestations of tertiary syphilis?

1. Gummas (granulomatous lesions) of skin and bones
2. Cardiovascular lesions, e.g., aneurysm of ascending aorta
3. Tabes dorsalis (neurosyphilis)
4. Argyll-Robertson pupil

What is tabes dorsalis?

Damage to the dorsal root and posterior column (dorsal column medial lemniscus) resulting in compromised vibration, proprioception, pain, and temperature sensation

What is Argyll-Robertson pupil?

A pupil that constricts to accommodation but not to light

What are the clinical manifestations of latent syphilis?

Absence of symptoms lasting 3–30 years that can ultimately progress to secondary or tertiary syphilis

How is syphilis diagnosed?

Serologically

Which types of antibodies does syphilis elicit?

1. Nontreponemal antibodies
2. Antitreponemal antibodies

What are nontreponemal antibodies specific for?

Phospholipid components of mammalian membranes, e.g., cardiolipin

What are two examples of nontreponemal antibody tests?

1. Venereal Disease Research Laboratory (VDRL)
2. Rapid plasma reagent (RPR)
VDRL and RPR not specific for *T. pallidum*

What are antitreponemal antibodies specific for?

Treponemal surface proteins

Clinically, what is the most sensitive diagnostic test for syphilis?

Fluorescent treponemal antibody absorption (FTA-ABS) test which detects human antibodies to treponemes

What is first line treatment for syphilis?

Penicillin, intramuscular (IM) or intravenous (IV)

What is the Jarisch-Herxheimer reaction?

Fever, chills, myalgias, and influenza-like symptoms in patients with secondary syphilis lasting up to 12 hours after penicillin administration

BORRELIA

What are two pathogenic *Borrelia* species?
   Which diseases do they cause?

1. *B. burgdorferi*
2. *B. recurrentis*
1. Lyme disease (*B. burgdorferi*)
2. Relapsing fever (*B. recurrentis*)

What is the vector for ...
   B. burgdorferi?

Deer tick (*Ixodes* tick)

   B. recurrentis?

Human body louse

How common is Lyme disease?

It is the most common tick-borne bacterial disease

What is the time course for Lyme disease...

Stage 1?

Days to weeks after tick bite

Stage 2?

Weeks to months after tick bite

Stage 3?

Months to years after tick bite

What are the clinical manifestations of Lyme disease...

Stage 1?

1. *Erythema chronica migrans*— a clear center surrounded by a spreading circular red rash (see Fig. 15-3)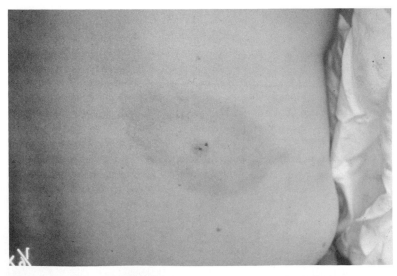
2. Flu-like symptoms including fever, chills, fatigue, and headaches

Stage 2?

1. Myocarditis or pericarditis
2. Bell's palsy (7th cranial nerve palsy)
3. Aseptic meningitis

Stage 3?

1. Arthritis of the large joints
2. Chronic central nervous system (CNS) disease

Figure 15-3. Erythema migrans (see also Color Photo 18).

What are the drugs of choice for Lyme disease?	Doxycycline or amoxicillin
What component of B. recurrentis causes relapsing fever?	*B. recurrentis* surface antigens
How does it cause relapsing fever?	*B. recurrentis* has the capability to alter surface antigens, making old host antibodies ineffective, thus causing relapses until new antibodies are synthesized
What are the symptoms of relapsing fever?	Cycle of high fever, headaches, muscle pain, and general malaise followed by 8 days of remission, which repeat up to 10 times
What is the treatment for relapsing fever?	Doxycycline or erythromycin

LEPTOSPIRA INTERROGANS

What disease is caused by *Leptospira interrogans*?	Leptospirosis
How is the disease transmitted?	The organism enters water sources via urine of rats, domestic livestock, and pets; humans are infected by drinking or swimming in contaminated water
What is the clinical presentation of leptospirosis in... **Phase 1?**	Symptoms 2 weeks postinfection characterized by a period of fever, chills, headaches, and resolution of symptoms
Phase 2?	Symptoms 1 week after resolution characterized by aseptic meningitis, liver damage (jaundice), and impaired kidney function
How is leptospirosis diagnosed in... **Phase 1?**	Culturing blood or cerebrospinal fluid (CSF)
Phase 2?	Culturing urine
What is the treatment of choice?	Doxycycline or penicillin G

Section II

Mycology

16

Introduction to Fungal Infections

What are fungi?

Eukaryotic organisms that have membrane-bound nuclei, unlike viruses or bacteria, and are heterotrophic

What are heterotrophic organisms?

Organisms that require preformed organic carbon sources for growth

What are the two morphologic forms of fungi?

1. Filamentous molds
2. Unicellular yeasts

What are three general structural components of filamentous moulds?
What is the function of each of these structures?

1. Mycelium/hypha
2. Septa
3. Thallus
1. A mycelium is a mass of filamentous threads that resembles a "cotton ball" composed of intercommunicating individual threads of tubular cells called hyphae
2. Septa forms partitions between cells within a hypha
3. Thallus is the vegetative body; a simply fungus body

What is the morphology of yeast-like fungi?

Single, unconnected spheroid cells (see Figs. 16-1 and 16-2)

What is the difference between yeasts and filamentous molds?

Yeasts reproduce by budding or fission
Filamentous molds grow by branching and tip elongation of hyphae

What are dimorphic fungi?

Fungi with the ability to grow in two forms, most commonly as yeast-like organisms in certain environments (37°C [98.6°F]) but can also grow as mold-like in others (25°C [77°F] or room temperature)

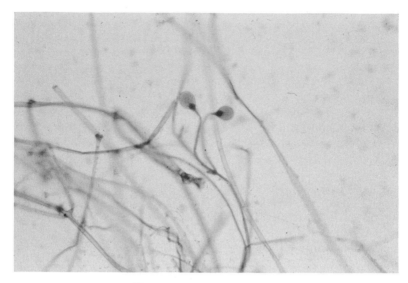

Figure 16-1. Filamentous molds.

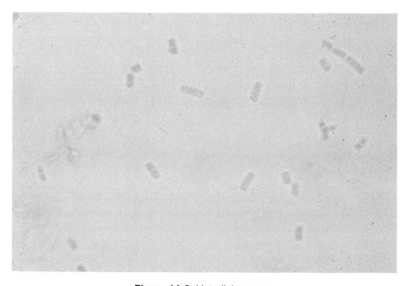

Figure 16-2. Unicellular yeasts.

"Mold in the cold, yeast in
  the heat"
Systemic mycoses are dimorphic
  fungi

**What are the two
mechanisms by which fungi
reproduce?**

1. Asexual sporulation
2. Sexual sporulation

**Which is more common
among human
pathogens?**

Asexual sporulation

**What is sporulation?
What are they?**

Production of fungal spores
Metabolically dormant, protected cells
capable of germinating and establishing
colonies

**What is asexual
sporulation?**

Asexual formation of spores through
mitosis (Fig. 16-3)

**What are asexually
produced spores called?**

Conidia or spores; although spores are
technically distinct from conidia, the
term spore is often used to encompass
both

What is sexual sporulation?

Sexual formation of spores through
meiosis between two haploid nuclei of
compatible strains (see Fig. 16-4)

**What are sexually
produced spores called?**

Ascospores, zygospores, and basidiospores

**What are two predominant
components of fungal cell
walls?**

1. Chitin
2. Glucans

**What is chitin composed
of?**

N-acetylglucosamine polymers

**What is glucan composed
of?**

Polymers of glucose

**What is one difference
between the cell wall of
fungi and bacteria?
  What is the clinical
  significance of this?**

Fungal cell walls are composed of
N-acetylglucosamine and glucose
polymers instead of peptidoglycan
β-Lactam antibiotics that interfere with
bacterial cell wall production and
subsequently have no effect on fungi

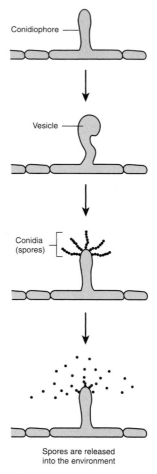

Figure 16-3. Production of conidia (spores) through asexual sporulation.

What is a standard medium for fungal culture?	Sabouraud dextrose agar
What type of medium is this?	A low pH beef-broth agar
How are human fungal diseases typically classified?	Based on their level of involvement and depth of invasion
What are four classifications of fungal disease?	1. *Superficial* when limited to hair and stratum corneum 2. *Cutaneous* when limited to the epidermis

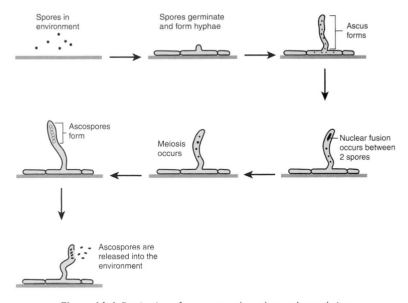

Figure 16-4. Production of ascospores through sexual sporulation.

3. *Subcutaneous* when the epidermis is breached
4. *Systemic* when there is significant penetration or dissemination to internal organs (see Fig. 16-5)

What are three cutaneous fungal pathogens?

1. *Epidermophyton*
2. *Microsporum*
3. *Trichophyton*

What are four subcutaneous fungal pathogens?

1. *Sporothrix schenckii*
2. *Madurella grisea*
3. *Cladophialophora*
4. *Phialophora*

What are four systemic fungal pathogens?

1. *Coccidioides immitis*
2. *Histoplasma capsulatum*
3. *Blastomyces dermatitidis*
4. *Paracoccidioides brasiliensis*

How else are fungal infections classified?

Based on their infectivity in regards to the host's immune status

What is one group of fungal infections based on this distinction?

Opportunistic fungal infections

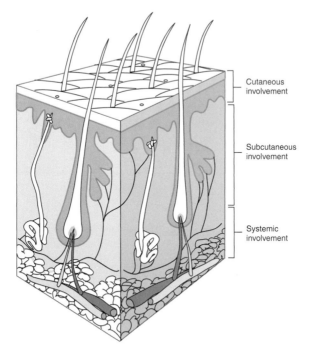

Cutaneous involvement

Subcutaneous involvement

Systemic involvement

Figure 16-5. Relationship of skin layer and fungal involvement

What property do these organisms have in common?

Opportunistic organisms cause clinically significant disease in the immuno-compromised, but rarely in the immunocompetent

What are six opportunistic fungal pathogens?

1. *Candida* species (yeast)
2. *Cryptococcus neoformans* (yeast)
3. *Aspergillus fumigatus* (mold)
4. *Rhizopus* species (mold)
5. *Fusarium* species (mold)
6. *Pneumocystis carinii* (yeast), now called *P. jiroveci*

How are pathogenic fungi classified?
Table 16-1

Table 16-1.   Pathogenic Fungi

Superficial and Cutaneous Pathogens	Subcutaneous Pathogens	Systemic Pathogens	Opportunistic Pathogens
	Sporothrix schenckii	*Coccidioides immitis*	*Candida spp.*
Microsporum spp.	*Madurella grisea*	*Histoplasma capsulatum*	*Cryptococcus neoformans*
Epidermophyton spp.	*Cladophialophora spp.*	*Blastomyces dermatitidis*	*Aspergillus fumigatus*
Trichophyton spp.	*Phialophora spp.*	*Paracoccidioides brasiliensis*	*Rhizopus spp.*
			Mucorales spp. (cause mucormycosis)
			Pneumocystis carinii (*P. jiroveci*)

Spp. = species

17   Superficial & Cutaneous Fungal Infections

What is the level of involvement of cutaneous mycoses?

Cutaneous involvement is limited to the epidermis

What is the general name given to cutaneous fungal pathogens?

Dermatophytes

   What do these pathogens cause?

Dermatophytosis

What are the three main genera of cutaneous fungal pathogens?

1. *Epidermophyton*
2. *Microsporum*
3. *Trichophyton*

Where are cutaneous fungi found?

Human skin (anthropophilic)
Domestic animal skin (zoophilic)
Soil (geophilic)

What are the modes of dermatophytosis transmission?

Contact with soil, human to human or animal to human transmission by direct contact or inoculation with infected skin scales

How do dermatophytoses present clinically?

Depends on part of body infected
The classic presentation is an annular, sharply marginated, raised lesion that may be erythematous and pruritic with a clear or scaly center

How are dermatophytoses classified?

According to the affected tissue or region

What are six common dermatophytoses?

1. Tinea corporis (ringworm)
2. Tinea pedis (athlete's foot)
3. Tinea capitis (scalp ringworm)
4. Tinea barbae (beard)
5. Tinea cruris (jock itch)
6. Tinea unguium (nails)

Which genus of dermatophytes does not infect hair?

Epidermophyton

Which genus of dermatophytes does not usually infect nails?

Microsporum

What are two cutaneous manifestations of dermatophytoses?

1. Kerion
2. *Id* reaction

What is a kerion?

Highly inflammatory pustular lesion secondary to scalp or beard dermatophytoses

What is an *id* reaction?

Sterile skin vesicle formation distant from primary dermatophytoses site secondary to hypersensitivity response to circulating fungal antigens; it is commonly seen in tinea pedis with subsequent hand lesions

What are four ways in which a clinical diagnosis of dermatophytosis can be confirmed?

1. Application of potassium hydroxide (KOH) to tissue sample with active fungal growth revealing fungal filaments by direct microscopy
2. Green fluorescence visualization of dermatophyte hyphae invasion of hair shafts under long-wave ultraviolet (UV) light (Wood lamp)
3. Culture on Sabouraud agar at room temperature demonstrating characteristic hyphae and conidia
4. Positive skin test with fungal extracts, e.g., trichophytin

How is dermatophytosis treated?

1. Removal of infected hairs
2. Topical antifungals for most infections
3. Oral/systemic antifungal therapy for hair and nail infections
4. Keep skin cool and dry

What causes pityriasis tinea versicolor?

Malassezia species

How does pityriasis versicolor present clinically?

Noninflamed patches of fine brown scaling, particularly on the trunk and upper arms

How does lesion appear?

The affected area may appear uniformly darker or uniformly lighter than the person's overall skin tone

What is the pathophysiology of this?

Melanocyte toxicity

What commonly predisposes one to pityriasis versicolor infection?

Systemic steroid therapy, suntan lotions and other lipid-containing lotions

How is a clinical diagnosis of pityriasis versicolor confirmed?

1. KOH treatment of skin scrapings revealing clusters of round, thick-walled yeasts budding from a medium base with a collar, and fragmented thick-walled hyphae
2. Yellow fluorescence under long-wave UV light (Wood lamp)

How is pityriasis versicolor treated?

2.5% selenium sulfide

18

Subcutaneous Fungal Infections

What is the level of involvement of subcutaneous mycoses?

Fungal infection in which the epidermis is breached

How are subcutaneous mycoses commonly acquired?

Traumatic laceration or puncture wound

What are four subcutaneous fungal pathogens?

1. *Sporothrix schenckii*
2. *Madurella grisea*
3. *Cladophialophora*
4. *Phialophora*

What does S. schenckii cause?

Sporotrichosis

What is this also known as?

"Rose gardener's" disease because infection is commonly associated with thorn pricks

What is the natural habitat of this fungus?

Soil and decaying or live vegetation, most commonly in tropical or subtropical areas

What is the morphology of S. schenckii?

Dimorphic, cigar-shaped yeasts, septate mold (see Fig. 18-1)

How does sporotrichosis present clinically?

1. Granulomatous ulcer with irregular, friable edges at a puncture site (primary lesion)
2. Nodular or ulcerative lesions can occur along draining lymphatics (secondary lesion), i.e., ascending, "cord-like" lymphangitis

What is the most reliable method used to confirm a clinical diagnosis of sporotrichosis?

Culture of biopsy material on Sabouraud agar

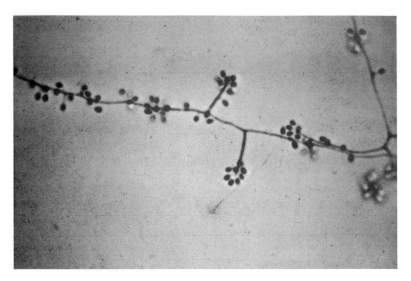

Figure 18-1. *Sporothrix schenckii.*

What is the treatment for sporotrichosis?	Most lesions heal spontaneously with scarring; otherwise, oral itraconazole or potassium iodide can be used
What does *Madurella grisea* cause?	Mycetoma
What is this also known as?	Madura
How does this present clinically?	Localized abscess, usually on the feet, i.e., Madura foot, that discharges pus, serum, and blood through sinus tracts and is capable of spreading to bone
What is the defining feature of a mycetoma?	Presence of white or colored grains composed of compacted hyphae in the exudates
What is the treatment for mycetoma?	Surgical excision, which is more effective than antifungals
What do *Phialophora* and *Cladophialophora* cause?	Chromoblastomycosis
How does this present clinically?	Warty nodule that slowly infects the lymphatic system, resulting in crusty abscesses

How do fungal cells appear?

As "copper pennies," i.e., fungal cells appear somewhat round and may have one to two transverse septa

What is the treatment for chromoblastomycosis?

Surgical excision, which is more effective than antifungals

Systemic Fungal Infections

OVERVIEW

What is the level of involvement of systemic mycoses?

Fungal infection in which there is significant penetration or dissemination to internal organs

What are four common systemic fungal pathogens affecting individuals?

1. *Coccidioides immitis*
2. *Histoplasma capsulatum*
3. *Blastomyces dermatitidis*
4. *Paracoccidioides brasiliensis*

What are four fungal characteristics of systemic mycoses?

1. Uniformly dimorphic
2. Exist as molds at lower temperatures (25°C [77°F]), e.g., in soil
3. Exist as yeasts or spherule at higher temperatures (37°C [98.6°F]), e.g., in hosts
4. Geographical/regional distribution (see Fig. 19-1)

"Mold in the cold, yeast in the heat."

How do systemic mycoses begin?

Inhaled fungal spores convert into yeasts or spherule in the lungs and initiate a lower respiratory tract infection with potential for dissemination within the host

What predisposes one to disseminated systemic mycoses?

Defective cell-mediated immunity

Which cells, when infected cause disseminated systemic mycoses?

Cells of the reticuloendothelial system, e.g., macrophages, become infected and disseminate throughout the body

Are systemic mycoses communicable?

No

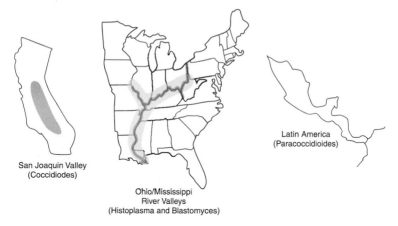

Figure 19-1. Classic geographical distribution patterns of systemic fungal pathogens.

How are disseminated systemic mycoses treated?

Amphotericin B
Amphotericin B has many side effects

How are localized systemic mycoses treated?

Itraconazole or voriconazole

COCCIDIOIDES

What are the two species of Coccidioides?
What do they cause?

1. *C. immitis*
2. *C. posadasii*
Coccidioidomycosis

Where is Coccidioides endemic?

1. Southwestern United States, e.g., San Joaquin Valley
2. Central and South America

What is the pathogenesis of Coccidioides species?

1. *Coccidioides* species generate spores in soil by hyphal filaments septation (arthroconidia)
2. Spores aerosolize and are inhaled, especially when the soil is disturbed and in dry environments
3. Spores swell in lungs and develop into endospores filled with large spherules
4. Spherules rupture releasing endospores
5. Endospore dissemination to the central nervous system (CNS), bone, or other tissues

What are four symptoms of acute pulmonary coccidioidomycosis?	Cough, fever, arthralgia, and rash
What is this quadrad of symptoms called?	San Joaquin Valley Fever or desert rheumatism
What is the characteristic chest x-ray finding?	Infiltrates and hilar lymphadenopathy
What type of rash is seen with *C. immitis* infection?	Erythema multiforme, erythema nodosum, or toxic erythema
When does this develop?	1–2 weeks after exposure
What is the prognostic value of developing erythema nodosum?	Erythema nodosum is a good prognostic indicator because it represents a delayed, cell-mediated hypersensitivity response to fungal antigens
What is the most common outcome of acute pulmonary coccidioidomycosis?	Recovery within 10–21 days
What are three uncommon outcomes?	1. Solid-lung granuloma (coccidioidoma) formation 2. Cavitary coccidioidomycosis in apical or mid-lung fields 3. Dissemination
What are three sites of dissemination and their manifestations for coccidioidomycosis?	1. CNS, resulting in meningitis 2. Skin, resulting in ulcers or crusted granulomas 3. Bone, resulting in lytic lesions of long bones, skull, and joint cavities
What percentage of patients infected with *C. immitis* develop disseminated disease?	1%
What populations have a higher percentage of disseminated disease?	Filipinos and African Americans have a roughly 10% chance of developing disseminated disease
What cerebrospinal fluid (CSF) findings are consistent with coccidioidal meningitis?	1. Lymphocytosis ($>10/\mu$L), eosinophilia 2. Increased protein 3. Decreased glucose 4. *C. immitis* can rarely be seen directly with microscopy of CSF

How can you tell if a person has produced adequate cell-mediated immunity to prevent disseminated *C. immitis* disease?	A positive skin test to fungal extracts, i.e., 5 mm induration developing within ~48 hours; although false positives do occur because of cross reactivity and/or past exposure
Which serological tests suggest *C. immitis* infection?	Immunoglobulin (IgM and IgG) precipitins within 2–4 weeks of infection
Which serological tests suggest *C. immitis* dissemination?	Increasing complement fixing antibody titer
What are three treatment options for coccidioidomycosis?	1. No treatment for asymptomatic or mild primary pulmonary infection 2. Amphotericin B for persistent lung disease or disseminated disease 3. Fluconazole is the drug of choice for *C. immitis* meningitis

HISTOPLASMA CAPSULATUM

What does *H. capsulatum* cause?	Histoplasmosis
What is unique about its life cycle?	1. It is an intracellular fungus 2. *H. capsulatum* has *no* capsule
What cells do *H. capsulatum* show tropism for?	Reticular endothelial cells, e.g., macrophages
What are the endemic areas for *H. capsulatum*? **Where is it most commonly found?**	Ohio and Mississippi River Valleys Bird and bat droppings
What is the pathogenesis of *H. capsulatum*?	1. Soil laden with bird or bat droppings rich in *H. capsulatum* microconidia (spores) aerosolize and are inhaled 2. Spores germinate in lungs into yeast-like cells 3. Yeast cells are engulfed by macrophages 4. Dissemination secondary to intracellular yeast cells division and macrophage movement throughout the body

What is the characteristic chest x-ray finding?

Infiltrates and hilar lymphadenopathy

What are seven symptoms of acute epidemic histoplasmosis?

Chills, fever, cough, headache, pneumonia, arthralgia, and rashes

What is the common clinical course of acute epidemic histoplasmosis in healthy individuals?

Spontaneous resolution

What are two uncommon clinical manifestations?

1. Chronic pulmonary histoplasmosis
2. Disseminated histoplasmosis

What type of patient is at increased risk for chronic pulmonary histoplasmosis?

Patients with preexisting lung disease, particularly emphysema

What are the sites for disseminated histoplasmosis infection?

Liver, spleen, lymph nodes, and bone marrow

What are four useful laboratory tests for diagnosing histoplasmosis?

1. Tissue biopsy or bone marrow aspiration demonstrating oval yeast cells within macrophages
2. Culture on Sabouraud agar showing hyphae with macroconidia
3. *Histoplasma* antigen detection by radioimmunoassay, especially in urine
4. Complement fixation assay

What tests are not diagnostically useful?

Skin and serologic tests because they lack specificity

What are four treatment options for histoplasmosis?

1. No treatment for asymptomatic or mild primary pulmonary infection
2. Oral itraconazole in treating progressive lung lesions
3. Amphotericin B for disseminated disease

What is the treatment for chronic suppression of histoplasmosis in acquired immune deficiency syndrome (AIDS) patients?

Oral itraconazole

BLASTOMYCES DERMATITIDIS

What does *B. dermatitidis* cause?	Blastomycosis
What is the classic histologic finding of *B. dermatitidis*?	Broad-based buds (see Fig. 19-2)

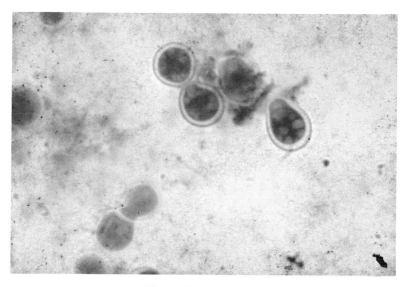

Figure 19-2. *Blastomyces.*

What are the endemic areas for *B. dermatitidis*?	Mississippi and Ohio River Valleys
Where is it commonly found?	Moist soil with decomposing wood
What is the pathogenesis of blastomycosis?	1. Soil-laden spores aerosolize and are inhaled 2. Spores germinate in lungs into thick-walled yeast cells, often with buds
What are six symptoms of acute blastomycosis?	Headache, cough, fever, chills, signs of pulmonary consolidation, and possibly pleural effusion
What is the characteristic chest x-ray finding?	Infiltrates and hilar lymphadenopathy

Does gender influence the presentation of systemic mycoses?

Yes

How does gender influence presentation?

Symptomatic infection is much more common in adult males than in adult females

What are sites for disseminated blastomycosis infection?

Bone, skin, and genitourinary tract Blastomycosis causes granulomatous lesions

How can a clinical diagnosis of blastomycosis be confirmed?

1. Tissue biopsy specimens demonstrating thick-walled yeast cells with single broad-based buds
2. Cultures of hyphae with small pear-shaped conidia are diagnostic

What are three treatments options for blastomycosis?

1. No treatment for asymptomatic patients
2. Itraconazole for mild, primary pulmonary infection or progressive lung lesions
3. Amphotericin B for disseminated disease or life-threatening disease

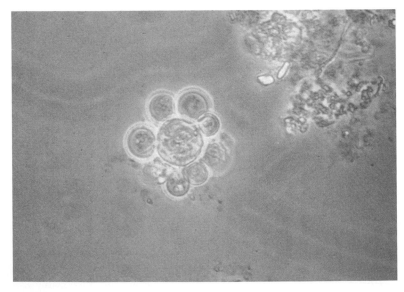

Figure 19-3. *Paracoccidioides brasiliensis.*

PARACOCCIDIOIDES BRASILIENSIS

What are the endemic areas for *P. brasiliensis*?

Latin America

What is the morphology of *P. brasiliensis*?

P. brasiliensis has a pilot-wheel appearance
(see Fig. 19-3)

    What is the clinical manifestation?

Similar to histomycosis and blastomycosis with a distinct predilection to cause secondary oral and nasal mucosal painful lesions

Opportunistic Fungal Infections

OVERVIEW

What are opportunistic organisms?

Organisms that cause clinically significant disease in the immunocompromised, but rarely in the immunocompetent

What are six opportunistic fungal pathogens?

1. *Candida* species (yeast/mold)
2. *Cryptococcus neoformans* (yeast)
3. *Aspergillus fumigatus* (mold)
4. *Rhizopus* species (mold)
5. *Mucor* (mold)
6. *Pneumocystis carinii/jiroveci* (yeast-like)

What is the relationship between the morphology assumed by a fungus in tissue and the pathogenesis it causes?

Fungal morphology determines which component of host defense is needed to fight infection

What five risk factors lead to systemic fungal infections?

1. Infection with human immunodeficiency virus (HIV)
2. Endocrinopathies, e.g., diabetes
3. Neutropenia, e.g., secondary to chemotherapy
4. Systemic corticosteroids
5. Systemic broad-spectrum antibiotics

What is the most common fungal infection encountered in immuno-compromised patients?

Candidiasis

CANDIDA

What are five species of *Candida*?

1. *C. albicans*
2. *C. tropicalis*

3. *C. parapsilosis*
4. *C. krusei*
5. *C. glabrata*

What is the most clinically important species of *Candida*?

C. albicans

Do immunocompetent individuals typically develop candidiasis?

Yes, e.g., vaginal candidiasis or oral thrush in young children

Do they typically develop systemic candidiasis?

No

How does candidiasis commonly present in immunocompromised, e.g., acquired immune deficiency syndrome (AIDS), patients?

Candida infection is almost exclusively mucosal in AIDS patients because helper T-cell deficiency predisposes to mucosal infection

Intact polymorphonuclear function in AIDS patients precludes disseminated, deepseated candidiasis

How is a diagnosis for *Candida* infection made on microscopy?

Oval yeasts, single or multiple buds, and pseudohyphae in tissue (see Fig. 20-1)

What two observations are used to distinguish *C. albicans* from other *Candida* species?

1. Germ tube formation in serum at body temperature (37°C [98.6°F]) (see Fig. 20-2)
2. Formation of dormant asexual spores, i.e., chlamydospores, at room temperature (25°C [77°F] to 28°C [82.4°F])

What is the role of skin tests in the diagnosis of candidiasis in immunocompetent versus immunosuppressed individuals?

Skin tests with *Candida* antigens are uniformly positive among immunocompetent adults capable of mounting a cellular immune delayed type hypersensitivity response

Patients who do not respond to *Candida* antigens have deficient cell-mediated immunity and are considered anergic

Note: Other skin tests, e.g., purified protein derivative (PPD), cannot be correctly interpreted in anergic patients

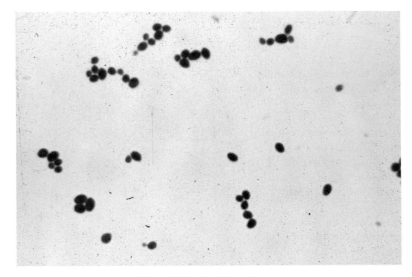

Figure 20-1. *Candida* oval yeast.

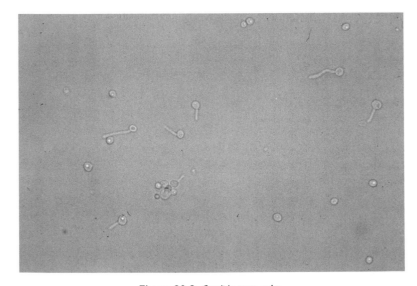

Figure 20-2. *Candida* germ tube.

What comorbidities are associated with ...

C. albicans?

Esophagitis, mucosal ulcerations, perforations, and abdominal surgery

C. tropicalis?

Cancer and leukemic patients with prolonged granulocytopenia

C. parapsilosis?

Prolonged total parenteral nutrition

CANDIDA ALBICANS

Is C. albicans part of the normal flora?

Yes; it is commonly found in the upper respiratory, gastrointestinal, and female genital tracts

What are six types of C. albicans infection (candidiasis)?

1. Oral thrush
2. Genitourinary (GU) mucocutaneous candidiasis
3. Gastrointestinal (GI) mucocutaneous candidiasis
4. Pulmonary candidiasis
5. Endocarditis
6. Cutaneous candidiasis

What is the most common site for superficial candidiasis?

Oral mucosa

What is thrush?

Inflammation of the oral mucosa and formation of superficial, white, elevated C. albicans plaques with possible ulceration

What are two common risk factors for this?

1. HIV infection
2. Patients receiving chemotherapy

How is this treated?

Nystatin "swish and swallow" or an oral azole

What two genitourinal sites are associated with candida?

1. Urinary tract
2. Vagina

What could predispose someone to candidiasis in each site?

1. Urinary tract candidiasis in the setting of a Foley catheter with superimposed antibiotic treatment

2. Vaginal candidiasis in the setting of being immunocompromised, e.g., diabetics, chronic steroid use, and pregnancy

What are the clinical manifestations of vaginal candidiasis?

Intense, burning, pruritic, erythematous vulva with abundant thick, white, and curd-like vaginal discharge

Which patient population is especially predisposed to hepatosplenic candidiasis?

Leukemic patients recovering from remission-induction treatment

What are three situations associated with candidal peritonitis?

1. Peritoneal dialysis complication
2. GI perforation secondary to ulcers, colitis, trauma, or neoplasia
3. Contamination during or after abdominal surgery

How common is dissemination following candidal peritonitis?

Rare

What are two manifestations of cardiovascular candidiasis?

1. Candidal blood infection (fungemia)
2. Candidal endocarditis

What are four dissemination sites for candidal fungemia?

1. Pulmonary
2. Renal
3. Ocular
4. Cardiac valves

What types of patients are likely to contract pulmonary candidiasis?

Patients with phagocytic cell defects such as chronic granulomatous disease or myeloperoxidase deficiencies

How is candida endocarditis treated?

Systemic antifungals and often surgery

Which two cutaneous sites are associated with candidiasis?

1. Skin folds (intertrigo), e.g., diaper rash
2. Fingernails

How does intertrigo present clinically?

Pruritic, erythematous vesicopustules between skin folds

What activity predisposes to finger and nail candidiasis?

Repeated immersion of hands in water, e.g., restaurant dishwashers

How is disseminated candidiasis treated?	Intravenous (IV) amphotericin B Recent evidence suggests that IV caspofungin may be effective

CRYPTOCOCCUS NEOFORMANS

What does *C. neoformans* cause?	Cryptococcosis
How is cryptococcosis acquired? Where is it found?	Inhalation of aerosolized soil enriched with pigeon droppings Worldwide distribution
What five diseases predispose one to cryptococcosis?	1. AIDS 2. Sarcoidosis 3. Lymphoma (mainly Hodgkin) 4. Systemic lupus erythematosus 5. Diabetes
What four sites are commonly infected by *C. neoformans*?	1. Meninges 2. Lungs 3. Skin 4. Bone
How does pulmonary cryptococcosis present? What other clinical manifestations are possible?	Usually asymptomatic Fever, moderately productive cough, and blood-tinged sputum
What are five possible chest x-ray findings suggestive of pulmonary cryptococcosis?	1. Hilar lymphadenopathy 2. Dense infiltrates in mid to lower lung fields 3. Single or multiple discrete nodules 4. Cavitation of upper lobes 5. Calcification
What is the treatment for pulmonary cryptococcosis?	Most cases resolve without treatment, although amphotericin B and flucytosine can be used
What are the clinical manifestations of cryptococcal meningitis?	Slow onset symptoms including frontal or temporal headache, mental status changes, nuchal rigidity, focal neurological deficits, and a mild fever

What is a common complication of *Cryptococcus*-caused meningitis?

Hydrocephalus

Does cryptococcal meningitis only occur in the immunosuppressed?

No; cryptococcal meningitis can occur in a small subset of immunocompetent individuals, but a thorough workup for an immunologic defect should still be performed

What is used for prophylaxis in AIDS patients against cryptococcal meningitis?

Indefinite prophylaxis with oral fluconazole

What is the mean survival for cryptococcal meningitis in AIDS patients?

~6 months from time of diagnosis

What cerebrospinal fluid (CSF) findings are consistent with cryptococcal meningitis?

High CSF opening pressure, high protein, low glucose, and lymphocytosis

What are three tests are available for *Cryptococcus* diagnosis?

1. India ink staining of CSF
2. Serologic testing for antigen, e.g., cryptococcal antigen latex particle agglutination testing
3. Culture

What does India ink staining demonstrate?

Thick, clear-appearing polysaccharide-encapsulated yeast cells resistant to India ink staining (see Fig. 20-3)

How is cryptococcal meningitis treated?

IV amphotericin B and flucytosine for 4–6 weeks

What is the most reliable test for assessing remission from creptococcosis?

Negative cryptococcal antigen tests

How common is relapse in non-AIDS–related cases?

Up to 30%

How are patients monitored?

Serial lumbar punctures

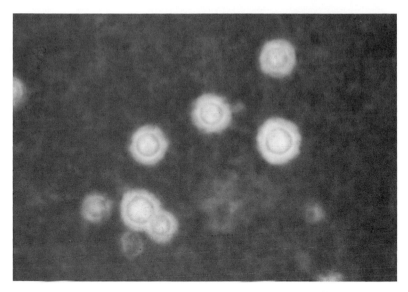

Figure 20-3. India ink staining of Cryptococcus (see also Color Photo 19).

What are three clinical manifestations of cutaneous cryptococcosis?	1. Painless, soft, and fluctuant subcutaneous swellings 2. Hard, occasionally purpuric, dermal plaques or nodules 3. Raised granulomata that can be papular or pustular
Which three studies are indicated in patients with cutaneous cryptococcus?	1. Lumbar puncture to rule out cryptococcal meningitis 2. X-ray for bone involvement of overlying cutaneous lesions 3. Serology to rule out disseminated cryptococcosis

ASPERGILLUS FUMIGATUS

What does *A. fumigatus* cause?	Aspergillosis
What other organisms cause aspergillosis?	Other *Aspergillus* genus members, e.g., *A. flavus*
What is unique about *A. flavus*?	*A. flavus* is carcinogenic because it produces aflatoxin, which is implicated with hepatomas

What foods are associated with *A. flavus*?

Moldy peanuts and grains

What three morphologic features of *Aspergillus* distinguish it from other opportunistic organisms?

1. *Aspergillus* and Zygomycetes (*Mucor* spp.) exist only as molds, whereas *Candida, Cryptococcus,* and *P. carinii* exist as yeast-like forms
2. *Aspergillus* has septate hyphae with parallel walls and typically V-shaped, dichotomous, 45-degree branching, whereas Zygomycetes (*Mucor* spp.) and *Rhizopus* species have nonseptate hyphae with irregular walls and right-angle branching
3. *Aspergillus* conidia form radiating chains, whereas *Rhizopus* and Zygomycetes (*Mucor* spp.) conidia are enclosed within a sporangium (see Fig. 20-4)

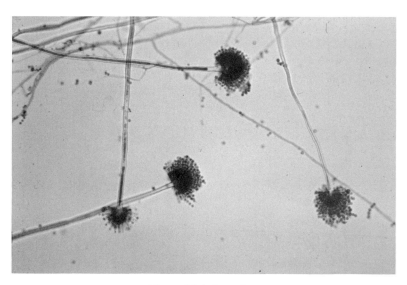

Figure 20-4. *Aspergillus.*

What is the pathogenesis of aspergillosis?

1. Inhalation of airborne conidia/environmental spores
2. Primary pulmonary infection
3. Colonization of skin, wounds, burns, cornea, external ear, or paranasal sinuses secondary to epidermal invasion

What is the most common cause of fungal sinusitis?

Aspergillus

What are four other clinical manifestations of aspergillosis?

1. Pulmonary hypersensitivity syndromes, e.g., extrinsic asthma, extrinsic allergic alveolitis, or allergic bronchopulmonary aspergillosis (ABPA)
2. Acute invasive and chronic necrotizing pulmonary aspergillosis
3. Aspergilloma ("fungus ball")
4. Miscellaneous infections, e.g., central nervous system (CNS), cardiac, cutaneous, ocular, bone, GI, and GU involvement

Which two host defense mechanisms are responsible for combating aspergillosis?

1. Pulmonary alveolar macrophages, which ingest inhaled spores and inhibit germination
2. Neutrophils, which destroy hyphae

What conditions predispose one to developing invasive aspergillosis?

1. High-dose corticosteroid treatment
2. Neutropenia

Would you expect *Aspergillus* to be a major opportunist in HIV infection?

No

Why wouldn't you expect it to be a major opportunist?

Aspergillosis is not commonly associated with T-cell deficiencies such as in HIV HIV patients can effectively defend against aspergillus infection because alveolar macrophages and neutrophils are unaffected by the virus

What are five common manifestations of pulmonary aspergillosis?

Lobar pneumonia, abscesses, hemorrhagic infarction, necrotizing bronchopneumonia, and aspergilloma

What is an aspergilloma?

Aspergilloma, or fungus ball, is a noninvasive mass of hyphal tissue that forms in lung cavities from prior necrotizing lung disease, such as tuberculosis

What clinical features suggest invasive pulmonary aspergillosis?	1. Persistent fever while on antibiotic therapy 2. Rales without fluid overload 3. Pleuritic chest pain
What is the chest x-ray finding seen with aspergilloma?	Radiopaque structure that changes position when the patient is moved from an erect to a supine position
What is ABPA?	Allergic reaction that arises from inhalation of *Aspergillus* spores without subsequent extensive spore germination or hyphal invasion
What symptoms do ABPA patients present with?	Asthmatic symptoms
What lab test is diagnostic for ABPA?	High IgE titer against Aspergillus antigens
What are four manifestations of intracranial aspergillosis?	1. Subcortical hemorrhagic infarct 2. Solitary or multiple abscesses 3. Meningitis 4. Granuloma
Why is pulmonary and cerebral infarction a hallmark of *Aspergillus* infection?	*Aspergillus* is angioinvasive, leading to thrombosis and infarction of distal tissues *Rhizopus, Aspergillus,* and *Mucor*—"R.A.M."—are angioinvasive!
What CSF findings are associated with *Aspergillus* meningitis?	Normal CSF in up to 50% of patients, i.e., isolation of *Aspergillus* from CSF is rare; however, may result in modestly elevated protein, monocytosis or neutrophilia, and normal glucose
What is the most common manifestation of paranasal sinus aspergillosis?	Aspergilloma
How does paranasal aspergillosis present clinically?	Headache or facial pain with periorbital swelling and visual disturbance
What is a complication of paranasal aspergillosis?	Local extension of infection from the paranasal sinuses to the brain

What is the x-ray finding seen with paranasal aspergillosis?	Opacification of the sinuses and, occasionally, local bone destruction
What are two clinical manifestations of cardiac aspergillosis?	1. Endocarditis secondary to heart surgery 2. Myocarditis secondary to hematogenous dissemination
Which patient population is particularly at risk for this?	IV drug users
What is the clinical manifestation of cutaneous aspergillosis?	Macule, nodule, or area of cellulitis that slowly develops into black necrotic eschars
What is the gold standard for diagnosis of aspergillosis?	Histologic evidence of tissue invasion by fungus with *Aspergillus* morphology; however, diagnosis is often difficult
What is the drug of choice for treatment of aspergillosis?	Amphotericin B

RHIZOPUS **AND MUCORMYCOSIS**

What three genera of fungi cause mucormycosis?	1. *Rhizopus* 2. *Absidia* 3. *Rhizomucor*
How is mucormycosis commonly acquired?	1. Inhalation of spores 2. Germination and invasion of mucosal membranes 3. Less commonly, infection can follow ingestion, direct inoculation through traumatic breaks in skin, or through IV injection
What is one characteristic that the pathogens that cause mucormycosis, especially *Rhizopus*, share with *Aspergillus*?	All are angioinvasive *Rhizopus*, *Aspergillus*, and *Mucor*—"R.A.M."—are angioinvasive!
What is the pathogenesis of *Rhizopus*- and *Mucor*-mediated vasculopathy?	1. Invade vessel walls 2. Form a tangled fibrin mesh inside the vessel lumen with rapid extension 3. Thrombosis and resultant infarction of distal tissue follow

What are five major clinical manifestations of mucormycosis?

1. Rhinocerebral mucormycosis (most common)
2. Pulmonary mucormycosis
3. Disseminated mucormycosis
4. Cutaneous mucormycosis
5. Gastrointestinal mucormycosis (rare)

What is the major risk factor for rhinocerebral mucormycosis?

Conditions associated with acidosis such as diabetes, renal failure, and diarrhea
Rhinocerebral mucormycosis rarely occurs in normal hosts

What other patient groups are at increased risk for mucormycosis?

Conditions associated with immunosuppression, e.g., leukemia, lymphoma, diabetics, and organ transplantation

How does rhinocerebral mucormycosis evolve?

1. Inhaled spores germinate and invade nasopharyngeal, palatal, or paranasal sinus mucosa
2. Extension spreads from these primary sites along vessels to secondarily infect the frontal lobes of the brain

How does rhinocerebral mucormycosis present clinically?

In early stages, patients present with facial or sinus pain and stuffiness, headache, and serosanguinous discharge
Most patients are not seen this early and more than two thirds present in stupor or coma caused by spread to frontal lobes. Proptosis, eye pain, conjunctival and eyelid swelling, and injection, as well as gangrenous changes of the skin of nose, eyelid, and face, suggest impending CNS involvement

What clinical scenario raises the concern for possible rhinocerebral mucormycosis?

Mental status changes in patients with acidosis secondary to uncontrolled diabetes who do not improve with correction of electrolyte abnormalities

How is rhinocerebral mucormycosis diagnosed?

Presence of nonseptate hyphae with right-angle branching in necrotic tissue
However, swab cultures of nose and palate are usually negative

How are imaging studies useful?

To delineate the extent of infection and evaluate for therapeutic debridement

What is the characteristic pulmonary lesion associated with mucormycosis?	Pulmonary infarction secondary to vessel invasion
Does the inflammatory reaction to *Rhizopus* and *Mucor* result in granuloma formation?	No
What are two methods used to diagnose pulmonary mucormycosis?	1. V/Q scan demonstrating multiple segmental perfusion defects resembling multiple pulmonary emboli 2. Biopsy of open lung or metastatic skin lesions
Who is at highest risk for cutaneous mucormycosis?	Patients with extensive burn wounds
What is the treatment for mucormycosis?	1. Acidosis correction 2. Debridement when possible 3. Amphotericin B
What is the outcome of untreated mucormycosis?	Death

PNEUMOCYSTIS CARINII (P. JIROVECI)*

What type of organism causes pneumocystis pneumonia?	Unicellular eukaryote
How does *P. carinii* (*P. jiroveci*) differ from fungi?	Lacks essential components of fungi, e.g., ergosterol
Why has deciphering the classification of *P. carinii* (*P. jiroveci*) been difficult?	*P. carinii* (*P. jiroveci*) has not been successfully grown in culture
How is *P. carinii* (*P. jiroveci*) transmitted?	Respiratory route

---

*Terminology of *P. carinii* has changed to *P. jiroveci*.

By what age have most humans been exposed/ become immune to *P. carinii* (*P. jiroveci*)?

3 years of age

How does *P. carinii* (*P. jiroveci*) infection most commonly present?

Pneumonia, pneumocystis pneumonia (PCP)

What is the triad of PCP symptoms?

1. Fever
2. Exertional dyspnea
3. Nonproductive cough

What is the pathogenesis of *P. carinii* (*P. jiroveci*)?

1. Attachment to type I alveolar cells
2. Proliferation
3. Formation of eosinophilic foamy exudates secondary to host inflammatory response
4. Occlusion of alveolar air spaces causing desaturation and respiratory distress
5. Interstitial thickening and fibrosis

What four factors predispose one to PCP?

1. Defective T-cell immunity with CD4 count <200/mL
2. Previous PCP or another AIDS defining illness
3. Primary immunodeficiency disease, especially severe combined immunodeficiency disease (SCID)
4. Protein malnutrition

What is a life-threatening complication of PCP?

Spontaneous pneumothorax

How is PCP diagnosed?

1. Silver stain of bronchial alveolar lavage revealing thick-walled cysts containing 6–8 intracystic sporozoites or extracystic trophozoites
2. Direct fluorescent antibody of sputum or bronchoalveolar lavage

What is the characteristic chest x-ray finding in PCP?

None
PCP can mimic many disease processes including normal

What is the treatment for PCP?

Trimethoprim-sulfamethoxazole (Bactrim) and corticosteroids

Why these drugs?

Trimethoprim-sulfamethoxazole is an antibiotic and kills the organism
Administration of corticosteroids within first 72 hours of initiating antipneumocystis treatment decreases respiratory failure and death by attenuating the inflammatory response in AIDS patients

Should treatment be stopped if patients desaturate more when trimethoprim-sulfamethoxazole is initiated?

No, desaturation is often secondary to inflammatory reaction to *P. carinii* cell death and treatment should not be changed for 5–7 days

What is the mortality of patients treated for PCP?

9–20% mortality despite full course of treatment

What are the indications for PCP prophylaxis with trimethoprim-sulfamethoxazole?

1. Patients with CD4 count <200/mL
2. Patients receiving aggressive immunosuppressive therapy

What other pathogen does trimethoprim-sulfamethox-azole protect against?

Toxoplasma gondii infection

Section III

Virology

21

Viral Structure & Replication

STRUCTURE

What are viruses?

Obligate intracellular parasites incapable of independent replication, protein synthesis, or energy production

What are obligate intracellular parasites?

Organisms that can only reproduce within cells because they cannot synthesize proteins or generate energy

What is the normal range for the size of a virus?

20–300 nanometers

How does this compare to other organisms?

100 times smaller than bacteria
1,000 times smaller than eukaryotic cells

What is the significance of this?

They are too small to be seen with light microscopy, but can be visualized with electron microscopy

What are two basic components common to all viruses?

1. Genome (nucleic acid)
2. Capsid

What additional component is seen with some viruses?

Envelope

What nucleic acid is found in viruses?

Either deoxyribonucleic acid (DNA) or ribonucleic acid (RNA), but not both

What type of genome do most DNA viruses contain?
What is the exception?

Double-stranded genome (dsDNA)

Parvoviridae, which contain a single-stranded DNA (ssDNA)

What type of genome do most RNA viruses contain?
What is the exception?

Single-stranded genome (ssRNA)

Reoviridae, which contain double-stranded RNA (dsRNA)

What types of ssRNA genomes exist?

1. Positive ssRNA (+ssRNA)
2. Negative ssRNA (−ssRNA)

What is the significance of +ssRNA?

Nucleic acid that can be directly translated by host machinery, thus making it analogous to host mRNA
Positive single-stranded RNA viruses do not require RNA-dependent RNA polymerase in the virion for viral replication

What is the significance of −ssRNA?

How is this achieved?

Nucleic acid that is incapable of being translated directly as messenger RNA (mRNA) and must synthesize a positive strand by serving as a template
The virus must contain its own RNA-dependent RNA polymerase to synthesize the positive strand
RNA-dependent RNA polymerase is found in the virion of negative single-stranded RNA viruses because it is required for viral replication

What is a capsid?

A protein coat that surrounds and protects viral nucleic acid

What is a capsomer?

The functional subunit of a capsid consisting of one or more proteins that determine the viral geometrical symmetry

What are two forms of geometrical symmetry found in viral capsids?

1. Icosahedral
2. Helical

What is icosahedral symmetry?

A sphere-shaped structure composed of 20 triangular faces and 12 vertices (see Fig. 21-1)

What is helical symmetry?

A rod-shaped structure composed of capsomers arranged in a hollow coil (see Fig. 21-2)

What are two functions of capsid proteins?

1. Protect nucleic acid containing genetic material
2. Mediate viral attachment to host cell receptors

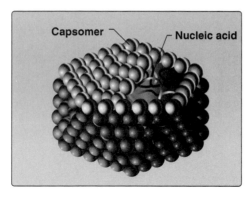

Figure 21-1. A viral capsid with icosahedral symmetry.

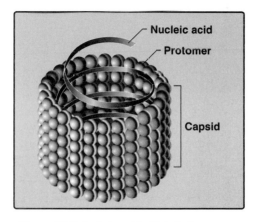

Figure 21-2. A viral capsid with helical symmetry.

What is an unintentional effect of capsid proteins?	Contain antigens that may stimulate an immunological response
What is a viral envelope?	A lipoprotein membrane surrounding the capsid
From where is it derived?	Host cell membranes
Do all viruses possess an envelope?	No
What families are nonenveloped?	DNA viruses: "PAP" 1. Papovaviridae (dsDNA) 2. Adenoviridae (dsDNA) 3. Parvoviridae (ssDNA)

RNA viruses: "CPR"
1. Caliciviridae (+ssRNA)
2. Picornaviridae (+ssRNA)
3. Reoviridae (dsRNA)

What is a name for nonenveloped viruses?

A nucleocapsid or a "naked" virus

What are defective viruses?

Viruses with nucleic acid and proteins that are able to invade but incapable of replication

What is an example?

Hepatitis D virus

UNCONVENTIONAL INFECTIOUS AGENTS

What are three unconventional infectious agents?

1. Prions
2. Viriods
3. Pseudovirions

What are prions?

Potentially infectious agents that are composed solely of proteins and lack nucleic acid

What diseases are caused by prions?

Transmissible spongiform encephalopathies, including Creutzfeldt-Jakob disease and kuru

What are viroids?

Small infectious agents that consist solely of RNA that do not code for proteins
Viroids only cause diseases in plants

What are pseudovirions?

Agents with a capsid containing host cell DNA instead of viral DNA incapable of replication

VIRAL REPLICATION

What are the two stages of the viral growth curve?

1. Eclipse period
2. Exponential growth period

What is the eclipse period?

The period of time when no intact virus is found inside the cell, from initial entry and disassembly of the virus to the assembly of the first progeny virus

How long is this period for most human viruses?

1–20 hours

What is the exponential growth period?

The period of time when the number of progeny virus produced within the infected cell increases exponentially and then plateaus

How long is this period for most human viruses?

8–72 hours

What is the incubation period for a virus?

The period of time between initial infection and onset of symptoms

What is the burst size?

The number of virions released from an infected cell

What is the typical range for the burst size of a virus?

100–10,000 virions per infected cell

What are the eight stages of the viral growth cycle?

1. Adsorption
2. Penetration
3. Uncoating
4. Early transcription and translation
5. Viral genome replication
6. Late transcription and translation
7. Assembly
8. Release (see Fig. 21-3)

What is adsorption?
How is this achieved?

Attachment of virion to host cell receptors
1. Viral envelope glycoprotein interaction with host cell receptors
2. Folding of capsid proteins creating a site for host cell receptor interaction

What is penetration?

Passage of virion from the cell surface into the cytoplasm

What are the two main mechanisms of penetration?

1. Direct membrane fusion
2. Receptor-mediated endocytosis

What is direct membrane fusion?

Fusion of the viral envelope with the host cell membrane enabling the nucleocapsid to enter the cell

What is receptor-mediated endocytosis?

Host cell membrane invagination after viral adsorption, creating an intracellular virion-containing endocytic vesicle (endosome) (see Fig. 21-4)

How is the virion released into the cytoplasm from the endosome?

1. Direct membrane fusion between the virion and endosome
2. Virion proteins create pores within

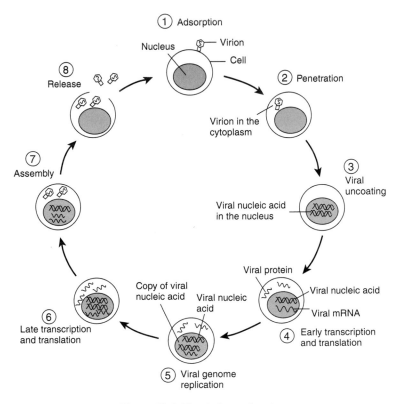

Figure 21-3. The viral growth cycle.

the endosome or cause the membrane to dissolve, facilitating viral entry into the cytoplasm

What must occur for a virion in an endosome to be pathogenic?

Release of virus into the cytoplasm before the endosome fuses with the lysosome

    Why must release occur first?

Lysosomes contain degradative enzymes

    What family of viruses is the one exception to this rule?

Reoviridae (dsRNA) can survive and partially uncoat within lysosomes

What is uncoating?

Disassembly of the virion

What is early transcription and translation?

Nucleic acid is transcribed into mRNA, which is then translated into proteins used for viral genome replication

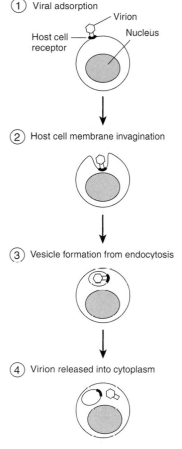

Figure 21-4. Receptor-mediated endocytosis.

What is the first step in viral gene expression?

Synthesis of mRNA

Where do most DNA viruses replicate?

In the nucleus

What family of DNA viruses is the exception?

Poxviridae, which replicate in the cytoplasm

What is the advantage of viruses replicating in the nucleus?

They can use host cell enzymes for viral replication

What is the general mechanism of replication for DNA viruses?

See Fig. 21-5

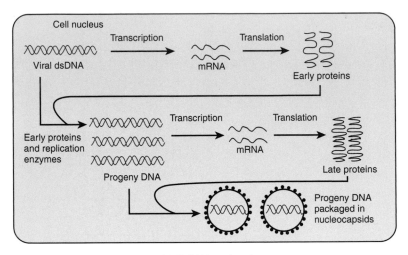

Figure 21-5. DNA viral replication.

Where do most RNA viruses replicate?	In the cytoplasm
What RNA viruses are the exceptions?	Retroviruses and influenza virus which have replication steps in the nucleus
What are two challenges that RNA viruses must overcome for replication?	1. Host cells that lack RNA polymerase used to synthesize complementary RNA strands from the RNA genome 2. RNA viruses frequently contain only one molecule of RNA, but must express two or more proteins
What are three groups of RNA viruses that have different patterns of replication to overcome these challenges?	1. +ssRNA 2. −ssRNA 3. dsRNA
What are two mechanisms by which +ssRNA replicate	1. Replication with a complementary −ssRNA intermediate 2. Replication with a DNA intermediate
What are two roles of +ssRNA that replicate with a complementary negative-strand intermediate?	1. Serves as mRNA for translation by host machinery 2. Template for synthesis of complementary negative strand

What is the product of translation?	A single protein
How are multiple proteins generated from this?	The protein contains protease domains that allow it to be cleaved into multiple proteins, e.g., RNA-dependent RNA polymerase and structural proteins (see Fig. 21-6)

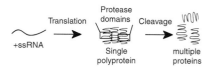

Figure 21-6. Translation of +ssRNA.

How does this type of RNA replicate?	1. The +ssRNA serves as a template for generating a complementary −ssRNA with RNA-dependent RNA polymerase 2. The −ssRNA can serve as a template for generating progeny +ssRNA via RNA-dependent RNA polymerase (see Fig. 21-7)
What is the initial step in replication of +ssRNA which replicate with a DNA intermediate?	Conversion of the positive-strand RNA to dsDNA
How is this achieved?	By RNA-dependent DNA polymerase, which is found within the virion and must be transferred into the host cell along with the viral genome for replication to occur
What is another name for this enzyme?	Reverse transcriptase
What step is required before the intermediate can generate viral progeny and proteins?	The dsDNA must integrate into the cell genome
What enzyme catalyzes this step?	Integrase
What unique challenge do −ssRNA viruses face?	The negative ssRNA strand cannot be directly translated by host machinery
How do −ssRNA viruses overcome this problem?	They contain RNA-dependent RNA polymerase within the virion that must be transferred into the host cell along with

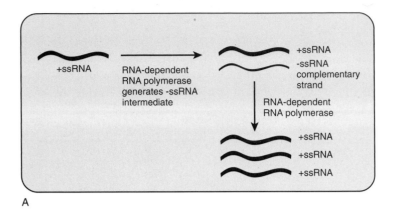

A

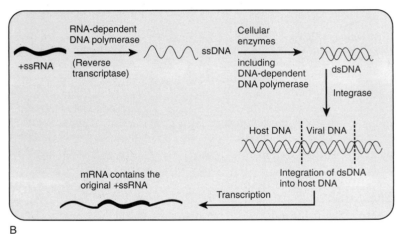

B

Figure 21-7. A. Replication of +ssRNA with a −ssRNA intermediate. **B.** Replication of +ssRNA with a DNA intermediate.

the viral genome for replication to occur

What is the first step of infection with −ssRNA viruses?	Synthesis of +RNA by the virion-encoded RNA-dependent RNA polymerase using the −ssRNA as a template
What are two roles of intermediate positive-strand RNAs?	1. Serve as mRNA for translation by host machinery 2. Template for synthesizing −ssRNA which is incorporated into progeny virions
What are two categories of −ssRNA viruses?	1. Viruses with a single, linear strand of RNA

2. Viruses with a segmented RNA genome
Remember "BOAR" for the segmented RNA viruses: Bunyaviridae, Orthomyxoviridae, Arenaviridae, and Reoviridae

How are multiple proteins translated from these two categories of −ssRNA viruses?

1. Linear RNA genomes may be polycistronic, generating multiple mRNAs specific for single proteins
2. Segmented RNA genomes produce multiple positive-strand mRNAs that usually encode single proteins (see Fig. 21-8)

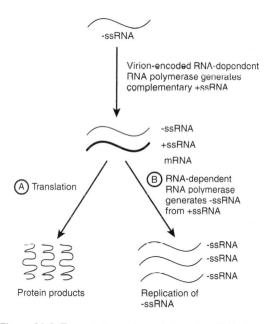

Figure 21-8. Transcription and translation of −ssRNA viruses.

What is the genome structure for dsRNA viruses?

All dsRNA viruses contain a segmented genome

How is mRNA synthesized in dsRNA viruses?

Because host cell machinery is unable to generate positive-strand mRNA from dsRNA, the virion must contain its own RNA-dependent RNA polymerase to generate positive-strand RNA from the negative strand (see Fig. 21-9)

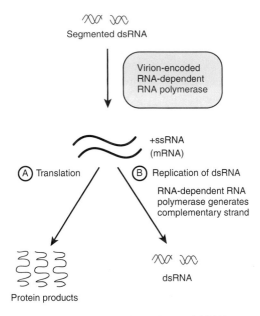

Figure 21-9. Transcription and translation of dsRNA viruses.

What is late transcription and translation?	Translation of nucleic acid into proteins that are either incorporated into the progeny virus particle or are required for viral assembly
What is assembly?	Construction of viral progeny from the necessary nucleic acids and proteins
Where does assembly occur?	In the cellular compartment where viral nucleic acid replicates
	DNA viruses that replicate in the nucleus assemble in the nucleus, and therefore require proteins to be transported from the cytoplasm
	RNA viruses that replicate in the cytoplasm assemble in the cytoplasm
What are two methods of viral release from the host cell?	1. Lysis of the host cell 2. Budding from the host cell
What types of viruses are released by budding?	Enveloped viruses

What are the six steps of budding? (See Fig. 21-10)

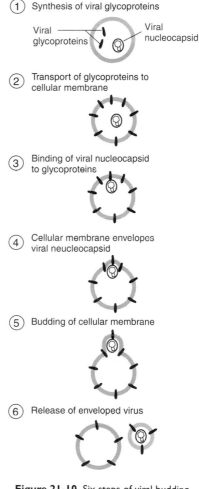

① Synthesis of viral glycoproteins

Viral glycoproteins

Viral nucleocapsid

② Transport of glycoproteins to cellular membrane

③ Binding of viral nucleocapsid to glycoproteins

④ Cellular membrane envelopes viral neucleocapsid

⑤ Budding of cellular membrane

⑥ Release of enveloped virus

Figure 21-10. Six steps of viral budding.

How long does one viral growth cycle typically last?

20 hours for human viruses
30 minutes for bacteriophage viruses

What is the lytic growth cycle?

A growth cycle in which the virus enters the cell, replicates, and is released by host cell lysis

What is the lysogenic growth cycle?

A growth cycle in which viral DNA becomes integrated into the host's genome, replicates autonomously under certain conditions, and then is released by host cell lysis or is simply passed along when the host cell multiplies

What are viruses called that replicate with a lysogenic growth cycle?

Temperate phages

What are viruses called that infect bacteria and replicate via the lysogenic growth cycle?

Bacteriophages

What is the integrated viral DNA called?

Prophage

What are two conditions that result in prophage entry into the lytic cycle?
What is this process called?

1. Ultraviolet (UV) light
2. Metabolic stress

Induction

What is the mechanism behind UV light induction?

Induces synthesis of a protease, which inhibits a viral repressor protein, allowing expression and excision of prophage DNA

Once this DNA has been expressed, the phage completes its replicative cycle and synthesizes progeny virions (see Fig. 21-11)

Induction of prophage

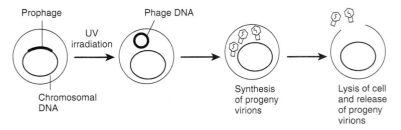

Figure 21-11. Induction into the lytic cycle.

22

Viral Genetics, Pathogenesis, & Phylogeny

VIRAL GENETICS

What is a wild-type organism?

A standard to which genetic mutants are compared

What is a mutant?

An organism that deviates from normal in some recognizable characteristic (phenotype)

What is a mutation?

A change in the base sequence of deoxyribonucleic acid (DNA)

What is an unstable mutation?

A mutation that frequently changes back to its original state

How are nucleotides classified?

Purines: adenine (A), guanine (G) have two rings
Pyrimidines: cytosine (C), thymine (T) have one ring
Pyrimidines contain the letter "Y"

What is a point mutation?

A mutation that only affects 1 base pair

What are two types of point mutations?

1. Transition substitution
2. Transversion substitution

What is a transition substitution?

A point mutation where a purine is substituted for a purine or a pyrimidine is substituted for a pyrimidine

What is a transversion substitution?

A point mutation where a purine replaces a pyrimidine or vice-versa

What is ...

An inversion mutation?

A mutation where a string of base pairs are deleted and reinserted in the same position, but in the opposite direction

A silent mutation?

A mutation that alters base pairs, but not the specific amino acid they encode

A missense mutation?

A mutation that alters base pairs resulting in the replacement one amino acid residue for another

A nonsense mutation?

A mutation resulting in a stop codon, prematurely terminating the elongation of a polypeptide chain

A frame-shift mutation?

A mutation that changes the reading frame of the genetic code, resulting in a misreading of all downstream nucleotides and altering the encoded amino acids of the polypeptide chain, often resulting in early stop codons (see also Chapter 2, Figure 2-7)

What are conditional-lethal mutations?

Mutations that allow gene expression and protein formation under permissive conditions, but fail to replicate or allow gene expression under restrictive conditions

What is their clinical significance?

These mutations allow for identification of specific genes responsible for viral properties and can be used to create live-attenuated vaccines that take advantage of these mutations

What are defective-interfering particles?

Deletion mutants that are incapable of replication unless the deleted function is supplied by a "helper" virus

What is their clinical significance?

They interfere with growth of normal viruses and stimulate cellular immune responses, thereby limiting spread of the virus

What are four interactions that occur when two different viral strains infect the same cell?

1. Recombination
2. Reassortment
3. Complementation
4. Phenotypic mixing

What is recombination?

Exchange of genes between two chromosomes by crossing over of regions with base pair homology

What viruses display a higher rate of recombination?

Double-stranded DNA (dsDNA) viruses

What is reassortment?

Exchange of gene segments between viruses with segmented genomes
Reassortment results in a higher frequency of gene exchange than recombination

What is a clinically important example of this?

Influenza virus undergoes major antigenic changes (antigenic shift) via reassortment that causes devastating worldwide epidemics

What is complementation?

A process by which a virus is able to assist a mutated virus by providing functional proteins for the defective virus

What is an important example of this?

Hepatitis B virus provides surface antigen for defective hepatitis delta virus (HDV), allowing HDV to replicate in coinfected cells causing a more severe form of hepatitis

What is phenotypic mixing?

A process by which the genome of virus type A can be coated with the surface proteins of virus type B, producing a phenotypically mixed virus

What is the significance of this?

Phenotypically mixed viruses infect cells based on the cells' type B protein coat

What is the genetic makeup of the progeny virions?

Progeny virions have the genome and protein coat of the type A virus (progeny virions will contain the protein coating of the virus whose genome is present)

PATHOGENESIS

What are five effects of viral infection on the cell?

1. No morphologic or physiologic change
2. Fusion of cells to form multinucleated giant cells
3. Malignant transformation
4. Death by lysis
5. Death by apoptosis

What are multinucleated giant cells?

Enlarged cells that are formed by membrane fusion of infected cells Multinucleated giant cells are also called syncytial cells (see Fig. 22-1)

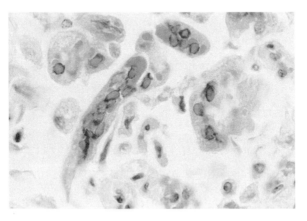

Figure 22-1. Multinucleated giant cells (see Color Photo 20).

Which two families of viruses typically cause multinucleated giant cell formation?

Herpesviridae and Paramyxoviridae

What is malignant transformation?

A process causing virus-infected cells to have altered morphology, abnormal growth control, and distinct cellular and biochemical properties, i.e., cells become cancerous

How is their morphology altered?

Cells lose their defined shape and appear more rounded

How is their growth control abnormal?

Cells have unrestrained growth, prolonged survival, and lose contact inhibition resulting in a pile of cells

How are cellular properties altered?

Cells have mutated genomes and DNA synthesis is induced

How are biochemical properties altered?

Cells produce less cyclic adenosine monophosphate (cAMP), have increased anaerobic metabolism, and produce altered sugar moieties on membrane-bound glycoproteins

What causes cell death?	Inhibition of protein and/or nucleic acid synthesis or stimulation of apoptosis
What is the cytopathic effect (CPE)?	A hallmark change in the appearance of virus-infected cells with rounding and darkening of the cell, eventually leading to lysis or giant cell formation and apoptosis
What are inclusion bodies?	Areas of the cell that contain viral proteins or particles that have a characteristic appearance, depending on the virus
Where are they located?	Either intranuclear or intracytoplasmic, depending on the virus
What is the name of the inclusion bodies found in rabies virus-infected neurons?	Negri bodies **USMLE**
What are they?	Eosinophilic cytoplasmic inclusions (see Fig. 22-2)

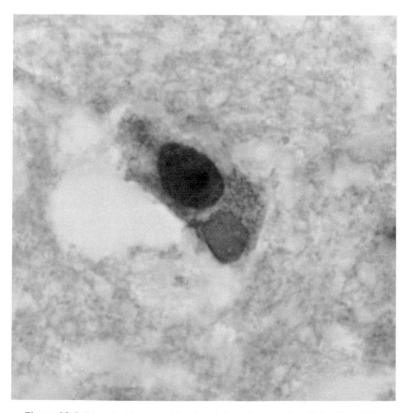

Figure 22-2. Negri bodies in a rabies virus-infected neuron (see Color Photo 21).

How do the inclusion bodies seen with cytomegalovirus infection appear microscopically?

As owl's-eye nuclear inclusions (see Fig. 22-3)

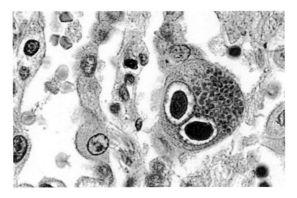

Figure 22-3. Owl's-eye nuclear inclusions in CMV-infected cells.

What are four stages in a typical viral infection?

1. Incubation period during which the patient is asymptomatic
2. Prodromal period during which the patient has nonspecific symptoms
3. Viral-specific illness period
4. Recovery period

What are two methods of transmission?

1. Vertical transmission
2. Horizontal transmission

What is the difference?

Vertical transmission involves the spread of a virus from parent to offspring either *in utero* or during the birth process, e.g., cytomegalovirus

Horizontal transmission involves the spread of a virus between two people other than during the birth process or while the fetus is *in utero*, e.g., influenza virus

What are two ways a virus can spread from a site of entry resulting in a disseminated infection?

1. Hematogenous spread
2. Neural spread

Which viruses use the . . .

Respiratory tract as a portal of entry?

1. Influenza virus (flu)
2. Rhinovirus (common cold)

3. Respiratory syncytial virus
(bronchiolitis)
4. Epstein-Barr virus (infectious
mononucleosis)
5. Varicella-zoster virus (chickenpox)
6. Herpes simplex virus type 1 (herpes
labialis)
7. Cytomegalovirus (mononucleosis)
8. Measles virus (measles)
9. Mumps virus (mumps)
10. Rubella virus (rubella)
11. Hantavirus (pneumonia)
12. Adenovirus (pneumonia)

**Gastrointestinal tract as
a portal of entry?**

1. Hepatitis A virus (hepatitis A)
2. Poliovirus (poliomyelitis)
3. Rotavirus (diarrhea)

Skin as a portal of entry?

1. Rabies virus (rabies)
2. Yellow fever virus (yellow fever)
3. Dengue virus (dengue)
4. Human papillomavirus (common
warts)

**Genital tract as a portal
of entry?**

1. Human papillomavirus (genital warts)
2. Hepatitis B virus (hepatitis B)
3. Human immunodeficiency virus
(AIDS)
4. Herpes simplex virus type 2 (herpes
genitalis and neonatal herpes)

**Blood as a portal of
entry?**

1. Hepatitis B virus (hepatitis B)
2. Hepatitis C virus (hepatitis C)
3. Hepatitis D virus (hepatitis D)
4. Human T-cell leukemia virus
(leukemia)
5. Human immunodeficiency virus
(AIDS)
6. Cytomegalovirus (mononucleosis
syndrome or pneumonia)

**Which viruses are
transmitted
transplacentally?**

1. Rubella
2. Cytomegalovirus
3. Herpes simplex virus
4. Human immunodeficiency virus (HIV)

**Which bacteria are trans-
mitted transplacentally?**

1. *Treponema pallidum*
2. *Listeria monocytogenes*

Which protozoa are transmitted transplacentally?

Toxoplasma gondii
"TORCHES" represents the most common infections transmitted transplacentally: Toxoplasmosis, Rubella, Cytomegalovirus, Herpes simplex virus/HIV, Syphilis (*T. pallidum*)

Which viruses are transmitted during parturition?

1. Hepatitis B virus
2. Hepatitis C virus
3. Herpes simplex virus-2
4. Human immunodeficiency virus (HIV)
5. Human papillomavirus

What is an attenuated virus?

A mutant virus that has diminished ability to cause disease in immunocompetent individuals

What is their clinical significance?

Attenuated viruses may be used in vaccines to induce an appropriate immune response to the wild-type virus

What are three viruses that cause hepatocellular pathology mainly by inducing an inappropriate immune response?

1. Hepatitis A virus
2. Hepatitis B virus
3. Hepatitis C virus

What are five factors that predispose one to chronic viral infections?

1. Immunosuppression
2. Formation of antigen–antibody complexes that remain infectious
3. Antigenic variation
4. Infection in an area that is isolated from an immune response, e.g., central nervous system (CNS) and testes
5. Integration of the viral genome with the host cell genome

What are three types of clinically important chronic viral infections?

1. Chronic carrier infections
2. Latent infections
3. Slow virus infections

What are chronic carrier infections?

Infections with viruses that continue to produce significant amounts of viral progeny for extended periods of time

What are examples of viruses with this trait?

Hepatitis B and C viruses, congenital rubella virus, HIV, and cytomegalovirus infections

What are latent infections?

Infections with viruses where the patient recovers from the initial infection and production of viral progeny ceases; however, the patient never clears the virus
A future stimulus can cause the virus to replicate and symptoms to recur

What families of viruses have this characteristic?

Herpesviridae family demonstrate latent infections

What are slow virus infections?

Infections with a prolonged period between the initial infection and the onset of disease

What is an example of a virus with this trait?

JC virus

VIRAL PHYLOGENY

How are DNA viruses classified? (See Fig. 22-4)

How are RNA viruses classified? (See Fig. 22-5)

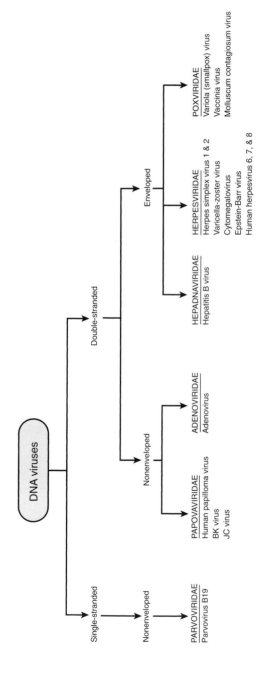

Figure 22-4. Classification of DNA viruses.

All DNA viruses have Icosahedral capsid geometry except for Poxviridae, which have complex capsid geometry.

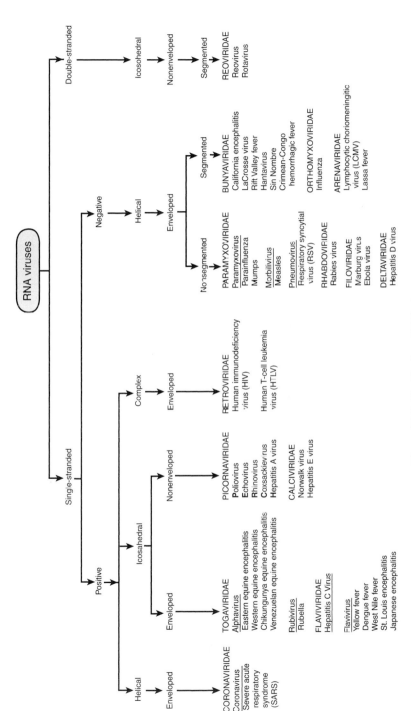

Figure 22-5. Classification of RNA viruses.

23

Nonenveloped DNA Viruses

OVERVIEW

What are two clinically relevant families of double-stranded, nonenveloped deoxyribonucleic acid (DNA) viruses?

1. Papovaviridae
2. Adenoviridae

What is the only clinically relevant family of single-stranded, nonenveloped DNA viruses?

Parvoviridae

PAPOVAVIRIDAE

What does the acronym "papova" stand for?

<u>Pa</u>pilloma, <u>po</u>lyoma, and simian <u>va</u>cuolating viruses

What type of nucleic acid do Papovaviridae contain in their genome?

Supercoiled, double-stranded, circular DNA

  What is their capsid geometry?

Icosahedral

  Do they contain an envelope?

No, they are nonenveloped

What are the two subfamilies of Papovaviridae?

1. Papillomaviridae
2. Polyomaviridae

  What clinically relevant viruses are associated with each family?

Papillomavirus:
1. Human papillomavirus (HPV)
Polyomavirus:
1. BK virus
2. JC virus

PAPILLOMAVIRIDAE

What type of lesions do all papillomaviruses cause?	Papillomas, e.g., warts
What are warts?	Hyperplastic epithelial lesions
How is HPV transmitted?	By direct contact, including sexual transmission
What type of tissue does HPV show tropism for?	Skin epithelium and mucous membranes
Which layer of the skin is initially infected?	Basal layer
Is there a high viral load in this layer?	No, there are only a few virions in the nuclei of basal cells
What does HPV do to cells in this layer?	Induces cell multiplication (mitogenic effect)
What is unique about the life cycle of HPV?	The viral life cycle progresses with increasing differentiation of the epithelium
In which layers of the skin are HPV early genes expressed?	Early genes are expressed in the undifferentiated stratum spinosum
In which layers of the skin are HPV late genes expressed?	Late genes are expressed in the differentiated stratum corneum (the outer layer) (see Fig. 23-1)

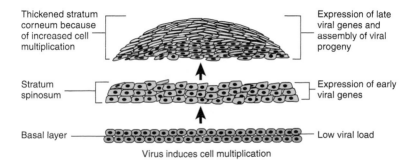

Thickened stratum corneum because of increased cell multiplication — Expression of late viral genes and assembly of viral progeny

Stratum spinosum — Expression of early viral genes

Basal layer — Low viral load

Virus induces cell multiplication

Figure 23-1. HPV life cycle in the layers of the skin.

How many different serotypes of HPV have been discovered?	More than 70
What is the characteristic histologic finding in papillomavirus infection?	Koilocytes
What is this?	Cytoplasmic vacuoles found in infected squamous epithelial cells (see Fig. 23-2)

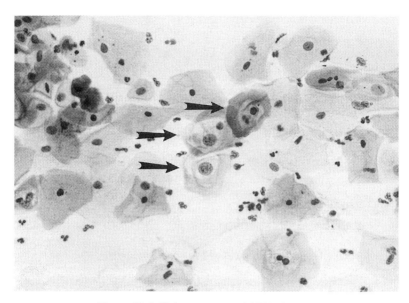

Figure 23-2. Koilocytes seen with HPV infection.

What are three clinical manifestations of genital warts?	1. Condyloma accuminata (genital warts) 2. Benign papillomas 3. Cancers of the anogenital region
What is condyloma acuminata?	A commonly acquired sexually transmitted infection (STI) caused by HPV Condyloma acuminata is caused by HPV and condyloma lata is caused by *Treponema pallidum*
What HPV serotypes are associated with this disease?	HPV-6 and HPV-11
What are five benign papillomas caused by HPV?	1. Common skin warts on the fingers and hands

2. Flat warts on the arms, face, and knees
3. Plantar warts on the soles of feet
4. Laryngeal papillomas
5. Epidermodysplasia verruciformis

What HPV subtypes are associated with skin and plantar warts?

HPV-1 through HPV-4

What are laryngeal papillomas?

Most common benign epithelial tumor of the larynx

What is epidermodysplasia verruciformis?

A condition characterized by multiple warts that spread to multiple sites and do not regress

What is thought to be the cause of this condition?

Inherited deficiency in cell-mediated immunity

What is a complication of this disease?

Squamous cell cancer

HPV infection has been linked to what types of cancer?

Cancer of the cervix, penis, and anus

Which HPV genes are implicated in carcinogenesis?

E6 and E7, two of the early genes

Which cellular proteins do these genes inactivate?

E6 inactivates proteins encoded by p53

E7 inactivates proteins encoded by Rb

p53 and Rb are both tumor-suppressor genes

Which HPV subtypes are implicated in cervical cancer?

HPV-16 and HPV-18

How is HPV infection diagnosed?

1. Presence of koilocytes
2. Hybridization of viral DNA to identify specific subtypes
3. Papanicolaou (Pap) smear to screen for dysplastic changes induced by HPV infection

What tests are not useful for diagnosis?

Serologic tests because exposure to many of the different HPV serotypes is common

How are warts treated?

Common warts usually regress on their own and removal is unnecessary
Warts in uncomfortable places may be removed surgically or destroyed with liquid nitrogen, laser vaporization, or cytotoxic chemicals, including salicylic acid, podophyllin, and trichloroacetic acid, all of which must penetrate the basal layer to eradicate the virus

What are two additional treatments for genital warts?

1. Injected interferon treats half of all genital warts
2. Topical cidofovir

How are laryngeal papillomas treated?

Oral interferon is effective for regression

POLYOMAVIRIDAE

What are two polyoma-viruses that infect humans?

JC and BK

How are JC and BK viruses transmitted?
  At what age does trans-mission usually occur?

Via respiratory droplets or urine of infected individuals
In childhood

What cells does JC virus show tropism for?

Oligodendrocytes

What disease does JC virus cause?
  What is this?

Progressive multifocal leukoencephalopathy (PML)
A rare demyelinating disease occurring only in immunocompromised patients

USMLE

What are symptoms of this disease?

Impaired speech and mental capacity rapidly followed by paralysis and death within 3–6 months

What disease does BK virus cause?

Cystitis in immunocompromised patients, otherwise it rarely has clinical consequences

How is JC or BK viral infection diagnosed?
  What tests are not useful for diagnosis?

DNA hybridization of PML lesions (JC virus) or urine samples (BK virus)
Serologic tests

ADENOVIRIDAE

What type of nucleic acid do Adenoviridae contain in their genome?	Double-stranded, linear DNA
What is their capsid geometry?	Icosahedral
Do they contain an envelope?	No, they are nonenveloped
How many different serotypes of Adenoviridae exist?	More than 40
What is unique about the structure of adenoviruses?	Contain hemagglutinin fibers protruding from each of 12 capsid vertices
What is their purpose?	Aid in viral attachment to host cells
How do viral early genes allow cells to progress through the cell cycle?	Inactivate cell regulatory proteins including p53 and pRB
What other enzyme do viral early genes encode?	DNA polymerase
How are newly replicated adenoviruses released?	Cell lysis
How are adenoviruses transmitted?	1. Respiratory transmission 2. Fecal–oral transmission 3. Direct inoculation of the eye, e.g., swimming in infected water
What are four clinical manifestations of adenovirus infection?	1. Upper and lower respiratory tract infections 2. Ocular disease 3. Infantile gastroenteritis 4. Hemorrhagic cystitis
What respiratory infections do adenoviruses cause?	1. Acute febrile pharyngitis in young children presenting as cough, sore throat, fever, and nasal congestion 2. Pharyngoconjunctival fever in school-aged children 3. Acute respiratory distress 4. Viral pneumonia

What ocular diseases do adenoviruses cause?	"Pink eye" 1. Follicular conjunctivitis 2. Keratoconjunctivitis
How does infantile gastroenteritis present?	Nonbloody diarrhea
What percentage of viral diarrheal disease in children is caused by adenoviruses?	5–15%
How are adenovirus infections most commonly diagnosed?	By clinical presentation
How are adenovirus infections diagnosed in the laboratory?	Cell culture, enzyme-linked immunoabsorbent assay (ELISA), neutralization or hemagglutination inhibition with type-specific antisera Laboratory diagnosis is rarely performed
What is the treatment for adenovirus infections?	Supportive treatment and quarantine because the virus is highly transmissible
What vaccines are available for adenoviruses?	Live-attenuated vaccines containing four serotypes are used only by military personnel

PARVOVIRIDAE

What type of nucleic acid do Parvoviridae contain in their genome?	Single-stranded, linear DNA Parvoviruses are the only family of single-stranded DNA (ssDNA)
What are two additional unique characteristics of the Parvoviridae genome?	1. It is the smallest of the DNA viruses 2. Contains terminal hairpin loops
What is the purpose of the terminal hairpin loops? **What is their capsid geometry?**	To initiate host-mediated viral genome synthesis Icosahedral
Do they contain an envelope?	No, they are nonenveloped

What is the most clinically important parvovirus?	Parvovirus B19
How is parvovirus transmitted?	Respiratory transmission and transplacental infection
What percentage of adults have antibodies to parvovirus B19?	Half of all adults
Which cells are susceptible to damage from parvovirus B19?	Mitotically active cells
Why?	The ssDNA must be converted to dsDNA before viral replication and transcription can occur The enzymes that can convert ssDNA to dsDNA are only found in mitotically active cells
What two types of cells do parvovirus B19 show tropism for?	1. Red blood cell precursors (erythroblasts) 2. Endothelial cells
What disease does parvovirus B19 infection cause in healthy children?	Erythema infectiosum
What are two additional names for this disease?	1. Fifth disease 2. Slapped-cheek syndrome
What are the clinical manifestations of fifth disease?	1. Bright red rash prominent on the cheeks 2. Low-grade fever 3. Runny nose 4. Sore throat 5. Acute symmetrical arthritis that occurs 2 weeks after infection
What is the cause for the rash?	Thought to be an immune-mediated response because the rash develops when the virus is no longer detectable in the blood
What is the risk of parvovirus B19 infection in patients with sickle cell, thalassemia, spherocytosis, or an immunocompromised state?	Aplastic anemia

How can parvovirus B19 infection affect a fetus?

1. First trimester: serious fetal infections may cause spontaneous abortion
2. Second trimester: hydrops fetalis resulting in neonatal death
3. Third trimester: no clinically significant disease

How is parvovirus infection diagnosed?

1. Serologically by immunoglobulin (Ig) M antibody detection
2. Polymerase chain reaction (PCR) of viral DNA from blood or amniotic fluid
3. Isolation of virus from throat swabs (rare)

How is parvovirus B19 treated?

Supportive treatment and limit contact with pregnant females

24

Enveloped DNA Viruses

OVERVIEW

What are three clinically
relevant families of
enveloped double-stranded
deoxyribonucleic acid
(dsDNA) viruses?

1. Hepadnaviridae
2. Herpesviridae
3. Poxviridae

HEPADNAVIRIDAE

What type of nucleic acid
do Hepadnaviridae contain
in their genome?

Incomplete circular dsDNA

What is their capsid
geometry?

Icosahedral

Do they contain an
envelope?

Yes, they are enveloped viruses

What is the main human
pathogen of the
Hepadnaviridae family?

Hepatitis B virus (HBV)
Not all viruses causing hepatitis
  in humans are members of
  Hepadnaviridae

What is the viral DNA
structure of HBV?

Long, negative strand with a
complementary short, positive strand

What are two unique
characteristics of HBV
replication?

1. Use of an ribonucleic acid (RNA)
   intermediate
2. Use of reverse transcriptase to create a
   template DNA strand inside the
   progeny capsid
Hepadnaviridae are the only
DNA viruses to replicate via an
RNA intermediate

What enzyme creates the RNA intermediate?

RNA polymerase II from the host cell

Where in the cell is the RNA intermediate synthesized?

In the nucleus

Where in the cell is the DNA template created by reverse transcriptase?

In the cytoplasm

What are the steps of HBV replication?

1. Incomplete circular viral DNA moves into the nucleus
2. The virus produces complete circular DNA in the nucleus
3. Viral DNA is transcribed into messenger RNA (mRNA) by host RNA polymerase II
4. mRNA migrates to the cytoplasm where it is translated into proteins using host enzymes
5. mRNA is reverse transcribed into a template strand by viral-encoded reverse-transcriptase enzyme
6. Template strand migrates into progeny capsid and is used to create a complementary DNA strand by host DNA-dependent DNA polymerase to form circular dsDNA progeny genomes

What is the Dane particle?

Infectious HBV particle

What are the four proteins encoded by HBV?

1. Hepatitis B surface antigen (HBsAg) encoded by gene S
2. Hepatitis C core antigen (HBcAg) encoded by gene C
3. Protein X encoded by region X
4. Reverse transcriptase/DNA polymerase encoded by region P

What is hepatitis B e antigen (HBeAg)?

A truncated form of HBcAg associated with the HBV nucleocapsid that circulates in the serum

What is the significance of this antigen?

Presence of HBeAg indicates increased transmissibility

What are three modes of HBV transmission?

1. Blood-to-blood transmission (intravenous [IV] needles, infected blood transfusions)
2. Sexual transmission
3. Perinatal transmission, including breastfeeding

What is the risk of becoming infected with HBV, hepatitis C virus (HCV), or human immunodeficiency virus (HIV) from a needle stick with contaminated blood?

20% chance of HBV infection
2% chance of HCV infection
0.2% chance of HIV infection

What are the signs and symptoms of acute HBV infection?

Jaundice, fatigue, nausea, vomiting, abdominal and joint pain, pruritus

What laboratory test anomalies are associated with acute HBV infection?

Elevated serum aminotransferases (aspartate aminotransferase [AST]/alanine aminotransferase [ALT]), bilirubin, and alkaline phosphatase

What is the prognosis for a patient with acute hepatitis B?

90% of patients clear infection
9% progress to chronic hepatitis
1% develop fulminant hepatitis and death

What are three complications of chronic HBV infection?

1. Chronic hepatitis
2. Cirrhosis
3. Hepatocellular carcinoma

Why is hepatocellular carcinoma common in chronic carriers of HBV?

Chronic hepatocyte damage secondary to the immune response to the virus causes chronic cellular regeneration and an increased opportunity for mutagenesis
HBV is not oncogenic by itself

Coinfection with what virus increases the risk of chronic and fulminant hepatitis in people infected with HBV?

Hepatitis D virus

What type of virus is this?	A defective RNA virus dependent on HBV for replication and its protective envelope
Who is at greatest risk for chronic carriage of HBV?	Individuals infected as infants 90% of infected infants will progress to chronic HBV infection if not treated with vaccine and hepatitis B immune globulin
Is there a vaccine for HBV? Who is this administered to?	Yes, a recombinant HBsAg Routinely given in three doses to all children and those at high risk for exposure (health care workers) *For more information on hepatitis B virus see Chapter 29, "Viral Hepatitis"*

HERPESVIRIDAE

What type of nucleic acid do Herpesviridae contain in their genome?	Linear dsDNA
What is their capsid geometry?	Icosahedral
Do they contain an envelope?	Yes, they are enveloped viruses
What unique structure lies between the envelope and capsid in Herpesviridae?	The tegument
What is this?	A proteinaceous material containing virus-encoded enzymes and transcription factors
How does this structure contribute to the pathogenicity of the virus?	One of the tegument proteins is involved in activation of immediate early HSV-1 gene expression
Where does replication of a herpesvirus occur?	In the nucleus
What are the three phases of herpesvirus gene expression?	1. Immediate-early 2. Early 3. Late
What do immediate-early genes code for?	Initiation of gene transcription in addition to a variety of regulatory functions

What do early genes code for?

Enzymes that are necessary for replication of viral DNA including DNA polymerase, helicase, and thymidine kinase

Why do herpesviruses require production of viral DNA polymerase?

They often infect nonreplicating cells (G_0), i.e., cells that do not contain the necessary enzymes for replication, e.g., neuronal cells

What do late genes code for?

Structural proteins and proteins involved in assembly and maturation of viral progeny

Where do Herpesviridae assemble?

In the nucleus

How do Herpesviridae acquire their envelope?

Part of the envelope is acquired from the nuclear membrane, which is unlike most enveloped viruses that acquire their envelope from the plasma membrane

What concept is a major characteristic of Herpesviridae?
What is this?

Latent viral infections

A persistent infection with replication-competent virus that does not produce viral progeny

What are the three classes of the herpesvirus family?

How are these classes differentiated?

1. Alphaherpesvirinae
2. Betaherpesvirinae
3. Gammaherpesvirinae
By their biologic characteristics, not by their morphology

What are three clinically relevant Alphaherpesviruses?

1. Herpes simplex virus 1 (HSV-1)
2. Herpes simplex virus 2 (HSV-2)
3. Varicella-zoster virus (VZV)

What are the characteristics of the growth cycle of Alphaherpesviruses?

A rapid, cytocidal growth cycle

Where do Alphaherpesviruses establish latency?

Nerve ganglia

What are three clinically relevant Betaherpesviruses?

1. Cytomegalovirus (CMV)
2. Human herpesvirus 6 (HHV-6)
3. Human herpesvirus 7 (HHV-7)

What are the characteristics of the growth cycle of Betaherpesviruses?

A slow replication cycle resulting in formation of multinucleated, giant host cells

Where do Betaherpesviruses establish latency?

Nonneural tissues, mainly macrophages and glandular tissue

What are two clinically relevant Gammaherpesviruses?

1. Epstein-Barr virus (EBV)
2. Human herpesvirus 8 (HHV-8), e.g., Kaposi sarcoma-associated herpesvirus (KSHV)

Where do Gammaherpesviruses establish latency?

Mucosal epithelium, where they also induce proliferation of lymphoblastoid cells

For more on Herpesviridae, see Chapter 28, "Herpesviridae"

POXVIRIDAE

What type of nucleic acid do Poxviridae contain in their genome?

Linear, dsDNA with a large coding capacity

What is their capsid geometry?

Complex; it is neither icosahedral nor helical

Do they contain an envelope?

Yes, they contain a double envelope

Where does replication of poxviruses occur?

Cytoplasm

Poxviridae are the only DNA viruses that replicate entirely in the cytoplasm

How is it able to do this?

The virus encodes all enzymes necessary for replication, including a DNA-dependent RNA polymerase

How large are the poxviruses?

They are the largest viruses in size and are visible under the light microscope

What are three clinically relevant viruses of the Poxviridae family?

1. Variola
2. Vaccinia
3. Molluscum contagiosum

What disease is caused by variola infection?

Smallpox

How does it present clinically?	Sudden onset of fever and malaise, followed by papular rash beginning on face and spreading to the extremities
What is the vaccine for smallpox?	Live-attenuated vaccinia virus
How effective is the vaccine for smallpox?	It was so effective that smallpox was the first infectious disease to be declared eradicated worldwide

What makes the vaccine so effective?

1. Smallpox has only one stable serotype
2. There is no animal reservoir
3. The antibody response is prompt, so exposed people are protected
4. Subclinical disease is very rare; therefore most people infected with the virus are easily identified
5. There is no carrier state

What disease is caused by vaccinia?	Cowpox or "milkmaid's blisters"
How does molluscum contagiosum present clinically?	Small, pink, wart-like benign tumors of skin or mucous membranes

25

Positive Single-Stranded RNA Viruses

OVERVIEW

What is single-stranded ribonucleic acid (ssRNA)?

Ribonucleic acid (RNA) that has 1 strand of nucleic acid

What are two classifications of ssRNA?

1. Positive ssRNA
2. Negative ssRNA

What is positive ssRNA?

Positive ssRNA is a form of RNA which can be translated into proteins using host cell machinery, thus being directly infectious

What is it similar to?

Messenger ribonucleic acid (mRNA)

What is negative ssRNA?

Negative ssRNA must first be used as a template for positive strand synthesis
The positive stand is then translated into proteins or used as a template to synthesize progeny genomic RNA

What enzymes do positive ssRNA need for replication?

Virus-encoded RNA-dependent RNA polymerases

What is the general site of nucleic acid replication of RNA viruses?

Cytoplasm

What RNA viruses are the exceptions?

1. Retrovirus (+ssRNA)
2. Orthomyxoviridae (−ssRNA)

Where do they replicate?

Nucleus

What is an enveloped virus?

A virus which has a lipid bilayer outer membrane surrounding its nucleic acid which plays an important role in viral penetration

Where do viruses acquire this envelope?

From host cell membranes secondary to viral host cell budding

How do enveloped viruses enter host cells?

Fusion of the viral envelope with the host cell membrane

What is a nonenveloped virus?

A virus without an outer membrane

What are two mechanisms by which nonenveloped viruses enter host cells?

1. Injection of nucleic acid through the cytoplasmic membrane of host cells
2. Receptor-mediated endocytosis of the virus

What are capsids?
What are two conformations that they assume?

Proteinaceous shells that surround viruses
1. Icosahedral
2. Helical

What are the three nonenveloped positive ssRNA families?
What is their capsid geometry?

1. Picornaviridae
2. Caliciviridae
3. Astroviridae
Icosahedral

What are the four enveloped positive ssRNA virus families and capsid geometry?

1. Coronaviridae, helical
2. Togaviridae, icosahedral
3. Flaviviridae, icosahedral
4. Retroviridae, complex (see Fig. 25-1)

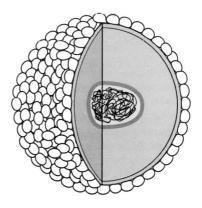

Figure 25-1. Complex capsid

What are the arthropod borne viruses?

1. Flaviviridae (+ssRNA)
2. Togaviridae (−ssRNA)
3. Bunyaviridae (−ssRNA)

What viral RNA genomes are translated immediately by host cell machinery upon entry into a cell and are analogous to mRNA?

Positive-strand RNA

PICORNAVIRIDAE

What type of nucleic acid do Picornaviridae contain in their genome?

Positive ssRNA
Picornaviridae has the smallest RNA genome; think "Pico equals small"

What is their capsid geometry

Icosahedral

Do they contain an envelope?

No

What are five genera of Picornaviridae?

1. Polio
2. Echovirus
3. Rhinovirus
4. Coxsackievirus
5. Hepatitis A virus (HAV)
"P.E.R.C.H."

What are enteroviruses?

Viruses that affect the gastrointestinal tract

Which picornaviruses are enteroviruses?

1. Polio
2. Echovirus
3. Coxsackievirus
4. Hepatitis A virus (HAV)
Enteroviruses are a major cause of central nervous system (CNS) disease, especially acute aseptic meningitis

POLIOVIRUS

How does the poliovirus attach to cells?

Via the polio virus receptor (PVR)

What is the virus's defense mechanism?

Proteolytic degradation of PKR

What is PKR? What is its function?

An RNA-activated protein kinase
PKR activation temporarily halts host cell protein synthesis, preventing viral use of

	host machinery and decreasing viral protein synthesis
Which cells does the poliovirus target?	1. Peyer patch 2. Motor neurons
What are three clinical outcomes of infection with poliovirus?	1. No illness (95%) 2. Minor illness (4%) 3. Major illness (1%)
What are the clinical manifestations of a minor illness?	Nonspecific symptoms of headache, sore throat, and nausea
What are two clinical manifestations of the major illness?	1. Nonparalytic poliomyelitis 2. Paralytic poliomyelitis
What are characteristics of each?	Nonparalytic polio is characterized headache, muscular spasms, nausea and abdominal pain, lethargy, and irritability; often indistinguishable from aseptic meningitis Paralytic polio is usually characterized by asymmetric proximal paralysis of the lower/ upper limbs, abdomen, and sometimes can spread cranially causing respiratory paralysis
How does the poliovirus replicate and ultimately penetrate the CNS?	1. Viral replication in tonsils and Peyer patches 2. Hematogenous spread allowing virus exposure to the blood–brain barrier 3. Attachment and penetration of anterior horn motor neurons of the spinal cord
How is poliovirus transmitted?	Fecal–oral transmission
What are the two forms of polio vaccines?	Salk and Sabin
What types of vaccines are they?	Salk is a killed poliovirus vaccine Sabin is a live-attenuated poliovirus vaccine "Salk is a killed vaccine, Sabin is not."

What type of immunoglobulin is produced in response to both vaccines?	IgG
What type of immuno-globulin is initially induced by the Sabin vaccine but not by the Salk vaccine?	Intestinal IgA
What is the risk of the Sabin vaccine that is not seen with the Salk vaccine?	Reversion to a virulent form The attenuated vaccine's (Sabin) genome is only 2 point muta-tions different from the wild-type virus
Why?	Killed vaccines cannot revert to a more virulent form and cause disease
What is an advantage of the Sabin vaccine?	Induces herd immunity

COXSACKIEVIRUS VIRUS

What four clinical features are common to coxsackievirus viruses and echoviruses?	1. Mild febrile infections 2. Respiratory infections 3. Rashes 4. Aseptic meningitis
What are two pathogenic coxsackievirus viruses?	1. Coxsackievirus virus A 2. Coxsackievirus virus B
What are three clinical manifestations of coxsackievirus virus A?	1. Herpangina 2. Hand-foot-and-mouth disease 3. Acute hemorrhagic conjunctivitis
What is herpangina?	Disease entity characterized by fever and sore throat with red vesicles on back of throat
What is hand-foot-and-mouth disease?	Disease entity characterized by vesicular eruptions restricted to the hands and feet and in the mouth; generally seen in children
What are three clinical manifestations of coxsackievirus virus B?	1. Myocarditis 2. Pericarditis 3. Pleurodynia

What is pleurodynia?	Disease entity characterized by pleuritic pain upon breathing, fever, and headache, which is life-threatening for infants
What are other names for this disease?	Bornholm disease, epidemic myalgia, and "devil's grip"

ECHOVIRUS

What does "Echo" stand for?	<u>E</u>nteric <u>c</u>ytopathic <u>h</u>uman <u>o</u>rphan

What diseases do echoviruses cause?	Echoviruses rarely cause disease

What are four rare clinical manifestations of echovirus?	1. Viral meningitis 2. Pericarditis 3. Rashes 4. Cold-like symptoms

HEPATITIS A VIRUS

How many serotypes of HAV exist?	1

How is HAV transmitted?	Fecal–oral transmission, commonly from eating uncooked shellfish harvested from sewage-contaminated water

What other hepatitis virus is transmitted fecal–orally?	Hepatitis E virus

Does HAV predispose one to hepatocellular carcinoma?	No; hepatitis A and E viruses are not linked to hepatocellular carcinoma

What percentage of those infected with HAV develop fulminant hepatitis?	< 1% HAV does not cause chronic disease

What is the overall death rate from HAV infection?	< 1%
What patient population is at highest risk for death?	Pregnant women

What is the typical incubation period after exposure to HAV?	15–40 days
What are three clinical manifestations of HAV?	1. Painful hepatomegaly 2. Jaundice 3. Fever
What is the treatment for HAV?	Patients with HAV infection should receive pooled immunoglobulin and supportive treatment
Is there a vaccine for HAV?	Yes, an inactivated viral vaccine is administered in two doses to those at risk

RHINOVIRUS

How many serotypes of rhinovirus exist?	More than 100
What does rhinovirus cause?	Common colds
What makes rhinovirus different from other enteroviruses?	1. Replicate in cooler body temperatures (e.g., 33°C [91.4°F]) such as found in the nose 2. Rhinoviruses are acid labile Rhino = <u>c</u>ommon <u>c</u>old in <u>c</u>ooler areas
What is the usual treatment for a rhinovirus infection?	Supportive care
What group of drugs is often incorrectly prescribed to patients with a common viral cold?	Antibiotics

CALICIVIRIDAE

What type of nucleic acid do Caliciviridae contain in their genome?	Positive ssRNA
What is their capsid geometry	Icosahedral
Do they contain an envelope?	No

What viruses are in the Caliciviridae family?	1. Norwalk virus (Calicivirus) 2. Hepatitis E virus (HEV)

NORWALK VIRUS (CALICIVIRUS)

What are clinical manifestations of Norwalk virus infection?	Gastroenteritis with explosive diarrhea without blood or pus, in addition to fever, vomiting, and abdominal pain
How is Norwalk virus transmitted?	Fecal–orally
Which patient population is affected by acute epidemic gastroenteritis from Norwalk virus?	Adults in close quarters, e.g., military bases, retirement communities, and cruise ships, and school-age children
What is the disease course?	24–48 hours of self-limited symptoms
What causes death in patients with Norwalk virus?	Dehydration and electrolyte losses
What is the treatment for Norwalk virus infection?	Supportive treatment including fluid replacement

HEPATITIS E VIRUS (HEV)

What are the clinical manifestations of HEV?	Similar to HAV: 1. Painful hepatomegaly 2. Jaundice 3. Fever Although HEV and HAV have similar clinical manifestations, they are two genetically distinct viruses
How is HEV transmitted?	Fecal–orally
Does HEV predispose one to hepatocellular carcinoma?	No, hepatitis E and A viruses are not linked to hepatocellular carcinoma
What patient population is HEV infection especially severe?	Pregnant women

Where is HEV responsible for epidemic outbreaks of hepatitis?	Asia
What is the treatment for HEV?	Supportive treatment
Is there a vaccine for HEV?	No

CORONAVIRIDAE

What type of nucleic acid do Coronaviridae contain in their genome?	Positive ssRNA
What is their capsid geometry	Helical
Do they contain an envelope?	Yes
What does Coronaviridae cause?	Common colds, severe acute respiratory syndrome (SARS)

TOGAVIRIDAE

What type of nucleic acid do Togaviridae contain in their genome?	Positive ssRNA
What is their capsid geometry	Icosahedral
Do they contain an envelope?	Yes
What genera are in the Togaviridae family?	1. Alphaviridae 2. Rubivirus

ALPHAVIRIDAE

How are alphaviruses transmitted?	Mosquitos transmit to humans and domestic animals
What name is given to viruses that are transmitted in this manner?	Arboviruses—arthropod borne viruses

What are four viruses in this genera?	1. Eastern equine encephalitis viruses 2. Western equine encephalitis viruses 3. Chikungunya viruses 4. Venezuelan equine encephalitis viruses
What are three clinical manifestations of this genera?	1. Eastern/Western equine encephalitis viruses—acute encephalitis 2. Chikungunya viruses—acute arthropathy 3. Venezuelan equine encephalitis viruses—febrile illness with flu-like symptoms

RUBIVIRIDAE

What virus belongs to the Rubiviridae genus?	Rubella virus (German measles)
What are the clinical features of rubella?	General maculopapular rash beginning on the face and progressing to extremities, along with posterior auricular/occipital lymphadenopathy
How is rubella most commonly transmitted?	1. Respiratory droplets 2. Transplacentally
What are the clinical complications of rubella infection during pregnancy?	Teratogenic effects on the developing fetal CNS, liver, heart, and eye in the first trimester of pregnancy Rubella is the "r" in TORCHEs, i.e., the mnemonic given to remember common congenital infections: Toxoplasmosis, Other (e.g., HIV), Rubella, Cytomegalovirus (CMV), Herpes, Syphilis
What are the CNS complications of congenital rubella?	Deafness, microcephaly, and mental retardation
What are the heart complications of congenital rubella?	Patent ductus, interventricular septal defects, and pulmonary artery stenosis
What are the eye complications of congenital rubella?	Cataracts and chorioretinitis

When are these complications most severe?	When rubella infection occurs during the first trimester

FLAVIVIRIDAE

What type of nucleic acid do Flaviviridae contain in their genome?	Positive ssRNA
What is their capsid geometry	Icosahedral

Do they contain an envelope?	Yes

What genera are in the Flaviviridae family?	1. Flavivirus 2. Hepatitis C virus (HCV)

What six diseases are associated with flavivirus?	1. Yellow fever 2. Dengue fever 3. Hepatitis C Virus (HCV) 4. West Nile Fever 5. St. Louis encephalitis 6. Japanese encephalitis

YELLOW FEVER

What is the historical significance of yellow fever?	First human virus discovered

What is the vector for yellow fever?	*Aedes aegypti* mosquito

What is the clinical presentation of Yellow fever?	Hepatitis, jaundice, fever, backache, and black vomitus 1 week postmosquito bite

What histologic finding is seen in liver specimens following yellow fever infection?	Councilman bodies
What do they look like?	Acidophilic inclusions

Is there a vaccine for yellow fever?	Yes, a live-attenuated vaccine

DENGUE FEVER

What is another name for dengue fever?	Break-bone fever
What is the vector for Dengue fever?	*Aedes aegypti* mosquito
How many serotypes of Dengue virus exist?	Four
What is the significance of this?	Dengue hemorrhagic fever results from an infection with a serotype different from a first infection
What are the clinical manifestations of dengue fever?	Hemorrhagic fever and shock syndrome, with painful crises, including backache, headache, muscle and joint pain
What is hemorrhagic fever?	High fever and increased vascular permeability
What is hemorrhagic shock syndrome?	A complication of dengue hemorrhagic fever with signs of circulatory failure
What are four warning signs of this syndrome?	1. Constant abdominal pain 2. Restlessness alternating with lethargy 3. Persistent vomiting 4. Change from fever to hypothermia
What causes the symptoms?	The immune response to the virus, including increased vascular permeability and disseminated intravascular coagulation (DIC) caused by circulating dengue antigen-antibody complexes and complement activation
What predisposes one to a more virulent form of dengue fever?	Previous episode with dengue fever
What causes this?	Because of the presence of memory cells to viral antigens there is a faster immune response than the initial response Although this is expected, the faster inflammatory response causes a more severe form of the disease

HEPATITIS C VIRUS (HCV)

What are three modes of HCV transmission?	1. Blood 2. Birth 3. Sex
What are two scenarios in which HCV is likely to have been transmitted by blood?	1. Posttransfusion hepatitis 2. Patient on hemodialysis with hepatitis
What is the increased risk factor for HCV infection?	Hepatocellular carcinoma
What percentage of those infected with HCV develop . . . **Chronic hepatitis?**	50%
Cirrhosis?	20%
What is the treatment for HCV?	Interferon-α
What is the success rate of interferon-α treatment for HCV?	50%
What effect does alcohol consumption have on an HCV positive patient?	Significantly increases the risk of hepatocellular cancer
Is there a vaccine for HCV?	No
What is the number one etiology for chronic hepatitis in the United States?	HCV
What is the number one etiology for chronic hepatitis worldwide?	HBV

WEST NILE FEVER

How is West Nile fever spread?	Mosquitoes
What is the reservoir?	Birds

How does West Nile fever present clinically? **What is the prognosis?**	Rash, lymphadenopathy, fever, and malaise Most people recover, but the elderly are more likely to develop meningitis or encephalitis which may be fatal
Where was the first U.S. West Nile fever breakout?	New York City (1999)

ST. LOUIS ENCEPHALITIS

Where is St. Louis encephalitis endemic?	Ohio, Gulf coast states (e.g., Mississippi, Florida) and western states
What is the vector for St. Louis encephalitis?	*Culex* spp. mosquitos

JAPANESE ENCEPHALITIS

Where is Japanese encephalitis endemic?	Mainly China, very little in Japan
What is the vector for Japanese encephalitis?	*Culex* spp. mosquitos

RETROVIRIDAE

What are Retroviridae?	Enveloped positive ssRNA with a complex capsid
What enzyme is unique to Retroviridae? **What is its function?**	Reverse transcriptase Produces a dsDNA intermediate during the replication of the positive ssRNA genome
What are three genera of Retroviridae?	1. Lentivirus 2. Oncomavirus 3. Spumavirus
What are three general components of the retrovirus structure?	1. Lipid membrane envelope (host-cell derived) 2. Complex capsid 3. Nucleoprotein

What are three envelope proteins associated with the lipid envelope?

1. Transmembrane glycoprotein (TM, fusion protein and gp41)
2. Surface glycoprotein (SU, attachment protein, and gp120)
3. Outer matrix protein (MA, and p17)

What is an important protein of the capsid?

Major capsid protein (p24)

What are three components of the nucleoprotein?

1. p7
2. Positive single-stranded RNA
3. Reverse transcriptase

Note: Please see Chapter 30, "Human Immunodeficiency Virus," for a more detailed discussion of HIV, and Chapter 31, "Oncogenic Viruses," for a more detailed discussion of human T-cell leukemia virus.

26

Negative Single-Stranded RNA Viruses

OVERVIEW

What is single-stranded ribonucleic acid (ssRNA)?

Ribonucleic acid (RNA) that has 1 strand of nucleic acid

What are two classifications of ssRNA?

1. Negative ssRNA
2. Positive ssRNA

What is unique about negative ssRNA?

Negative ssRNA must first be converted into positive ssRNA before it can be translated

What enzyme is needed to aid in the replication of negative-strand RNA?

RNA-dependent RNA polymerase

What is the general site of nucleic acid replication of RNA viruses?

Cytoplasm

What RNA viruses are the exceptions?
Where do they replicate?

1. Orthomyxoviridae (–ssRNA)
2. Retrovirus (+ssRNA)
Nucleus

What is an enveloped virus?

A virus that has a lipid bilayer outer membrane surrounding its nucleic acid, which, when present, plays an important role in viral penetration

How do viruses acquire this envelope?

From host cell membranes secondary to viral host cell budding

How do enveloped viruses enter host cells?

Fusion of the viral envelope with the host cell membrane

What are capsids?
What are two conformations that they assume?

Proteinaceous shells that surround viruses
1. Icosahedral
2. Helical

What are the enveloped negative ssRNA virus families?

1. Filoviridae
2. Orthomyxoviridae
3. Bunyaviridae
4. Arenaviridae
5. Rhabdoviridae
6. Paramyxoviridae

What is their capsid geometry?

Helical
All –ssRNA have:
1. Envelopes
2. Helical capsids

What are the arthropod borne viruses?

1. Flaviviridae (–ssRNA)
2. Bunyaviridae (–ssRNA)
3. Togaviridae (+ssRNA)

What is a segmented genome?

A genome that is physically separated into several segments (see Fig. 26-1)

What viruses have segmented genomes?

Bunyavirus (–ssRNA), Orthomyxovirus (–ssRNA), Arenavirus (–ssRNA), and Reovirus (double-stranded RNA [dsRNA])
Remember: B.O.A.R.

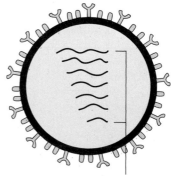

Segmented RNA genome

Figure 26-1. Segmented viruses

BUNYAVIRIDAE

What type of nucleic acid do Bunyaviridae contain in their genome?	Negative ssRNA with a three-part segmented genome
What is their capsid geometry?	Helical
Do they contain an envelope?	Yes
What four genera are associated with Bunyaviridae?	1. Hantavirus 2. Bunyavirus 3. Phlebovirus 4. Nairovirus
Which are arthropod borne?	All *except* hantavirus

HANTAVIRUS

What are two species of Hantavirus?	1. Sin Nombre 2. Hemorrhagic fever with renal syndrome (Korean fever)
What is the reservoir for hantavirus?	Deer mouse
Where in the United States is hantavirus endemic?	Southwestern states
How is hantavirus transmitted?	Aerosolized rodent excretions
What are the mild clinical manifestations of hantavirus?	Influenza-like illness
What are the severe clinical manifestations of hantavirus?	Hemorrhagic fever, acute renal failure, and a pulmonary syndrome with a high mortality
What is the mortality of hantavirus pulmonary syndrome?	80%

BUNYAVIRUS

What are two species of bunyavirus? What do they cause?	1. California Encephalitis 2. La Crosse Encephalitis
What is the reservoir for California encephalitis?	Rodents and rabbits
How is the virus acquired?	Animal bites
How does the virus reach the brain?	Hematogenously secondary to viral replication at entry point
What time of year does this virus commonly affect humans?	Summer
How common is death?	Rare

PHLEBOVIRUS

What are two species of Phlebovirus?	1. Rift Valley fever 2. Sandfly fever
What organisms are usually affected by Rift Valley fever?	Domesticated animals
What name is given to this form of infection?	A zoonosis, i.e., a disease that predominantly affects animals
How is the virus transmitted?	Via mosquitos, e.g., *Aedes* spp. that have fed on infected livestock
What is the most common complication of Rift Valley fever?	Retinitis
How common is death?	Death is rare
What are the clinical manifestations of sandfly fever?	Sudden onset of fever, frontal headache, low back pain, retro-orbital pain, and malaise

NAIROVIRUS

What is a species of Phlebovirus?	Crimean Congo hemorrhagic fever

How is the virus transmitted?	Ticks
What are the symptoms?	Initial fever, myalgia, vertigo, photophobia, and vomiting, followed by mental status changes

ORTHOMYXOVIRIDAE

What type of nucleic acid do Orthomyxoviridae contain in their genome?	Negative ssRNA with an eight-part segmented genome
What is their capsid geometry?	Helical
Do they contain an envelope?	Yes
What disease is caused by Orthomyxoviridae?	Influenza
What is the incubation period of influenza?	24–48 hours
What are the clinical manifestations of influenza?	Sudden onset of symptoms, i.e., fever, myalgia, headache, cough, and fatigue
What are three important glycoproteins associated with influenza virus?	1. Hemagglutinin (IIA) 2. Neuraminidase (NA) 3. M2
How does hemagglutinin contribute to pathogenesis?	Promotes viral entry into the cell by acting as the viral receptor resulting in viral–cell fusion
How does hemagglutinin promote viral-cell fusion?	1. Attaches to sialic acid receptors on host cell 2. Creates conformational changes at low pH inside the host cell endosome
How does neuraminidase contribute to pathogenesis?	1. Prevents binding of virus back to infected cells by cleaving host cell sialic (neuraminic) acid, allowing progeny virus to infect uninfected cells and not be "wasted" on previously infected cells 2. Disrupts the mucin of healthy mucosal epithelial cells, exposing new sialic acid binding sites for virions

How does M2 contribute to pathogenesis?

Acts as an ion channel within the endosome allowing H$^+$ to enter the virion and viral RNA to be released to the cytoplasm

What are the treatment implications of understanding these glycoproteins?

HA, NA, and M2 protein are cellular targets used to suppress influenza infections

What is different about influenza replication when compared to the majority of other RNA viruses?

Replication occurs in the nucleus Orthomyxoviridae and Retroviridae (+ssRNA) are the only RNA viruses that replicate in the nucleus

What is one defense mechanism of influenza virus?

Suppressing the host cell antiviral mechanism with viral NS1 protein preventing PKR activation

How does PKR work?

PKR activation temporarily halts host cell protein synthesis, preventing viral use of host machinery and decreasing viral protein synthesis (see Fig. 26-2)

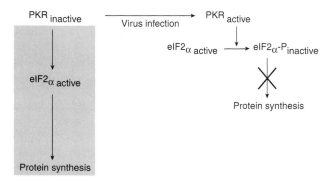

Figure 26-2. NS-1 and PKR

What does the body use to combat the destruction of respiratory epithelial cells by influenza virus?

Cytotoxic CD-8+ T cells

What are three strains of influenza viruses?	Influenza A, B, and C
Which strain causes worldwide flu pandemics at intervals of 10–20 years?	Influenza A
Which strain causes major seasonal outbreaks of influenza?	Influenza B
Which strain is associated with mild respiratory tract infections?	Influenza C
What is the distinguishing feature between influenza A, B, and C?	Each has different internal proteins, mainly matrix proteins (M) and nucleocapsid proteins (NP)
Which viruses are associated with Reye syndrome and liver degeneration?	1. Influenza B 2. Varicella
Which drug is associated with Reye syndrome?	Aspirin use in pediatric patients
What is Reye syndrome?	Noninflammatory encephalopathy with hepatic failure
What is the best site on the influenza virus to target an immune response?	Antibodies against the HA glycoprotein
What are two important changes occurring in influenza virus resulting in genetic diversity?	1. Antigenic shift 2. Antigenic drift
What is antigenic shift?	Major antigenic changes characterized by sudden replacement of a new strain with an antigenically different HA and NA occurring by reassortment of viral RNA segments (e.g., HA1NA1 to HA3NA2) Antigenic shift only occurs in type A

USMLE

How often does antigenic shift occur?	Every 10–40 years
What is antigenic drift?	Minor antigenic changes characterized by random point mutations in viral RNA leading to amino acid substitutions in HA glycoproteins
Which strains demonstrate antigenic drift?	Influenza A and B
How often does antigenic drift occur?	Every 2–3 years
Which two drugs are effective against both influenza A and B? **What is the mechanism of action?**	1. Zanamivir 2. Oseltamivir Inhibit NA
Which two drugs are only effective against influenza A? **What is the mechanism of action?**	1. Amantadine 2. Rimantadine Blocks viral uncoating by inhibition of influenza viral M2 membrane protein
What immunoglobulin mediates immunity against influenza virus?	Secretory IgA in respiratory tract

PARAMYXOVIRIDAE

What are Paramyxoviridae?	Enveloped, helical negative ssRNA virus
What four genera are in the Paramyxoviridae family?	1. Paramyxoviridae 2. Rubulavirus 3. Morbillivirus 4. Pneumovirinae
What are four clinical manifestations caused by Paramyxoviridae infection?	1. Parainfluenza/croup (Paramyxoviridae) 2. Respiratory syncytial virus (Pneumovirinae) 3. Mumps (Rubulavirus) 4. Measles (Morbillivirus)
Which Paramyxoviridae membrane glycoprotein is responsible for viral-cell fusion?	F protein

PARAINFLUENZA/CROUP

What is another name for croup?	Acute laryngotracheobronchitis
Do Paramyxoviridae have HA and NA?	Yes, both are present
How is it possible to distinguish between influenza and parainfluenza in regards to HA and NA?	In parainfluenza, HA and NA are on the *same surface spikes* In influenza, HA and NA are on *different surface spikes*
What are the clinical characteristics of parainfluenza?	Upper and lower respiratory tract infection without viremia

RESPIRATORY SYNCYTIAL VIRUS

In what patient population is respiratory syncytial virus (RSV) responsible for bronchiolitis?	Pediatric population
What is a specific pharmacologic treatment for RSV? **What is this?**	Palivizumab (Synagis) A monoclonal antibody to RSV

MUMPS

What is the clinical presentation of mumps?	Swollen parotid glands
What are three possible postinfection sequelae of mumps?	1. Parotitis 2. Orchitis 3. Aseptic meningitis
When is the yearly peak incidence of mumps?	Winter months
Are HA and NA present in mumps?	Yes, both are present

MEASLES

What is the cell receptor for measles?	CD46 molecule

How are measles transmitted?	Respiratory droplets
What are the clinical features of measles?	1. Prodromal period of fever 2. Upper respiratory symptoms 3. Maculopapular rash 4. Koplik spots 5. Conjunctivitis
How does the maculopapular rash associated with measles spread?	Cranial caudally, i.e., away from the head
What are Koplik spots?	White spots on bright-red oral mucous membranes
What is the characteristic cytopathology of measles?	Multinucleated giant cells due to fusion of F proteins (see color photo 20)
What is a severe complication of measles several years following infection?	Subacute sclerosing panencephalitis
Are HA and NA present in measles?	Only HA is present

RHABDOVIRIDAE

What are Rhabdoviridae?	Enveloped, helical, negative-ssRNA, bullet-shaped viruses
What genera are in the Flaviviridae family?	1. Lyssavirus 2. Vesiculovirus
What major human pathogen is in the Rhabdoviridae family?	Rabies virus (Lyssavirus)
What is the structure of the rabies virus?	Bullet-shaped capsid with an antigenic G-glycoprotein on envelope
What is the cell receptor for rabies?	Acetylcholine receptor

How does the rabies virus infection spread within the nervous system?	Retrograde axoplasmic transport from peripheral neurons to the central nervous system (CNS)
How long is the incubation period for rabies?	2 weeks to 1 year
What symptoms are associated with rabies?	Painful spasm of throat muscles upon swallowing and hydrophobia
What histologic finding is associated with rabies?	Negri bodies (see color photo 21)
What do they look like?	Eosinophilic cytoplasmic inclusion bodies
How is rabies infection prevented in individuals at high risk of exposure?	1. Avoidance of rabid animals 2. Preexposure prophylactic immunization with human diploid cell vaccine (HDCV)
What is the treatment for rabies infection?	Postexposure immunization with HDCV and rabies virus immune globulin Rabies virus vaccine and Hepatitis B virus vaccine are the only vaccines that can be given effectively postexposure
What is the cause of death once rabies symptoms become evident?	Respiratory center dysfunction and encephalitis
What is Vesiculovirus?	The best studied Rhabdoviridae, Vesiculovirus infects cattle and horse, causing vesicular stomatitis, but does not cause disease in humans

FILOVIRIDAE

What are Filoviridae?	Enveloped, helical, negative-ssRNA viruses
What are two Filoviridae that are human pathogens?	1. Marburg virus 2. Ebola virus
What are the clinical manifestations of Filoviridae infections?	Severe hemorrhagic fever with widespread bleeding from skin, mucous membranes, and visceral organs

What is the mechanism for hemorrhagic fever?	Virus contains proteins that mimic factors inducing the coagulation cascade, leading to the depletion of clotting factors

MARBURG VIRUS

What animal was the original source for Marburg virus?	African green monkey
What is the route of transmission for Marburg?	Airborne transmission and blood exposure
What is the incubation period for Marburg?	7–21 days
What is the clinical presentation of Marburg?	Muscle aches, mild fever, nausea, vomiting, rash, and bloodshot eyes with defecation of blood approximately 10 days later
What is the mortality rate of Marburg?	~25%

EBOLA

What is the mode of transmission for Ebola virus?	Direct contact with body fluids
What component of the Ebola virus is responsible for its cytotoxic effects?	Modified glycoprotein on the virus
What cells are most susceptible to these cytotoxic effects?	Endothelial cells
How was the Ebola virus initially isolated?	From patients with hemorrhagic fever in Zaire and Sudan
What are the clinical manifestations of Ebola virus?	Fever, diarrhea, weakness, and bleeding from mucous membranes
What is the mortality rate of Ebola?	~65%

ARENAVIRIDAE

What are Arenaviridae?	Enveloped, helical, negative-ssRNA viruses
What animal is associated with Arenaviridae?	Rodents
How is the virus transmitted?	Inhaling aerosolized virus particles or eating contaminated food
What are two diseases caused by Arenaviridae?	1. Lymphocytic choriomeningitis (LCM) 2. Lassa fever
What are the clinical manifestations of LCM?	Influenza-like illness sometimes associated with a viral meningitis that has a relatively benign course and low mortality
What are the clinical manifestations of Lassa fever?	Hemorrhagic fever with nausea, vomiting, severely bloodshot eyes, and a painful rash after rodent exposure
What is the mortality rate of Lassa virus?	~50%

DELTAVIRIDAE

What is the only virus found in this genus?	Deltaviridae or hepatitis D virus (HDV)
What type of virus is it?	A defective RNA virus
What causes detrimental HDV infections?	Liver cells already inhabited by the hepatitis B virus (HBV), a double-stranded deoxyribonucleic acid (dsDNA) virus
How does HDV replicate?	Using a HBV reverse transcriptase
What makes HDV dependent on HBV?	1. HDV uses HBV-encoded reverse transcriptase 2. HDV requires the protective HBV envelope
Where are three types of HDV and where do they exist?	Type I, which exists in North America and Italy Type II, which exists in Japan and Taiwan Type III, which exists in South America

What is the clinical consequence of HDV superinfection in HBV-infected individuals?

The superinfection causes a more aggressive form of hepatitis

How can one avoid detrimental HDV infections?

HBV vaccination

27

Double-Stranded RNA Viruses: Reoviridae

REOVIRIDAE

What does "reo" stand for in Reoviridae?

Respiratory and enteric orphan viruses

What type of nucleic acid do Reoviridae contain in their genome?

Double-stranded ribonucleic acid (dsRNA) with a 10- to 12-part segmented genome
Reoviridae are "orphan" viruses because they are the only double-stranded ribonucleic acid (RNA) viruses

USMLE

What is their capsid geometry?

Icosahedral

Do they contain an envelope?

No, they are nonenveloped

Which genus is clinically important?

Rotavirus

Where do they replicate?

Cytoplasm

What enzyme is needed to aid in the replication of the rotavirus genome?

Virus encoded RNA-dependent RNA polymerase

What is the characteristic morphology of rotaviruses?

Wheel-and-spoke structure (see Fig. 27-1)

How many viral coats does rotavirus have?

Three, which is why it is also called a triple-layered particle

What proteins are found in the outer coat?

Viral proteins (VP) 4, 6, 7, and integrins
VP4 is cleaved to form VP5 and VP8, which are important for cell adhesion

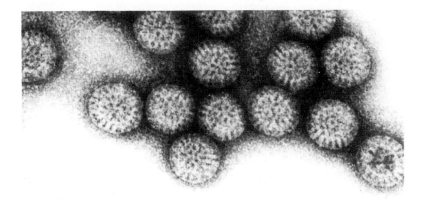

Figure 27-1. Electron microscopy of rotavirus demonstrating wheel-and-spoke structure.

How are newly synthesized rotaviruses released?
By cell lysis

How does this affect the structure of the virus?
Rotaviruses lack envelopes because they are released from cells by lysis, unlike enveloped viruses that acquire their envelope from cell budding

How is rotavirus transmitted?
Fecal–oral transmission

What does rotavirus cause?
Gastroenteritis in infants and young children

How does this present clinically?
Often as outbreaks of non-inflammatory, nonbloody diarrhea in day care centers or schools

How common are rotavirus infections?
Most common cause of gastroenteritis which accounts for approximately 40% of severe diarrhea in children younger than 2 years old

What cells do rotavirus show tropism for?
Epithelial cells of the small intestine, primarily the jejunum

What histologic changes occur with rotavirus infection?
1. Shortening and atrophy of villi
2. Flattening of epithelial cells
3. Denuding of microvilli

What clinical effect do these changes have?
They decrease surface area and production of brush-border enzymes resulting in malabsorption and diarrhea

What is the incubation period?	48 hours or less
How is rotavirus diagnosed?	Clinical diagnosis or by detection of virus in the stool with either radioimmunoassay or enzyme-linked immunoabsorbent assay (ELISA)
How is rotavirus treated?	Supportive treatment only, with rapid replacement of fluid and electrolytes
Is there a vaccine for rotavirus? Why is it not used?	Yes, RotaShield is a live-attenuated virus containing 4 serotypes It is associated with intussusception in infants

Herpesviridae

ALPHAHERPESVIRUSES

HERPES SIMPLEX VIRUS I AND 2

What percent nucleotide homology exists between herpes simplex virus (HSV)-1 and HSV-2?	50%
What percentage of U.S. adults has antibodies to HSV-1?	80%, but half of these individuals are completely asymptomatic
How are HSV-1 and HSV-2 acquired?	Direct contact with virus-containing secretions or lesions
Can virus be transmitted from infected individuals without visible lesions?	Yes, asymptomatic shedding of virus can occur
Where does HSV-1 and HSV-2 multiply?	In mucosal epithelial cells
How can HSV-1 and HSV-2 infection present clinically?	Most commonly as oral lesions for HSV-1 and genital lesions for HSV-2, but both viruses can infect either area Lesions are usually vesicles and painful shallow ulcers that are accompanied by fever, malaise, and myalgias
How else can HSV present clinically?	1. Gingivostomatitis (children) 2. Pharyngitis (adults) 3. Tonsillitis (adults) 4. Keratoconjunctivitis 5. Aseptic meningitis 6. Encephalitis
What part of the central nervous system (CNS) does HSV preferentially infect?	The temporal lobes by way of the trigeminal nerves

What are the major risks for newborns of mothers infected with HSV?	Herpes encephalitis and disseminated viral infection
What is the mortality rate for herpes encephalitis in children?	70%
What is the risk of pregnant women with genital herpes infecting their newborn during vaginal delivery?	30–40%
How can this risk be reduced?	Women with active HSV infection at the time of birth must undergo cesarean section to reduce exposure to HSV
Is the risk of transmission to a newborn greater during HSV-2 primary infection or reactivation? Why?	Primary infection More virus is shed during primary infection and the mother has not yet made anti-HSV antibody
What is the reservoir for HSV-1 and HSV-2?	Mature neurons, commonly the trigeminal ganglia for HSV-1 and the sacral or lumbar ganglia for HSV-2
What can cause reactivation of a virus?	Hormonal changes, fever, sunlight, stress, and damage to neurons
How does HSV-1 reactivation present?	As clusters of vesicles on the lips (known as herpes labialis, cold sores or fever blisters), which take approximately 10 days to heal Reactivation infections are typically less severe than primary infections
How is HSV infection diagnosed?	1. Clinical diagnosis 2. Cell culture 3. Tzanck smear 4. Serologic tests (in acute infection) 5. Polymerase chain reaction (PCR) of viral deoxyribonucleic acid (DNA) from spinal fluid to diagnose herpes encephalitis

What is the gold standard for diagnosis?

Cell culture

What does the Tzanck smear show?

Multinucleated giant cells with intra-nuclear inclusions (see color photo 20)

What is the drug of choice for treating all HSV infections?

Acyclovir, a guanine analog

How does it work?

Acyclovir is phosphorylated by viral thymidine kinase which activates it, enabling it to terminate replication of viral DNA

How is it specific for viruses and not for host cells?

Viral thymidine kinase phosphorylates acyclovir more effectively than cellular thymidine kinase, therefore there is a higher concentration of active drug in virus-infected cells

Does it cure HSV?

No, because it does not prevent recurrence of primary disease

What are the benefits of acyclovir treatment?

It can reduce the duration of lesions, as well as viral shedding, and if used prophylactically, it may reduce the number of recurrences
Acyclovir also reduces mortality and morbidity from herpes encephalitis

VARICELLA-ZOSTER VIRUS

What disease does primary varicella-zoster virus (VZV) infection cause?

Varicella (chickenpox)

How does this present clinically?

Rash that begins as pruritic macules that evolve into papules, which present simultaneously at all stages of evolution, in conjunction with a prodrome of chills, fever, malaise, headache, sore throat, and cough

How is VZV transmitted?

Respiratory droplets

How does initial infection result in disseminated disease?

The virus initially infects respiratory mucosa, then spreads hematogenously to internal organs, and finally spreads to the skin

Can asymptomatic individuals spread the virus?

Yes, an infected individual can transmit virus before infection becomes clinically apparent

What is the incubation period for primary VZV infection?

14–16 days

What is the reservoir for latent VZV infection?

Multiple sensory ganglia, most commonly trigeminal and dorsal root ganglia

Does asymptomatic viral shedding after primary infection occur?

No, VZV is the only herpesvirus in which asymptomatic shedding does not usually occur

What is reactivated VZV?

Herpes zoster or shingles

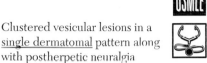

How does this present clinically?

Clustered vesicular lesions in a single dermatomal pattern along with postherpetic neuralgia (pain) and abnormal sensation over the affected dermatome

How often does VZV reactivation occur?

15% of individuals with varicella will develop zoster, usually later in life as immunity to VZV wanes

What are three complications of VZV infection?

1. Varicella pneumonia
2. Fulminant hepatic failure
3. Varicella encephalitis

What is Reye syndrome?

Encephalopathy and liver failure of unknown etiology associated with children given aspirin during VZV and influenza infection

For this reason, aspirin should be avoided in children younger than age 18

How is VZV diagnosed?

Usually by a clinical diagnosis; however, a laboratory diagnosis for atypical presentations or infections in immunocompromised patients can be performed with immunofluorescence or immunoperoxidase (which only takes 24 hours), cell culture (which takes several days), in situ DNA probe, or scraping vesicular cells and reacting with different stains

What does cell culture demonstrate in VZV infections?	Multinucleated giant cells with intranuclear inclusions (see color photo 20)
What is the treatment for varicella?	Intravenous (IV) acyclovir is preferred for varicella, but treatment is reserved only for severe cases Varicella immune globulin (VZIG) is also used in immunocompromised individuals
What is the treatment for zoster?	Famciclovir and valacyclovir (if given early in the course of infection) can reduce acute pain and shorten duration of zoster and postherpetic neuralgia Oral acyclovir is also effective for zoster, but has no effect on postherpetic neuralgia, which is often treated with tricyclic antidepressants or gabapentin
Is there a vaccine for VZV?	Yes a live-attenuated virus is routinely given to infants

BETAHERPESVIRUSES

CYTOMEGALOVIRUS

How is cytomegalovirus (CMV) transmitted?	By respiratory droplets, intrauterine infection, sexual contact, blood contact (transfusions and transplants), and breast milk
Can CMV cross the placenta?	Yes, it is the most common cause of intrauterine viral infection and congenital abnormalities in the United States CMV is one of the "TORCHES" organisms
What percent of the adult population is CMV positive?	More than 80%
What is the reservoir for latent CMV?	Unknown; possibly monocytes and macrophages

Does asymptomatic viral shedding occur?	Yes; CMV is characterized by repeated episodes of asymptomatic viral shedding for prolonged periods
What group of patients is at risk for symptomatic CMV infection?	Immunocompromised
How does CMV present clinically in children?	Usually asymptomatic
How does CMV present clinically in immuno-competent adults?	As heterophile-negative infectious mononucleosis causing fever, myalgias, and lymphadenopathy
How does infectious mononucleosis with CMV differ from that caused by Epstein-Barr virus (EBV)?	Unlike EBV, there is an absence of heterophile antibodies with CMV infection EBV–heterophile antibody positive CMV–heterophile antibody negative
What are heterophile antibodies?	IgM antibodies that agglutinate horse and sheep red blood cells
What are clinical manifestations of CMV infection in immunocompromised adults?	Pneumonia, retinitis, hepatitis, encephalitis, esophagitis, enterocolitis, and gastritis
What are clinical manifestations of CMV infection in neonates?	Mental retardation, microcephaly, hepatosplenomegaly, seizures, deafness, and purpura
During what stage of pregnancy does primary CMV infection result in the most severe symptoms?	First trimester
How is CMV diagnosed?	Cell culture and PCR
What does cell culture demonstrate?	"Owl's-eye" nuclear inclusion bodies in infected cells (see Fig. 22-3)
How is CMV treated?	Ganciclovir, foscarnet, or cidofovir

Is there a vaccine available for CMV?	There is no vaccine for CMV
Why is acyclovir ineffective against CMV infection?	CMV lacks thymidine kinase necessary for acyclovir activation

HUMAN HERPESVIRUS 6 AND 7

How are human herpesvirus (HHV)-6 and HHV-7 transmitted?	Oral secretions
What disease do HHV-6 and HHV-7 cause?	Roseola infantum
How does this present clinically?	High fever followed by erythematous macular rash and possibly febrile seizures
How often are HHV-6 infections symptomatic?	33–50% of infections are symptomatic
How often are HHV-7 infections symptomatic?	Rarely; generally asymptomatic
Where does viral replication take place?	Salivary glands
What percent of the population has been exposed to HHV-6 and -7?	90% of the population has detectable antibody by 3 years of age
How does HHV-6 coinfection with human immunodeficiency virus (HIV) accelerate progress to terminal acquired immune deficiency syndrome (AIDS)?	1. HHV-6 induces synthesis of CD4 on lymphocytes, allowing more cells to be infected with HIV 2. HHV-6 accelerates the rate of cell death by transactivating transcription of HIV
How does HHV-6 usually present in AIDS patients?	As encephalitis
How are HHV-6 and HHV-7 diagnosed?	No good single diagnostic test, but PCR amplification can be used to detect DNA in cerebrospinal fluid (CSF) or serum
How are HHV-6 and HHV-7 treated?	Ganciclovir, cidofovir, and foscarnet For AIDS patients, treatment of HIV helps treatment for HHV-6

Is there a vaccine available for HHV-6 or HHV-7?	No

GAMMAHERPESVIRUSES

EPSTEIN-BARR VIRUS

How is EBV transmitted?	Contact with respiratory secretions and saliva
What is the reservoir for latent EBV?	B lymphocytes
What is the B-cell receptor for EBV?	The complement C3b receptor
What do the early genes of EBV encode?	Unlike other herpesviruses, early genes of EBV induce cell multiplication and immortalization rather than cell death
How does EBV present clinically?	1. Infectious mononucleosis with fever, pharyngitis, and lymphadenopathy 2. Hepatitis (rare) 3. Encephalitis (rare)
When is the peak incidence of EBV infectious mononucleosis?	Between 15 and 19 years of age; because it is spread via close contact, it is often known as "kissing disease" Most EBV infections occur earlier in life but in contrast to late childhood infections, early childhood infections are usually asymptomatic
What is the typical incubation period for EBV?	4–7 weeks
How does infectious mononucleosis from EBV differ from infectious mononucleosis caused by CMV or toxoplasmosis?	The presence of IgM heterophile antibodies ("heterophile positive") that agglutinate sheep and horse red blood cells are found in EBV
What three malignancies are associated with EBV?	1. Burkitt's lymphoma 2. Nasopharyngeal carcinoma 3. B-cell lymphomas

What populations have a high rate of nasopharyngeal carcinoma caused by EBV?

Inuits (Eskimos) and people living in Southeast Asia and North Africa

What nonmalignant lesion does EBV cause in AIDS patients?

Hairy leukoplakia of the tongue

What percent of the population has been exposed to EBV?

90%

How is EBV diagnosed?

1. Presence of heterophile antibodies
2. Detection of EBV-specific antibodies such as viral capsid antigen (VCA), early antigen (EA), Epstein-Barr nuclear antigen (EBNA) (the Monospot test)
3. Presence of atypical lymphocytes on peripheral blood smear

What are "atypical lymphocytes"?

Cytotoxic T lymphocytes activated by EBV infection (see Fig. 28-1)

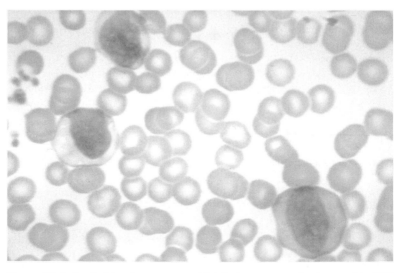

Figure 28-1. Atypical lymphocytes seen with infectious mononucleosis caused by EBV infection.

What is the treatment for EBV infection?	Supportive treatment only, because antiviral therapy has no effect on the course of typical EBV infection
Is there a vaccine for EBV?	No

HUMAN HERPESVIRUS 8/KAPOSI SARCOMA-ASSOCIATED HERPESVIRUS

What is the primary mode of transmission?	Sexual
What does HHV-8 cause?	Kaposi sarcoma and primary effusion lymphoma
What is Kaposi sarcoma?	A vascular neoplasm consisting of nodules in the skin, mucous membranes, and visceral organs usually with an indolent course
What are the clinical manifestations of Kaposi sarcoma?	Reddish-purple skin nodules, oral mucosa discolorations, lymphadenopathy, and organ failure
What population is at increased risk for developing Kaposi sarcoma?	Patients with HIV
How is HHV-8 identified?	Serologically by detection of antibody with enzyme-linked immunoabsorbent assay (ELISA) or immunofluorescence reaction or by PCR amplification with subsequent DNA hybridization

Viral Hepatitis

OVERVIEW

What is viral hepatitis?
Inflammation/infection of liver hepatocytes by one or more of many possible viruses, resulting in hepatocyte destruction and subsequent regeneration

What are the symptoms of viral hepatitis?
Constitutional symptoms, such as fever, malaise, myalgias, nausea, and vomiting, in addition to flank pain and jaundice

What can be detected on physical exam?
Tender and enlarged liver

What are the five major viruses that cause hepatitis?
1. Hepatitis A virus (HAV)
2. Hepatitis B virus (HBV)
3. Hepatitis C virus (HCV)
4. Hepatitis D virus (HDV)
5. Hepatitis E virus (HEV)

What other viruses may cause hepatitis?
1. Cytomegalovirus
2. Epstein-Barr virus
3. Herpes simplex virus
4. Yellow fever virus

What is the definition of chronic hepatitis?
Presence of the hepatitis antigen for more than 6 months

What viruses cause chronic hepatitis?
HBV, HCV, and HDV (if coinfected with HBV)

What is the most common cause of chronic hepatitis?
HBV infection: only 10% of HBV infections are chronic versus 75% of HCV infections; however, the total number of HBV infections is much greater than HCV

Which hepatitis virus is comprised of deoxyribonucleic acid (DNA)?
HBV

Which hepatitis virus is unable to replicate without the help of HBV?	HDV
What is the mode of transmission for the hepatitis viruses?	Hepatitis A and E are both transmitted via the fecal–oral route Hepatitis B, C, and D are transmitted parenterally (blood, semen, etc.) "ABCDE": A and E are at both ends and are transmitted by both ends of the gastrointestinal (GI) tract—fecal–oral; BCD are in the middle and are transmitted by blood

HEPATITIS A VIRUS

How is hepatitis A virus transmitted?	Fecal–oral route
What is the nucleic acid in HAV?	Linear (+) single-stranded ribonucleic acid (ssRNA) with a nonenveloped icosahedral capsid
What viral family does HAV belong to?	Picornaviridae
What is the incidence of HAV infection?	Approximately 150,000 new cases are reported in the United States each year; approximately 50–75% of U.S. adults have been infected at some point in their lives
What is the incubation period for HAV?	25–40 days
How is HAV infection diagnosed?	Serologic tests: anti-HAV IgM indicates active infection and anti-HAV IgG indicates prior infection that has since resolved
Is immunity possible?	Yes; anti-HAV IgG lasts indefinitely and will protect against future HAV infections
Is a vaccine available?	Yes, a formaldehyde-inactivated whole-virus vaccine is recommended for travelers to developing countries

Does HAV cause chronic hepatitis?

No

What is the treatment?

If given early during incubation, serum immune globulin is effective

Once infection is established, treatment is only supportive

HEPATITIS B VIRUS

How is hepatitis B virus transmitted?

Body fluids: blood, semen, saliva, milk

What is the nucleic acid in HBV?

Circular double-stranded DNA (dsDNA) with an enveloped icosahedral capsid

What is the viral family?

Hepadnaviridae

What is the incidence of HBV infection?

Approximately 300,000 new cases are reported in the United States each year

What is the incubation period of HBV?

60–90 days

What is a Dane particle?

Another name for the infectious HBV virion

What is the pathogenesis of HBV?

Most damage results from the cell-mediated immune response to the virus, not from the virus itself

What are three important antigens encoded by HBV?

1. Surface antigen (HBsAg)
2. Core antigen (HBcAg)
3. E antigen (HBeAg)

What is unique about replication of HBV virus?

It is the only DNA virus that produces DNA by reverse transcriptase from a ribonucleic acid (RNA) template

What is the prognosis for a patient with acute hepatitis B?

See Fig. 29-1

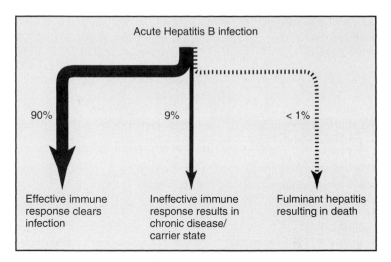

Figure 29-1. Typical course of HBV infection.

What are three complications of chronic HBV infection?	1. Chronic hepatitis 2. Cirrhosis 3. Hepatocellular carcinoma
Why is hepatocellular carcinoma common in chronic carriers of HBV?	Chronic hepatocyte damage secondary to the immune response to the virus causes chronic cellular regeneration and an increased opportunity for mutagenesis
What age group is most susceptible to chronic infection?	Neonates, because of an immature immune system
What percentage of neonates develops chronic infection?	Approximately 90% of HBV-infected neonates develop chronic infection as compared to 25% of infected children who develop chronic infection
How is HBV infection diagnosed?	Serologically
What are the first markers of HBV infection?	HBsAg and HBeAg
What is the window period?	The time period following infection when HBsAg levels are undetectable, but prior to the rise in concentration and detection of antibodies to HBsAg (anti-HBs)

What marker is still detectable during the window period?	Anti-HBc The anti-HBc must always be checked to rule out HBV infection in the window period because HBsAg and anti-HBs will be negative
What is found in the blood of a patient who has cleared HBV infection?	Anti-HBs, anti-HBc
What is found in the blood of a patient who has received a HBV vaccination?	Anti-HBs only
What is found in the blood of a patient to indicate chronic infection with HBV?	HBsAg present for greater than 6 months and the absence of anti-HBs (see Fig. 29-2)

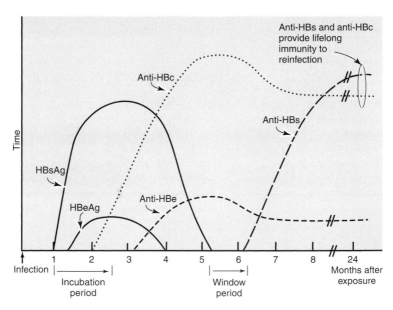

Figure 29-2. Presence of HBV antigens and antibodies in the blood during the course of acute infection with full resolution.

| What do the serologic markers indicate during the different stages of infection? | see Table 29-1 |

Table 29-1. Interpretation of HBV Serological Markers

	HBsAg	Anti-HBs	Anti-HBc
Acute disease	+	−	+ (IgM)
Window phase	−	−	+ (IgG)
Complete recovery	−	+	+ (IgG)
Vaccinated	−	+	−
Chronic carrier	+	−	+ (IgG)

What is a good indicator of high transmissibility?	HBeAg

| **Is a vaccine available?** | Yes, Recombivax, a recombinant subunit vaccine derived from HBsAg is given as a 3-dose regimen to all infants and to those at high risk (health care workers) Only vaccines for HBV and rabies are effective if given after exposure to the virus |

| **What is the treatment for acute HBV infection?** | Supportive therapy and passive–active immunization with both hepatitis B immunoglobulin and vaccine |

| **What is the treatment for chronic HBV infection?** | Lamivudine and interferon are moderately effective |

HEPATITIS C VIRUS

| **How is HCV transmitted?** | Via blood; sexual transmission can occur but is uncommon HCV is the most prevalent blood-borne pathogen in the United States |

| **What is the nucleic acid in HCV?** | Linear, (+) ssRNA with an enveloped icosahedral capsid |

| **What is the viral family?** | Flaviviridae |

| **What is the incidence of HCV infection?** | Approximately 50,000 new cases are reported in the United States each year |

What is the incubation period of HCV?	40–120 days
What are long-term sequelae of HCV infection?	75% of patients develop chronic hepatitis and a large percentage of these will progress to cirrhosis and hepatocellular carcinoma
Do HBV and HCV contain oncogenes in their genomes?	No, the mechanism of how HBV and HCV cause hepatocellular carcinoma is uncertain, but it is believed that fibrosis and necrosis accompanied by continuing regeneration of hepatocytes increases the risk of genetic mutation or rearrangement that leads to hepatocellular carcinoma
Who is at high risk for HCV?	Intravenous (IV) drug users and patients on hemodialysis
How is HCV infection diagnosed?	Enzyme-linked immunoabsorbent assay (ELISA) detection of antibodies to HBcAg
What is the treatment for HCV infection?	Combination treatment with ribavirin and interferon may be effective for some patients

HEPATITIS D VIRUS

How is HDV transmitted?	Body fluids: blood, semen, saliva, breast milk
What is the nucleic acid in HDV?	Circular, enveloped (–) ssRNA
What is unique about HDV replication? Why?	HDV is a defective virus and cannot replicate on its own. It lacks the genes for envelope protein and can only replicate when cells are coinfected with HBV
What is the one protein encoded by HDV?	Delta antigen
How is HDV infection diagnosed?	Detecting delta antigen or IgM antibody to delta antigen

What is the significance of HDV infection?	More severe acute disease and greater risk of fulminant hepatitis, cirrhosis, and hepatocellular carcinoma when coinfected with HBV
What is the treatment for HDV infection?	There is no specific therapy, although interferon-α can mitigate some of the effects of the virus and HBV immunization can prevent HDV infection

HEPATITIS E VIRUS

How is HEV transmitted?	Fecal–oral transmission HEV is a major cause of water-borne epidemics of hepatitis outside of the United States
What is the nucleic acid in HEV?	Linear, (+) ssRNA with a nonenveloped icosahedral capsid
What is the viral family?	Caliciviridae
What are long-term sequelae of HEV infection?	None because there is no chronic infection
How is HEV infection diagnosed?	It is a diagnosis of exclusion because no test for HEV antibody exists
What is the treatment for HEV infection?	Supportive therapy because there is no antiviral therapy
Is there a vaccine for HEV?	No
What group of patients shows increased mortality with HEV infection?	Pregnant women

30

Human Immunodeficiency Virus

OVERVIEW

What genera of retroviruses does human immunodeficiency virus (HIV) belong to?

Lentivirus

What enzyme is unique to retroviruses?

Reverse transcriptase
Of the ribonucleic acid (RNA) viruses, Retroviridae is the only family of RNA viruses to use a reverse transcriptase
Of the deoxyribonucleic acid (DNA) viruses, Hepadnaviridae is the only family of DNA virus to use a reverse transcriptase

USMLE

What is the role of this enzyme?

To convert a single-stranded RNA viral genome into a double-stranded DNA genome

Why are mutations common with reverse transcriptase?

The enzyme is "sloppy"

What is the implication of this?

Development of resistance secondary to increased mutation rate requiring changes in pharmacotherapy, e.g., triple-therapy drug regimens

What are the two identified serotypes of HIV responsible for?

HIV-1 is responsible for Acquired immune deficiency syndrome (AIDS)
HIV-2 is responsible for a similar illness as HIV-1, but overall has milder clinical manifestations

HUMAN IMMUNODEFICIENCY VIRUS STRUCTURE

What is the general structure of retroviruses?

An enveloped virus with a positive single-strand ribonucleic acid (ssRNA) genome

What is the viral envelope made from?	The host cell membrane
What are two surface glycoproteins found on the HIV envelope?	1. Transmembrane glycoprotein (TM; fusion protein, and gp41) 2. Surface glycoprotein (SU; attachment protein, and gp120)
Which surface glycoprotein is a transmembrane (fusion) protein?	gp41
Which surface glycoprotein is a surface (attachment) protein?	gp120
What additional protein is found on the IIIV envelope?	Outer matrix protein (MA; p17)
Where is it found?	Between the envelope and the capsid
What is it involved with?	Entry of the DNA provirus into the nucleus and virus assembly
What is the capsid geometry of HIV?	Complex, cone-shaped geometry (see Fig. 30-1)
What is the major capsid protein?	p24
Can p24 be used to detect IIIV infection?	Yes
When during the course of HIV is p24 expressed?	Throughout the infection
What are the five components of the HIV capsid?	1. Two identical copies of positive ssRNA genome 2. Nucleocapsid proteins 3. Reverse transcriptase 4. Protease 5. Integrase
What is p7? **What is its role?**	Nucleocapsid protein To complex with RNA within the capsid

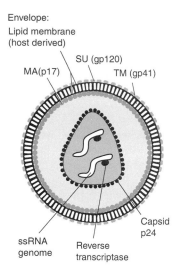

Envelope:
Lipid membrane
(host derived)

SU (gp120)

MA(p17)

TM (gp41)

Capsid
p24

ssRNA
genome

Reverse
transcriptase

Figure 30-1. HIV capsid

HUMAN IMMUNODEFICIENCY VIRUS GENOME

What are the three major HIV genes?	1. gag 2. pol 3. env
What does the gag gene code for?	1. Core proteins 2. Matrix proteins
What does the env gene code for?	1. Transmembrane 2. Surface proteins
Which does the pol gene code for?	1. Reverse transcriptase 2. Integrase 3. Protease 4. Ribonuclease
What are four additional coding regions found in the HIV genome?	1. U5 2. U3 3. R sequence 4. Long terminal repeats
What is U5?	Sequence of viral RNA found at the 5´ end which contains part of the site needed for viral integration into the host cell chromosome and contains the transfer

ribonucleic acid (tRNA) primer binding
site for reverse transcriptase

What is U3?

The sequence of viral RNA at the 3' end
which contains sequences used for control
of transcription of the DNA provirus

What is the R sequence?

The repeated sequence of viral RNA
found at both ends which is used during
reverse transcription

**What are long terminal
repeats?**

Two identical repeats that result from the
duplication of the U and R units during
the synthesis of the DNA provirus
(Fig. 30-2)

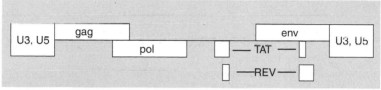

gag gene encodes p17, p24, MA, CA

env gene encodes gp120, gp41

Figure 30-2. HIV genome

HUMAN IMMUNODEFICIENCY VIRUS REPLICATION

**What are six steps of HIV
replication?**

1. Binding to host cell receptor
2. Viral entry
3. Reverse transcription
4. Integration into host cell DNA
5. Transcription and translation
6. Assembly and maturation

**Which three steps of HIV
replication are dependent
on viral proteins?**

1. Viral entry
2. Reverse transcription
3. Integration

**What parts of HIV
replication require use of
host cell machinery?**

Synthesis of viral genomes, messenger
ribonucleic acids (mRNAs), and structural
proteins

**Which host cell receptor
does HIV show tropism for?**

CD4 receptors

What are four types of cells that contain these receptors?

1. T-helper cells
2. Lymphocytes
3. Macrophages
4. Dendritic cells

Which cell type is usually the first cell to become infected?

Macrophages

What is a chemokine receptor?

Protein involved in the control of the immune response and inflammation

Is there only one type of chemokine receptor?

No, in fact different HIV strains prefer certain chemokine receptors over others

What occurs if HIV binds the chemokine receptor?

Fusion between the viral envelope and the cell membrane secondary to envelope glycoprotein (TM) activation

What host cell component serves as a primer for the initiation of reverse transcription?

tRNA, which binds a specific viral RNA sequence

What is the first product of reverse transcription?

A DNA-RNA hybrid

Which enzyme is involved in creating DNA from RNA?

Reverse transcriptase

    What is another one of its roles?

This enzyme also has RNAse activity which degrades the DNA-RNA hybrid's RNA while concurrently synthesizing the DNA strand

What is the double-stranded DNA molecule end product called?

The provirus

What protein then helps with the transport of the provirus to the nucleus?

Matrix protein (MA)

What enzyme then cleaves chromosomal DNA and inserts the provirus into the host genome?

Integrase

Is the insertion and integration of the provirus random?

Yes

What are the two genomic forms of HIV?

1. Positive ssRNA (extracellular)
2. dsDNA (proviral, intracellular)

Which enzyme transcribes the integrated provirus into full length mRNA?

Host cell RNA polymerase II

What are the three basic products of the mRNA transcribed from the virus?

1. Genome for viral progeny
2. gag proteins and gag-pol polyproteins
3. Spliced RNA

What is a gag-pol polyprotein?

The source of viral reverse transcriptase and integrase

How is gag-pol polyprotein formed?

In the process of translating a gag protein precursor, approximately 5% of the time the stop codon is missed, resulting in a gag-pol polyprotein

What components combine with each other during HIV assembly?

The genomes, uncleaved gag and gag-pol polyproteins, associate with the envelope glycoprotein (TM)-modified plasma membrane

How does the plasma membrane become associated with the env glycoproteins?

The env polyproteins are cleaved into SU and transmembrane (TM) proteins by the Golgi apparatus, which is subsequently transported to the host cell membrane

When is the viral protease that cleaves the gag and gag-pol polyproteins activated?

As the virion buds from the surface of infected cells

Which cell dies as a result of release of mature virions?

Lymphocytes

Which cell lives even after release of mature virions?

Macrophages

HUMAN IMMUNODEFICIENCY VIRUS TRANSMISSION

What are the four major routes of transmission?	1. Sexual contact 2. Blood transfusion 3. Contaminated needles 4. Perinatal transmission
Is HIV present in both semen and vaginal secretions?	Yes
Can other sexually transmitted diseases (STDs) increase the rate of transmission of HIV?	Yes; any disease that compromises the integrity of the skin can facilitate transmission
Which types of transfusions have resulted in HIV transmission?	All types resulting in the screening of the blood supply for the presence of HIV
What are three methods of HIV perinatal transmission?	1. Transplacentally 2. Passage of baby through the birth canal 3. Breast feeding
What can prevent perinatal transmission?	Azidothymidine (zidovudine, AZT)

THE PROGRESSION OF HUMAN IMMUNODEFICIENCY VIRUS INFECTION TO ACQUIRED IMMUNE DEFICIENCY SYNDROME

What are three general ways in which HIV leads to clinical manifestations?	1. Induction of an immunodeficient state 2. Host response to HIV-infected cells 3. Destruction of cells by virus
What percent of HIV-positive individuals take more than 20 years to develop AIDS?	10%
What unique finding was found to decrease the likelihood of acquiring HIV in Kenyan prostitutes?	Homozygously altered HIV coreceptors
Where does the virus usually proliferate to after the initial infection?	CD4+ T cells, macrophages, and dendritic cells

| **How do CD4+ lymphocytes generally become infected?** | By contacting infected follicular dendritic cells in the germinal centers of lymph nodes (see Fig. 30-3) |

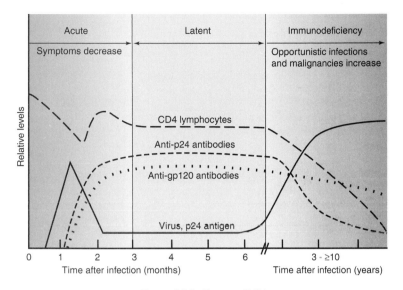

Figure 30-3. Course of HIV

ACUTE VIRAL ILLNESS

| **What percent of HIV-positive individuals suffer from an acute, mononucleosis-like viral illness several weeks after being first infected?** | 33%–66%
Patients are rarely diagnosed during the acute viral illness | |

| **What symptoms do these people report?** | Fever, malaise, lymphadenopathy, and pharyngitis |

| **What occurs during the acute viral illness?** | High rate of HIV replication in CD4+ lymphocytes leading to high levels of HIV (viremia) and presence of p24 |

| **What is the response to the acute phase viremia?** | HIV-specific cytotoxic T cells respond, followed by the humoral response 1 to 10 weeks after initial infection; this decreases the viral load and helps resolve the symptoms |

Does viral replication cease after the acute viral illness resolves?

No

LATENT VIRAL ILLNESS

What is "latent" during the latent period?

Clinical symptoms

What is not "latent" during the latent period?

Viral replication

What gradually results in a net loss during the latent period?

CD4+ T cell count

Why does the CD4+ T cell count only drop a little during the majority of the latent period?

Stem cell output compensates

What percent of HIV proviruses are transcriptionally inactive during the latent period?

90%

Why are there viremic episodes during the latent period?

When the person becomes infected by other pathogens

What are some of the possible clinical manifestations of HIV during the latent period?

Generalized lymphadenopathy, fevers, weight loss, and diarrhea, as well as bouts of herpes zoster and candidiasis

Generally speaking, what speeds the progression of HIV to AIDS?

A stimulus, e.g., infection, activating resting T cells, inducing HIV replication, increasing the chance for mutations, and promoting syncytium formation

What is a syncytium in the context of HIV?

Uninfected cells that become directly infected by an infected cell

Do T-cell precursors get infected?

Yes, and they eventually die

What is the problem with HIV mutations in terms of containing the infection?

Decreased ability of antibodies and cytotoxic T cells to detect new antigens

ACQUIRED IMMUNE DEFICIENCY SYNDROME

When is a patient said to have AIDS?

CD4 count < 200/mL with serologic evidence of HIV and/or the appearance of one or more AIDS-defining illnesses

What cells play a key role in spreading HIV to other organs?

Macrophages

What is responsible for AIDS encephalopathy?

Macrophages are responsible, not a decrease in CD4+ cells

How are macrophages linked with the wasting syndrome seen in AIDS?

Likely by the release of cytokines such as tumor necrosis factor (TNF)

Are the eye, skin, and bone marrow infected by HIV?

Yes

What are the malignancies commonly associated with AIDS?

1. Kaposi sarcoma
2. Lymphoma

What are the common bacterial opportunistic infections associated with AIDS?

1. *Mycobacterium avium complex* (MAC)
2. Tuberculosis
3. *Streptococcus pneumoniae*
4. *Salmonella*

What are the common viral opportunistic infections associated with AIDS?

1. Herpes simplex virus (HSV-1 and HSV-2)
2. JC virus
3. Epstein-Barr virus
4. Cytomegalovirus (CMV)
5. Kaposi sarcoma (human herpesvirus 8 [HHV-8])

Which virus is commonly associated with chorioretinitis?

CMV

What are the common fungal, parasitic, and protozoan opportunistic infections associated with AIDS?

1. *Candida* (common)
2. *Cryptococcus* (common)
3. *Pneumocystis carinii* (*P. jiroveci*)
4. *Histoplasma*
5. *Coccidioides*
6. *Cryptosporidium*
7. *Toxoplasma gondii*
8. *Isospora*

What are some of the many diseases caused by the these organisms?	Disseminated miliary disease, pneumonia, meningitis, encephalitis, esophagitis, diarrhea, osteomyelitis, retinitis, vaginitis, and thrush
What organism is responsible for the classically described pneumonia in AIDS patients?	*P. carinii* (*P. jiroveci*)

DIAGNOSIS OF HUMAN IMMUNODEFICIENCY VIRUS INFECTION

What method is commonly used to screen for HIV?	Enzyme-linked immunoabsorbent assay (ELISA)
What test is used to confirm the diagnosis if an ELISA test is positive for HIV?	Western blot for p24
What is the most sensitive method for early detection of HIV?	Polymerase chain reaction (PCR)
Why else is PCR helpful in managing HIV? **What is the viral load?**	Helps estimate viral load, drug response, and prognosis The level of replicating virus in plasma determined by PCR
What is the significance of the viral load?	Indicator of the rate of progression to AIDS
Why is PCR not used to screen for HIV?	Cost

TREATMENT OF HUMAN IMMUNODEFICIENCY VIRUS INFECTION

What are the three basic categories of antiviral drugs?	1. Nucleoside reverse-transcriptase inhibitors 2. Nonnucleoside reverse transcriptase inhibitors 3. Protease inhibitors
What are nucleoside reverse-transcriptase inhibitors (NRTIs)?	Agents that are phosphorylated by host cell kinases that terminate and/or inhibit reverse transcriptase

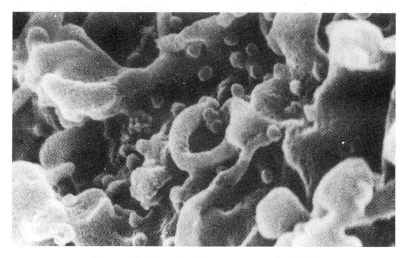

Figure 30-4. Scanning electron micrograph of HIV

What are some examples?	Lamivudine, stavudine, zalcitabine, zidovudine, didanosine, and abacavir
What are nonnucleoside reverse-transcriptase inhibitors (NNRTIs)?	Agents that inhibit the action of reverse transcriptase that bind to a site on reverse transcriptase that is different than NRTIs
What are some examples?	Delavirdine, efavirenz, and nevirapine
What are protease inhibitors?	Agents that inhibit HIV-1 protease which prevents cleavage of viral precursors
What are some examples?	Indinavir, nelfinavir, ritonavir, saquinavir, and amprenavir (see Fig. 30-4)
Why are anti-HIV drugs theoretically more effective early in the course of the disease?	There are fewer mutations and less resistance early in the course of the disease

31

Oncogenic Viruses

OVERVIEW

What are four chromosomal changes that occur in malignant cells?

1. Deletions
2. Duplications
3. Translocations
4. Insertions

What are three new antigens expressed as a result of malignant transformation?

1. Virus-encoded proteins
2. Modified preexisting cellular proteins
3. Previously repressed cellular proteins

Why do malignant cells appear rounded?

Disaggregation of actin filaments and decreased adhesion to surface

What term is applied to the disorganized, "piled-up" growth pattern of malignant cells?

Loss of contact inhibition

What term is applied to the infection of a cell by a tumor virus that enables it to continue growing past the lifetime of a normal cell?

Immortalization

What happens in regards to deoxyribonucleic acid (DNA) synthesis when cells resting in the G_0 phase are infected with a tumor virus?

They enter the S phase and go on to divide

Are the levels of cyclic adenosine monophosphate (cAMP) increased or decreased in malignant cells?

Decreased

HIGH-YIELD COLOR ATLAS

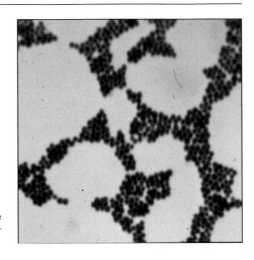

Color Photo 1. Gram-positive bacteria (*Staphylococcus aureus*)—see also Chapter 1

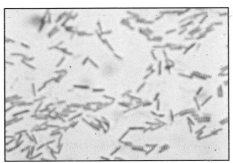

Color Photo 2. Gram-negative bacteria (*Escherichia coli*)—see also Chapter 1

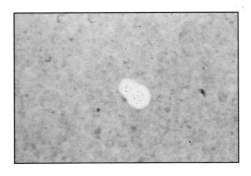

Color Photo 3. Positive Quellung reaction—see also Chapter 4

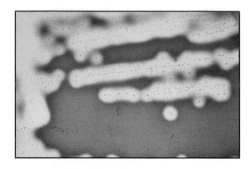

Color Photo 4. Beta hemolytic streptococci—see also Chapter 4

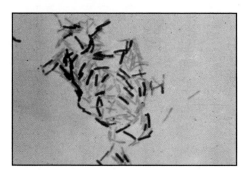

Color Photo 5. Gram-positive rod: *Bacillus cereus*—see also Chapter 5

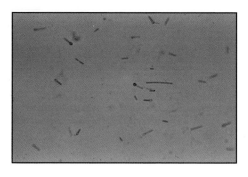

Color Photo 6. *Clostridium tetani*—see also Chapter 5

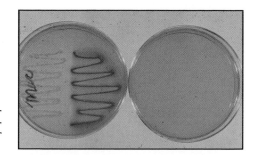

Color Photo 7. Lactose-fermenting bacteria on Mac-Conkey agar—see also Chapter 7.

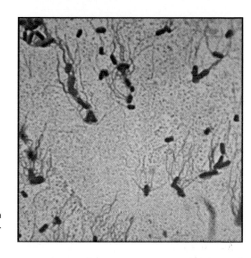

Color Photo 8. *Salmonella* with multiple flagella—see also Chapter 7.

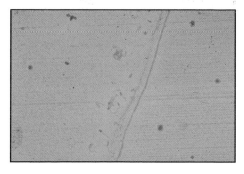

Color Photo 9. *Vibrio* with single polar flagellum—see also Chapter 7

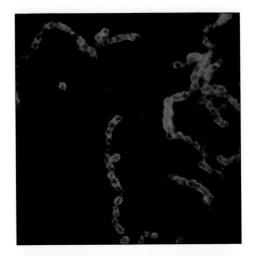

Color Photo 10. *Streptococcus pyogenes*

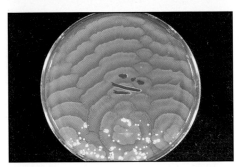

Color Photo 11. Swarming proteus—see also Chapter 7

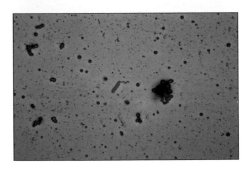

Color Photo 12. *Pseudomonas aeruginosa* with flagella stain—see also Chapter 9

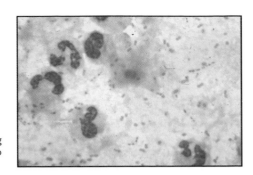

Color Photo 13. Bipolar staining seen with *Yersinia pestis*—see also Chapter 10

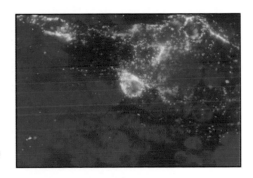

Color Photo 14. *Chlamydia*—see also Chapter 11

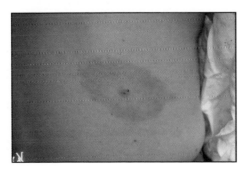

Color Photo 15. Erythema migrans—see also Chapter 11

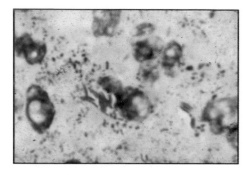

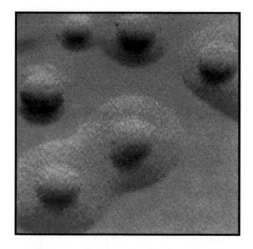

Color Photo 16. Mycobacteria—see also Chapter 12

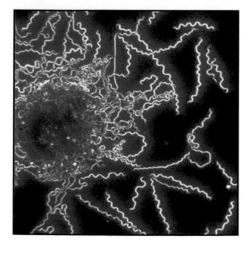

Color Photo 17. *Mycoplasma*—see also Chapter 13

Color Photo 18. Spirochete under darkfield microscopy—see also Chapter 15

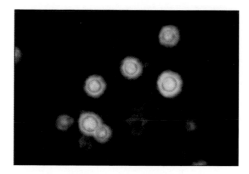

Color Photo 19. *Cryptococcus* and India ink—see also Chapter 20

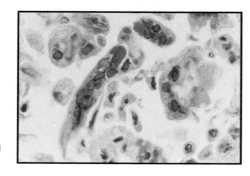

Color Photo 20. Multinucleated giant cells—see also Chapter 22

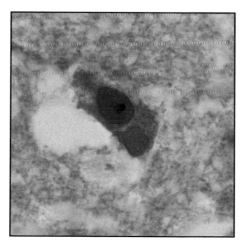

Color Photo 21. Negri bodies in a rabies virus-infected neuron—see also Chapter 22

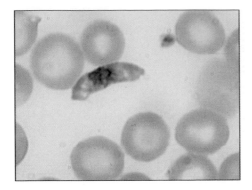

Color Photo 22. *Plasmodium falciparum* with characteristic banana-shaped gametocyte within red blood cell—see also Chapter 33

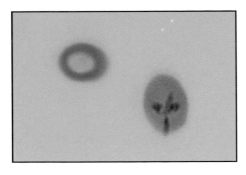

Color Photo 23. *Babesia microti* infection demonstrating a Maltese cross—see also Chapter 33

What is the phenomenon called whereby malignant cells have increased anaerobic glycolysis with increased lactic acid production?	Warburg effect

TUMORIGENESIS

What are two models for viral tumorigenesis?	1. Provirus model 2. Oncogene model
Which model explains viral tumorigenesis?	Both proviruses and oncogenes may play a role in malignant transformation
What is the provirus model?	Virion DNA is incorporated into host cell DNA seen with papillomavirus infection
What is the oncogene model?	Activation of viral oncogenes leading to a malignant transformation

ONCOGENES

What are oncogenes?	Genes encoding proteins involved in cellular growth which are present in oncogenic retroviruses
What are two types of oncogenes?	1. Cellular protooncogenes 2. Viral oncogenes
What is a difference between the cellular and viral oncogenes?	Cellular protooncogenes have exons and introns Viral oncogenes *do not* have exons and introns
How are cellular oncogenes activated?	1. Tumor viruses 2. Chemicals 3. Radiation
How are viral oncogenes acquired?	Cellular oncogenes are incorporated into retroviruses (transducing agents) that carry the cellular oncogenes from one cell to another
What are two functions of oncogenes?	1. Encode a protein kinase that specifically phosphorylates tyrosine 2. Encode for cellular growth factors

What do growth factors act on?	1. G proteins 2. Tyrosine kinases
How do the G proteins and tyrosine kinases affect DNA synthesis?	They interact with cytoplasmic proteins that interact with the cell membrane or produce secondary messengers that are transported to the nucleus and interact with nuclear factors
What are three examples of oncogenes?	1. *ras* gene 2. *myc* gene 3. *src* gene
On what part of the cell does the *ras* oncogene have its effect?	Cell membrane
On what part of the cell does the *myc* oncogene have its effect?	Nucleus
How do tumor viruses of the retrovirus family that do not contain oncogenes cause malignant transformation?	The DNA copy of the viral ribonucleic acid (RNA) integrates near a cellular oncogene increasing its expression

TUMOR-SUPPRESSOR GENES

What is a tumor-suppressor gene?	A gene encoding a protein product involved in the control of the cell cycle that, if mutated, can result in a malignant transformation, i.e., releasing the cells' "safety brake"
What is the most studied tumor-suppressor gene?	p53 Mutation of this tumor-suppressor gene has been found in malignant cells in more than half of all human cancers
What is the function of a normal, nonmutated p53 gene?	To encode a protein that promotes apoptosis of cells that have sustained DNA damage or that contain activated cellular oncogenes
Why are tumor-suppressor genes considered recessive?	They are considered recessive because two mutations are needed for carcinogenesis, i.e., the "two-hit model"

What are four diseases caused by tumor-suppressor gene inactivation?	1. Retinoblastoma 2. Wilms' Tumor 3. Neurofibromatosis 4. Li-Fraumeni syndrome These are all associated with inherited loss of the affected allele, also known as the "one-hit model"

TRANSMISSION OF ONCOGENIC VIRUSES

What is vertical transmission?	Tumor virus transmission involving movement of the virus from mother to offspring
What are three ways by which vertical transmission occurs?	1. Viral genetic material is present in the sperm and egg, i.e., prenatal 2. Virus is passed across the placenta, i.e., perinatal 3. Virus is transmitted in breast milk (see Fig. 31-1)

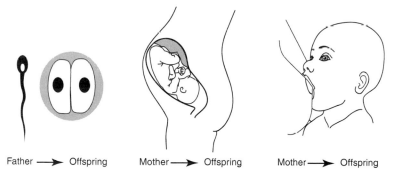

Father ⟶ Offspring   Mother ⟶ Offspring   Mother ⟶ Offspring

Figure 31-1. Vertical transmission

How does the immune system respond to a virus transmitted by vertical transmission?	The immune system does not eliminate the virus because it is exposed to it early in life and develops tolerance to the viral antigens
What is horizontal transmission?	Tumor virus transmission involving the passage of virus between animals that do not have a mother–offspring relationship (see Fig. 31-2)

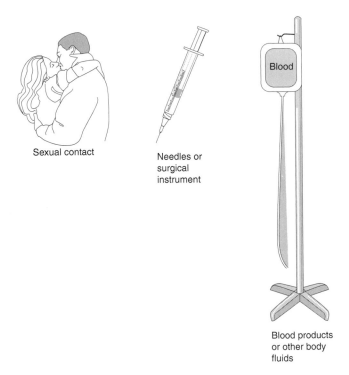

Sexual contact

Needles or
surgical
instrument

Blood

Blood products
or other body
fluids

Figure 31-2. Horizontal transmission

GENOMES OF TUMOR VIRUSES

What are nonpermissive cells?	Cells that do not permit viral replication
What are examples of nonpermissive cells?	Rabbit cells do not replicate human T-cell leukemia virus (HTLV)
What is required for malignant transformation in RNA and DNA tumor viruses?	Viral gene expression
Is replication of the viral genome required for malignant transformation?	No, only viral gene expression
What common intermediate do both DNA and RNA tumor viruses have?	Double-stranded DNA intermediate

What follows the production of this intermediate?	Integration into the host genome
What are three important DNA tumor virus families?	1. Papovaviruses, e.g., human papilloma virus (HPV) 2. Herpesviruses, e.g., Epstein-Barr virus (EBV) and Kaposi sarcoma herpesvirus 3. Poxviruses, e.g., molluscum contagiosum virus
What is an important RNA tumor virus family?	Retroviruses, e.g., HTLV

DISEASES AND TUMOR VIRUSES

What diseases are associated with the following viruses . . .	
HTLV?	1. Leukemia 2. Lymphoma
HPV?	1. Cervical cancer (types 16 and 18) 2. Plantar warts (types 1 and 4) 3. Condyloma acuminatum and laryngeal papillomas (types 6 and 11)
EBV?	1. Burkitt's lymphoma 2. Nasopharyngeal carcinoma
What chromosomal translocation occurs in Burkitt's lymphoma cells?	8;14
What cellular oncogene is juxtaposed to an active promoter as a result of the 8;14 translocation in Burkitt's lymphoma?	c-*myc*
Hepatitis B virus (HBV)?	Primary hepatocellular carcinoma
Hepatitis C virus (HCV)?	Primary hepatocellular carcinoma
Human herpesvirus (HHV)-8?	Kaposi sarcoma

HUMAN T-CELL LEUKEMIA VIRUS TYPE I

What type of virus is HTLV-1?	Retroviridae (+ ssRNA)
How is HTLV-1 transmitted?	1. Sexual contact 2. Exchange of contaminated blood
What type of cancer has HTLV-1 been found to cause?	1. Leukemia 2. T-cell lymphoma
How is the mechanism by which HTLV-1 causes cancer different from that of other retroviruses?	It has no viral oncogene
What types of T cells does HTLV-1 prefer to infect?	CD4-positive
What are the two unique HTLV-1 genes that play a role in oncogenesis?	*tax* and *rex*
How?	By regulating messenger ribonucleic acid (mRNA) transcription and translation
What are the two roles of the *tax* protein produced by HTLV-1?	1. It acts on the viral long terminal repeat (LTR) sequences to stimulate viral mRNA synthesis 2. It induces nuclear factor-kappa B (NF-κB), which stimulates the production of interleukin-2 (IL-2) and the IL-2 receptor
What is the role of the *rex* protein produced by HTLV-1?	It determines which viral mRNAs can exit the nucleus and enter the cytoplasm to be translated

HUMAN PAPILLOMAVIRUS

What type of virus is human papillomavirus (HPV)?	Papovavirus (dsDNA)
What types of epithelia does HPV infect?	Keratinizing or mucosal squamous epithelia
What does the term "papova" in papovaviruses represent?	<u>Pa</u>pillomaviruses, <u>po</u>lyoma viruses, <u>va</u>cuolating viruses

How are papillomaviruses classified?

DNA nucleocapsid viruses with circular supercoiled dsDNA and an icosahedral nucleocapsid

What papovavirus causes progressive multifocal leukoencephalopathy?

JC virus

Please see Chapter 28, "Herpesviridae," for a more detailed discussion of Epstein-Barr virus (EBV) and human herpesvirus 8 (HHV-8), and Chapter 29, "Viral Hepatitis," for a more detailed discussion of hepatitis B virus (HBV) and hepatitis C virus (HCV).

Section IV

Parasitology

32

Helminths

What are helminths?

Macroparasitic worms that range from 10 mm to 10 m in length and are classified as cestodes (tapeworms), nematodes (roundworms), or trematodes (flukes) (see Fig. 33-1B)

How do they replicate?
(5 steps)

1. Helminth enters the host from the environment through ingestion or through skin penetration
2. Matures and produces/sheds eggs or larvae within the host
3. Reenters the environment
4. Invades specific hosts, replicate asexually/sexually, and mature
5. Released into the environment ready to infect humans

How are most helminth infections diagnosed?

Microscopic examination of fecal samples for organisms

What are the three types of helminths?

1. Cestodes (i.e., tapeworms)
2. Trematodes (i.e., flukes)
3. Nematodes (i.c., roundworms)

What are the differences between helminths?

1. Segmented or nonsegmented body types
2. Presence or absence of a digestive system

When infected with a helminth, what changes are seen on a complete blood count (CBC)?

Eosinophilia, i.e., increase in eosinophils

  What are five additional conditions that are associated with this finding?

N.A.A.C.P.
1. Neoplasm
2. Allergic reaction
3. Asthma
4. Collagen vascular disease
5. Parasites

CESTODES (TAPEWORMS)

What type of organisms are cestodes?	Segmented, ribbon-like worms that are primarily intestinal parasites and lack a digestive system (see Fig. 32-1)

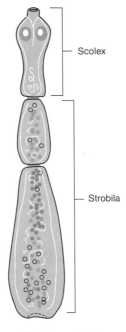

Figure 32-1. Example of a cestode

What are the cestodes?	1. *Taenia solium* (pig tapeworm) 2. *Taenia saginata* (beef tapeworm) 3. *Hymenolepis nana* (dwarf tapeworm) 4. *Echinococcus* sp. 5. *Diphyllobothrium latum* (fish tapeworm)
What are cestodes composed of?	1. Scolex (head) 2. Strobila (body)
What is the function of these structures?	1. Scoleces have hooks and suckers to anchor parasites to the intestinal wall 2. Strobilae are composed of hermaphroditic proglottids which each have the capacity to generate fertilized eggs

How is *T. solium* contracted?	Eating *T. solium* larvae from undercooked pork or by eating eggs found in human feces
What is cysticercosis?	When ingested, eggs of *T. solium* hatch in the small intestine and migrate to form cysts in tissues
What is neurocysticercosis? What are symptoms associated with this?	*T. solium* cysts in the brain Seizures, obstructive hydrocephalus, neurological deficits, meningitis (see Fig. 32-2)

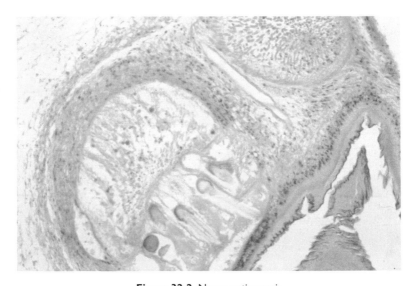

Figure 32-2. Neurocysticercosis

How is *T. saginata* contracted?	Eating *T. saginata* larvae from undercooked beef
Can *T. saginata* cause cysticercosis?	No, cysticercosis is a disease entity specific to *T. solium*
For which cestode are humans the only host? How is it acquired?	*H. nana* (dwarf tapeworm) Fecal–oral route
What diseases are associated with the *Echinococcus* species?	1. Hydatid cyst disease (*Echinococcus granulosis*) 2. Alveolar cyst disease (*Echinococcus multilocularis*)

Alveolar cyst disease caused by *E. multilocularis* is more aggressive than hydatid cyst disease, with invasion of tissue in a tumor-like fashion

What is hydatid cyst disease?

Infection affecting liver and lungs that is contracted from dogs

What are two clinical manifestations?

1. Anaphylactic reaction to parasite antigens
2. Mass effects of cyst enlargement or rupture

What complication can occur by removing cysts?

The fluid in the cysts is highly allergenic and accidental rupture can cause a fatal anaphylactic reaction. Therefore cysts are more commonly drained by ultrasound-guided needle aspiration

How is *D. latum* acquired?

By ingesting larvae in raw fish

What hematologic condition is *D. latum* associated with?

Cobalamin (vitamin B_{12}) deficiency

What is the treatment for tapeworm infections?

Praziquantel or niclosamide

NEMATODES

INTESTINAL NEMATODES

What type of organisms are nematodes?

Nonsegmented, elongated parasitic worms with a complete digestive system (see Fig. 32-3)

What are the intestinal nematodes?

"P. W. A. S. H."
1. Pinworm, i.e., *Enterobius vermicularis*
2. Whipworm, i.e., *Trichuris trichiura*
3. *Ascaris lumbricoides*, i.e., giant roundworm
4. *Strongyloides stercoralis*, i.e., small roundworm
5. Hookworm, i.e., *Necator americanus; Ancylostoma duodenale*

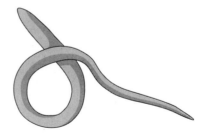

Figure 32-3. Example of a nematode

Which are acquired by ingestion?	1. Pinworm 2. Whipworm 3. *Ascaris*
Which are acquired by penetration through skin?	1. *Strongyloides* 2. Hookworm
What are the clinical manifestations of pinworm infection?	Perianal pruritus
How is pinworm infection diagnosed?	Morning Scotch® tape touch prep on perianal region
In what population is this infection common? **Why?**	All children, but especially those who attend day care centers Children are more prone to scratch themselves and less likely to wash hands in the heat of playtime
What are the clinical manifestations of whipworm infection?	Rectal prolapse with the worms seen on the rectum, i.e., "coconut cake"
Identify the manifestations of *Ascaris* infection: **Intestinal manifestations?**	1. Small-bowel obstruction 2. Pancreatitis 3. Hepatosplenomegaly
Extraintestinal manifestations?	1. Pulmonary eosinophilia 2. Retinal granuloma

How many people worldwide are infected by *Ascaris*?	More than 2 billion people affected worldwide
What condition is associated with dog *Ascaris*?	Visceral larval migrans (humans are a dead-end host) Cutaneous larval migrans is seen with dog hookworm while visceral larval migrans is seen with dog *Ascaris*
What are the clinical manifestations of *Strongyloides* infection?	Relatively benign in healthy individuals
What is hyperinfection syndrome?	Severe condition in an immuno-compromised host, resulting in pneumonitis and colitis, and potentially fatal septic shock and gram-negative meningitis
In what three ways is *Strongyloides* replication unique?	1. Can multiply in host 2. Only larvae are seen in stool; eggs are never seen 3. Infection can persist for 45 years
	Strongyloides is the only nematode that can replicate in the host
What are the clinical manifestations of hookworm infection?	1. Anorexia 2. Ulcer-like symptoms 3. Anemia secondary to continual intestinal blood loss
What condition is associated with dog or cat hookworm?	Cutaneous larval migrans secondary to penetration through skin and migration beneath epidermis Visceral larval migrans is seen with dog *Ascaris* whereas cutaneous larval migrans is seen with dog hookworm

TISSUE NEMATODES

What type of organisms are nematodes?	Nonsegmented, elongated parasitic worms with a complete digestive system

What are the tissue nematodes?	1. *Trichinella spiralis*, i.e., trichinosis 2. Filariae, i.e., *Brugia malayi*, *Loa loa*, *Onchocerca volvulus*, *Wuchereria bancrofti*
Which are acquired by ingestion?	*Trichinella*
Which are acquired by arthropod vector?	Filariae
What are the clinical manifestations of *Trichinella* infection?	1. Periorbital edema 2. Myositis 3. Abdominal pain
What is a risk factor for contraction?	Consumption of homemade pork sausage or undercooked pork
What causes significant clinical manifestations in filariae?	Occlusion of lymphatics by parasite (see Fig. 32-4)

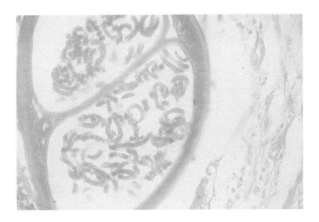

Figure 32-4. Lymphatic obstruction secondary to filariasis

What is the vector for each of the following? *Brugia malayi*?	Mosquitoes
Wuchereria bancrofti?	Mosquitoes
Loa loa?	Deer fly
Onchocerca volvulus?	Black fly

What are the clinical manifestations of *Brugia malayi* and *Wucheria bancrofti* infections?	1. Elephantiasis 2. Tropical pulmonary eosinophilia
What are the clinical manifestations of *Loa loa* infection?	1. Skin lesions 2. Conjunctivitis
What are the clinical manifestations of *Onchocerca volvulus* infection?	1. River blindness 2. Subcutaneous nodules with severe pruritus

TREMATODES (FLUKES)

What type of organisms are trematodes?	Nonsegmented, small, flat, leaf-like parasitic worms with complete digestive systems that infest various organs
What is the intermediate host for all trematodes?	Water snails (see Fig. 32-5)

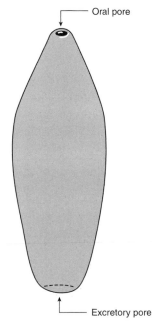

Oral pore

Excretory pore

Figure 32-5. Example of a trematode (liver fluke)

What are five trematodes?

1. Blood fluke, i.e., *Schistosoma mansoni*
2. Chinese liver fluke, i.e., *Clonorchis sinensis*
3. Liver fluke, i.e., *Opisthorchis, Fasciola hepatica*
4. Intestinal fluke, i.e., *Fasciolopsis buski, Heterophyes heterophyes*
5. Lung fluke, i.e., *Paragonimus westermani*

What are three diseases associated with schistosomiasis?

1. Dermatitis, e.g., "swimmer's itch"
2. Acute schistosomiasis, e.g., Katayama fever
3. Chronic schistosomiasis, e.g., "pipestem fibrosis" caused by granulomas in the liver and intestines

How is schistosomiasis transmitted? What is the pathogenesis?

Direct skin contact, often from swimming in fluke-infested freshwater
Inflammatory response to parasite

What are the long-term clinical manifestations?

1. Leading cause of portal hypertension worldwide
2. *Schistosoma haematobium* is associated with squamous cell carcinoma of the bladder

What are the clinical manifestations of liver fluke infection?

1. Cholangitis
2. Cholangiocarcinoma

What is the host for each of the following?
C. sinensis?

Fish or fish-eating mammals

Opisthorchis?

Cats or dogs

F. hepatica?

Sheep and aquatic plants, e.g., watercress

What enables pathogenesis by intestinal flukes?

High parasite load

Where can parasites be found for the following?
F. buski?

Aquatic plants of the Orient

H. heterophyes?

Freshwater or brackish fish

What are the clinical manifestations of *P. westermani*?

Pulmonary involvement resulting in fluke eggs in sputum

What is the host for *P. westermani*?

Crayfish and freshwater crabs

What is the treatment for trematode infections?

Praziquantel

33

Protozoa

What are protozoa?	Single-celled eukaryotic organisms, many of which have evolved organelles, including mitochondria, food vacuoles, nuclei, and an endoplasmic reticulum (see Fig. 33-1A)
How do they replicate?	Mainly by binary fission; however, some species undergo sexual reproduction
What is the clinical significance of protozoal infections?	The majority of protozoa are not human pathogens; however, many types of protozoal infections are more common in developing tropical and subtropical regions and thus may be a significant cause of morbidity and mortality in these regions
What are the two stages of the protozoan life cycle seen in many (but not all) protozoa?	1. Cyst stage 2. Trophozoite stage
How do the stages differ?	In the cyst stage, the protozoa are dormant and immotile, allowing for survival in harsh environments In the trophozoite stage, protozoa are actively feeding, reproducing, and mobile
What are the three main categories of protozoa that are classified according to the area of the body where they usually cause disease?	1. Intestinal 2. Urogenital 3. Blood and tissue
How are protozoa further classified within these main categories?	According to their mode of locomotion

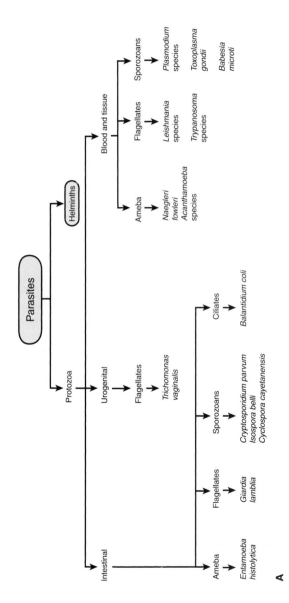

Figure 33-1. A and **B:** Protozoal phylogeny

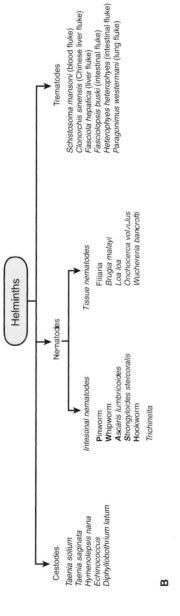

Figure 33-1. (Continued)

What are four groups of protozoa according to this classification?

1. Amebas
2. Flagellates
3. Sporozoans
4. Ciliates

What is the method of locomotion for each of the groups?

Amebas?

Extension of pseudopodia, i.e., cytoplasmic projections, outward from the main cell body

Flagellates?

Rotation of flagella, i.e., whip-like projections

Sporozoans?

Adult form is typically nonmotile

Ciliates?

Synchronous beating of cilia, i.e., hair-like projections

Why are protozoal infections difficult to treat?

Protozoa are eukaryotes with metabolic processes similar to humans, therefore, many of the drugs that are effective against protozoal infections are also toxic to the human host

Identify the major pathogenic intestinal species of each of the groups:

Ameba?

Entamoeba histolytica

Flagellate?

Giardia lamblia

Sporozoa?

Cryptosporidium parvum

Ciliate?

Balantidium coli

What are the minor pathogenic sporozoans?

Isospora belli
Cyclospora cayetanensis

Which is the major pathogenic urogenital flagellate?

Trichomonas vaginalis

What are the major pathogenic blood and tissue species in each of the following groups?

Amebas?	1. *Naegleria fowleri* 2. *Acanthamoeba* species
Flagellates?	1. *Leishmania* species 2. *Trypanosoma* species
Sporozoans?	1. *Plasmodium* species 2. *Toxoplasma gondii*
What is a minor pathogenic blood and tissue sporozoa?	*Babesia microti*

INTESTINAL PROTOZOA

ENTAMOEBA HISTOLYTICA

What diseases does *E. histolytica* cause?	1. Amebic dysentery (bloody diarrhea) 2. Liver abscess 3. Pulmonary abscess
What is the natural reservoir for *E. histolytica*?	Humans only
How is it transmitted?	Fecal–oral transmission of cysts from contaminated food or water
What is the pathogenesis of *E. histolytica* infection?	1. Ingestion of cysts 2. Formation of trophozoites in the small intestine 3. Passage of trophozoites to the colon where they feed on intestinal bacteria 4. Trophozoites invade epithelium and multiply, forming "flask-shaped" ulcers 5. Cysts form and are passed in the stool 6. Rarely (1% of cases), trophozoites spread to liver, resulting in abscess formation 7. Direct spread from liver through diaphragm to the lung, resulting in abscess formation
How does the infectious cyst appear under microscopy?	As a mature cyst with four nuclei (see Fig. 33-2)
How does the trophozoite appear under microscopy?	Organism with multiple pseudopodia, i.e., cytoplasmic projections, and a single nucleus with a central nucleosome (see Fig. 33-3)

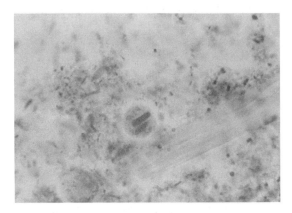

Figure 33-2. *Entamoeba histolytica* infectious cyst

Are most infections symptomatic?

No, only 10% of carriers develop symptoms

What are the symptoms of active disease?

Hemorrhagic colitis with bloody diarrhea or weight loss, fatigue, and right upper quadrant (RUQ) pain, suggesting liver abscess

What is the worldwide mortality from *E. histolytica* infection?

Third leading cause of death caused by parasitic infection, accounting for 100,000 deaths annually

How is *E. histolytica* infection diagnosed?

1. Microscopic observation of erythrophagocytic trophozoites

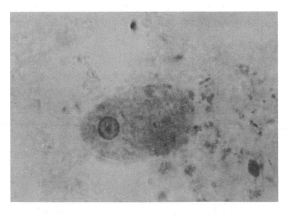

Figure 33-3. *Entamoeba histolytica* trophozoite

2. Stool antigen detection by enzyme-linked immunoabsorbent assay (ELISA)
3. Serologic tests

How is symptomatic *E. histolytica* infection treated?

Metronidazole (for parasites in the tissue) followed by paromomycin (for parasites in the intestinal lumen)

GIARDIA LAMBLIA

What disease does *G. lamblia* cause?
How is it transmitted?

Giardiasis, a diarrheal illness with no extraintestinal disease
Fecal–oral transmission of cysts from contaminated food or water

What is the classic history for *Giardia* infection?

Campers returning from a trip where they drank stream water

What is the pathogenesis of *Giardia* infection?

1. Ingestion of cysts
2. Formation of trophozoites in the duodenum
3. Trophozoites attach to epithelial wall causing villous atrophy and malabsorption

What are the symptoms of active disease?

Nonbloody diarrhea often with steatorrhea
Giardiasis is a noninvasive colitis that causes a nonbloody diarrhea, but may interfere with fat absorption resulting in steatorrhea

How common is *Giardia* infection?
How is it diagnosed?

Approximately 5% of Americans are infected; however, most are asymptomatic
1. Microscopic exam of diarrheal stool for trophozoites and cysts or of formed stool for cysts
2. ELISA immunoassay
3. String test, placing string down to the duodenum with removal after several hours and examination for cysts and trophozoites

How do *Giardia* cysts appear with microscopy?

Thick-walled oval cysts with four nuclei

How to trophozoites appear with microscopy?

Binucleate pear-shaped organisms with 4 flagella (see Fig. 33-4)

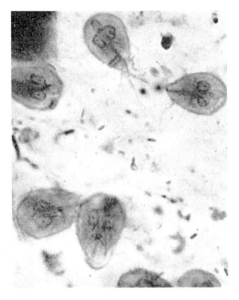

Figure 33-4. *Giardia lamblia* trophozoite

How is *Giardia* infection treated?

Metronidazole

CRYPTOSPORIDIUM PARVUM

What disease does C. parvum cause?

Cryptosporidiosis

How is it transmitted?

Fecal–oral transmission of cysts from contaminated food or water

Mini-outbreaks are seen in day care centers from person-to-person spread

What is the pathogenesis of *Cryptosporidium* infection?

1. Ingestion of cysts
2. Oocytes release sporozoites in small intestine
3. Sporozoites form trophozoites
4. Trophozoites attach and penetrate microvillous gastrointestinal (GI) mucosal surface

What are the clinical manifestations of active disease?

Watery, nonbloody diarrhea and abdominal pain, usually more severe in the immunocompromised

How common is *Cryptosporidium* infection?	25% of Americans have serologic evidence of previous infection; most, however, are asymptomatic
How is it diagnosed?	1. Presence of cysts on modified acid-fast stain of stool 2. Stool ELISA
How do the cysts appear?	As oocysts containing four motile sporozoites (see Fig. 33-5)

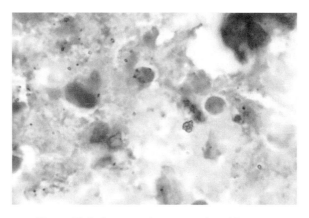

Figure 33-5. *Cryptosporidium* cysts with acid-fast stain

How is it treated?	Nitazoxanide

ISOSPORA BELLI

What disease does *I. belli* cause?	Coccidiosis
What is the reservoir for *I. belli*?	Dogs
How is it transmitted?	Fecal–oral transmission of oocysts
What are the clinical manifestations of active disease?	Fever, headache, diarrhea, abdominal pain
How does *I. belli* cause diarrhea?	Oocysts excyst in the upper small intestine and invade mucosa, destroying the brush border causing malabsorption and increased water loss
What is unique about the life cycle of *I. belli*?	Cysts need to develop outside of the host

How is it diagnosed?	Identifying oocysts in feces by acid-fast stain
How is it treated?	Trimethoprim-sulfamethoxazole

CYCLOSPORA CAYETANENSIS

What disease does C. cayetanensis cause?	Cyclosporiasis
How is it transmitted?	Fecal–oral transmission of cysts
What food is associated with Cyclospora infection?	Raspberries, especially those from Guatemala

What are the clinical manifestations of active disease?	Prolonged and relapsing diarrhea
What is unique about the life cycle of Cyclospora?	Cysts need to develop outside the host
How is Cyclospora infection diagnosed? **How is it treated?**	Identification of spherical oocysts in feces by acid-fast stain Trimethoprim-sulfamethoxazole

BALANTIDIUM COLI

What disease does B. coli cause?	Usually asymptomatic, but dysentery (diarrhea) may occur
What is unique about B. coli?	It is the only ciliated protozoan to cause disease in humans
How is B. coli infection diagnosed?	Microscopy can identify large ciliated trophozoites or large cysts with a "V-shaped" nucleus in the stool
How is it treated?	Tetracycline

UROGENITAL PROTOZOA

TRICHOMONAS VAGINALIS

What disease does T. vaginalis cause?	Trichomoniasis
How is T. vaginalis transmitted?	Sexually

**What are the stages of
T. vaginalis?**

Only exists as a trophozoite; there is no
cyst form

**What are the clinical
manifestations of active
disease?**

Profuse watery or foamy greenish
    vaginal discharge associated
    with severe itching/dysuria in
    females
Urethritis/prostatitis in males, although
    most males are asymptomatic

**How common is
T. vaginalis infection?**

Approximately 3 million women per year
in the United States are infected

**How is T. vaginalis
infection diagnosed?**

Wet mount of vaginal discharge
or urine microscopy demonstrates motile trophozoites

    **How do they appear with
    microscopy?**

Pear-shaped organisms with 1 central
nucleus and 4 anterior flagella and
undulating membranes (see Fig. 33-6)

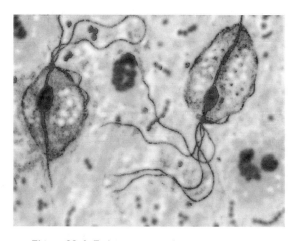

Figure 33-6. *Trichomonas vaginalis* on wet mount prep

    How is it treated?

Metronidazole

BLOOD AND TISSUE PROTOZOA

NAEGLERIA FOWLERI

**What disease does
N. fowleri cause?**

Meningoencephalitis

**How is N. fowleri
transmitted?**

Swimming in warm freshwater
lakes

How?

Trophozoites penetrate nasal mucosa and cribriform plate, directly infecting the overlying meninges and brain

What population is usually infected?

Normal healthy children

What are the clinical manifestations of active disease?

Headache, fever, nuchal rigidity, nausea, vomiting

What is the prognosis for a person with active disease?

Rapidly fatal

How common is symptomatic infection?

Rare, although many people are exposed to the organism

How is N. fowleri infection diagnosed?

Cerebrospinal fluid (CSF) wet prep demonstrating trophozoites

How is it treated?

No effective treatment, but intrathecal amphotericin B has sometimes resulted in recovery

ACANTHAMOEBA SPECIES

What diseases does Acanthamoeba cause?

1. Keratitis
2. Chronic granulomatous meningoencephalitis

How is Acanthamoeba transmitted?

Swimming in freshwater lakes

How does Acanthamoeba cause keratitis?

Direct inoculation of eyes or by inadequately cleaning of soft contact lenses

What are the clinical manifestations of this disease?

Eye pain, photophobia, visible lesion of cornea, and sometimes blindness

How is Acanthamoeba keratitis diagnosed?

1. History and physical
2. Rarely, a ring-shaped corneal infiltrate is present

What population usually develops meningoencephalitis?

Immunocompromised

What are the clinical manifestations of meningoencephalitis?	Headache, fever, seizures, focal neurologic signs
How is chronic granulomatous meningoencephalitis diagnosed?	CSF wet prep or brain-tissue biopsy demonstrating trophozoites and possibly granulomas
How is it treated?	Antifungal drugs and pentamidine are occasionally effective

LEISHMANIA SPECIES

What disease does the *Leishmania* species cause?	Leishmaniasis
What is the natural reservoir for the *Leishmania* species?	Wild rodents, dogs, and humans
How is *Leishmania* transmitted?	Sandfly
What is the life cycle of *Leishmania*?	1. Infected female sandfly bites human, transmitting promastigotes into the skin 2. Promastigotes lose flagella and turn into amastigotes 3. Amastigotes invade macrophages and reproduce, killing the host cell and releasing more amastigotes that infect other cells 4. Sandfly ingests amastigotes from an infected person during a blood meal 5. Amastigotes divide in the gut of the sandfly, producing promastigotes
What are the four types of leishmaniasis?	1. Cutaneous 2. Diffuse cutaneous 3. Mucosal 4. Visceral
What are the clinical manifestations of the following?	
Cutaneous leishmaniasis?	Ulcerating, pizza-like lesions that can be single or multiple and heal after months to years with scarring

Diffuse cutaneous leishmaniasis?	Nonulcerating nodules with a widespread distribution
Mucosal leishmaniasis?	Ulceration of mucous membranes of nose and/or mouth years after infection, which can obliterate the nasal septum and the buccal cavity; death can occur from secondary infection
Visceral leishmaniasis?	Splenomegaly, hepatomegaly, and jaundice; death can occur from secondary infection
What is another name for this condition?	Kala azar
What is the prevalence and incidence of *Leishmania* infection?	Approximately 500,000 new infections occur each year An estimated 12 million people are currently infected
How is *Leishmania* infection diagnosed?	1. Identification of amastigotes in Giemsa-stained tissue or fluid 2. Serological tests with ELISA, indirect fluorescent antibody, and complement fixation 3. Montenegro skin test for cutaneous and mucosal leishmaniasis
How is *Leishmania* infection treated?	Sodium stibogluconate, a pentavalent antimonial, and liposomal amphotericin

TRYPANOSOMA SPECIES

What are the three main human pathogenic strains of *Trypanosoma*?	1. *Trypanosoma cruzi* 2. *Trypanosoma brucei gambiense* 3. *Trypanosoma brucei rhodesiense*
What disease does *T. cruzi* cause?	Chagas disease
Where does this disease occur?	Southern United States and Central and South America
How is *T. cruzi* transmitted?	Reduviid or "kissing" bug; blood transfusions

What is the life cycle of
T. cruzi?

1. Reduviid bug ingests trypomastigotes in the blood of reservoir hosts, e.g., humans, domestic cats and dogs, wild armadillo, raccoons, and rats
2. Organisms multiply within the bug's gut and differentiate into epimastigotes and trypomastigotes
3. Reduviid bug bites are infected with feces containing trypomastigotes
4. Trypomastigotes enter blood and lose flagellae, forming amastigotes
5. Amastigotes infect myocardial, glial, and reticuloendothelial cells

What are the two symptomatic stages of Chagas disease?

1. Acute stage lasting 1–2 months
2. Chronic stage occurring years after initial infection

What are the clinical manifestations of the acute stage?

Skin nodule at the site of bite (chagoma) and periorbital swelling (Romaña sign) associated with fever, malaise, and lymphadenopathy

What are the clinical manifestations of the chronic stage?

1. Cardiac: myocarditis, dysrhythmias, and dilated cardiomyopathy
2. Gastrointestinal: megaesophagus and megacolon

How is *T. cruzi* infection diagnosed?

Acute stage—identification of "C"-shaped motile trypanosomes in blood (see Fig. 33-7)
Chronic stage—by clinical presentation, serologic evidence of previous infection, and xenodiagnosis by allowing lab-raised reduviid bug to feed on a patient and analysis of intestinal contents several weeks later

How is *T. cruzi* infection treated?

Acute stage—nifurtimox
Chronic stage—no treatment

What disease does *T. brucei gambiense* cause?

West African sleeping sickness

What disease does *T. brucei rhodesiense* cause?

East African sleeping sickness

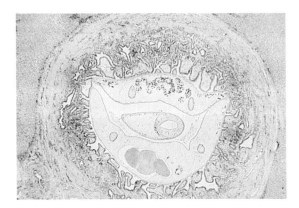

Figure 33-7. Peripheral blood smear demonstrating "C"-shaped trypanosomes in Chagas disease.

How are *T. brucei gambiense* and *T. brucei rhodesiense* transmitted?	Tsetse fly
What is the pathogenesis of infection with these species?	Organisms spread from inoculated skin to the blood and lymph nodes; eventually causing inflammation of the brain and spinal cord
What are the clinical manifestations of these infections?	1. Initial primary skin lesion, i.e., trypanosomal chancre 2. Intermittent fever and lymphadenopathy (Winterbottom sign) 3. Encephalitis characterized by lethargy, continuous sleep ("sleeping sickness"), mental status changes, and death
How do these infections differ?	*T. brucei gambiense* causes a low-grade chronic disease progressing over years *T. brucei rhodesiense* causes an acute, rapidly progressing disease that is usually lethal within several months
How are these infections diagnosed?	1. Peripheral blood smear demonstrating trypanosomes. Giemsa stain of CSF or lymph node aspirates 2. ELISA serologic tests 3. Brain biopsy demonstrates Morula or Mott cells

| **What is the treatment for T. brucei gambiense and T. brucei rhodesiense infections?** | Suramin and pentamidine for early stages of disease without central nervous system (CNS) involvement Melarsoprol and suramin for late-stage disease with CNS involvement |

PLASMODIUM SPECIES

What are the four major species of Plasmodium that are human pathogens?	1. *Plasmodium falciparum* 2. *Plasmodium vivax* 3. *Plasmodium malariae* 4. *Plasmodium ovale*
What disease does Plasmodium cause?	Malaria
How is Plasmodium transmitted? **How else may it be transmitted?**	*Anopheles* mosquito 1. Blood transfusions 2. Transplacental transmission
What is the life cycle of Plasmodium?	1. Infected female mosquito bites human, transmitting sporozoites from its salivary gland 2. Sporozoites infect liver cells and develop into merozoites 3. Merozoites invade red blood cells and become trophozoites 4. Trophozoites undergo asexual reproduction within red blood cells and form schizonts (large multinucleated masses) and more merozoites 5. Red cells lyse, releasing merozoites 6. Merozoites infect other red blood cells or become gametocytes 7. Gametocytes ingested by a female mosquito during a blood meal 8. Sexual reproduction with gametocytes occurs in the mosquito, forming sporozoites
What is the life cycle that occurs outside of red blood cells called?	Exoerythrocytic cycle
What is unique about the life cycle of P. vivax and P. ovale?	They form hypnozoites, dormant forms of *Plasmodium* in hepatocytes which can remain for up to 5 years

P. vivax and *P. ovale* form hypnozoites that are very old

What are the clinical manifestations of active *Plasmodium* infection?

Severe chills, high fevers, profuse sweating at 48- to 72-hour intervals with anemia, hepatosplenomegaly, and, in severe cases, splenic rupture

How do the clinical manifestations of *P. falciparum* differ from other species?

P. falciparum produces a more serious form of malaria with continuous high fever, orthostatic hypotension, and capillary obstruction causing hemorrhage and ischemia, particularly in the kidneys, lung, and brain

What is the worldwide incidence and mortality of malaria?

200–300 million people are infected annually and 1–2 million die

Which population is at an increased risk for developing serious infection?

Asplenic patients

Which conditions confer protection against malaria by increasing host resistance to *P. falciparum* and *P. vivax*?

Sickle cell trait and glucose-6-phosphate dehydrogenase (G6PD) deficiency protect against *P. falciparum*

Absence of Duffy blood group antigens A and B protects against *P. vivax*

How is malaria diagnosed?

1. Identification of parasitic ring within red blood cells on thick blood smear with Giemsa stain and/or on thin blood smear
2. Serologic tests

How is malaria treated?

Chloroquine, quinine, primaquine, mefloquine, doxycycline/tetracycline, atovaquone/proguanil, or pyrimethamine/sulfadoxine

Chloroquine, quinine, and primaquine all cause hemolysis in patients with G6PD deficiency

**What are differentiating
characteristics of . .**

P. falciparum?   High parasite load; multiple ring forms, including banana-shaped gametocytes, appear in red blood cells on smear; occurs in tropical areas and results in the most severe form of malaria (see Fig. 33-8)

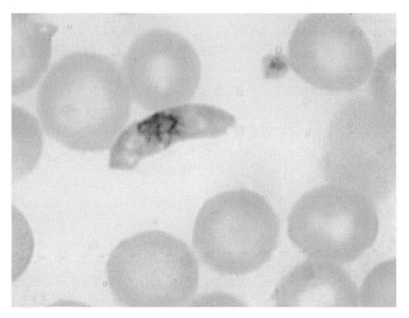

Figure 33-8. *Plasmodium falciparum* with characteristic banana-shaped gametocyte within red blood cell. (see also color photo 22)

P. vivax?   Forms large ameba-like red blood cells with Schüffner dots; all stages of growth are seen on blood smear; forms hypnozoites; more temperate distribution

P. malariae?   Milder form of disease; can be dormant in liver for years; may cause chronic problems like nephrotic syndrome, all stages of growth and band forms are seen on smear

P. ovale?   Large ovoid red blood cells with Schüffner dots; forms hypnozoites

BABESIA MICROTI

What disease does B. microti cause?	Babesiosis
Where does this disease commonly occur?	Northeastern coastal United States and upper midwest
How is B. microti transmitted?	*Ixodes scapularis* ticks
What other organism is transmitted by this vector?	*Borrelia burgdorferi*, the bacteria that causes Lyme disease
What is the pathogenesis of B. microti infection?	Infects red blood cells causing them to lyse
What are the clinical manifestations of B. microti infection?	Often asymptomatic and subclinical, but may cause influenza-like symptoms including fever, myalgias, fatigue, and muscle weakness
In what population can B. microti cause a potentially fatal infection?	Asplenic patients
What disease does babesiosis resemble? How are they similar?	Malaria Both are transmitted by blood-sucking insects, cause fever and hemolysis, and the organisms are within red blood cells
How do they differ?	*B. microti* is transmitted by a tick (vs. a mosquito), makes no pigment within red blood cells, produces no sexual forms, and has no exoerythrocytic cycle, and therefore has no reservoir in hepatocytes
How does B. microti appear on blood smear?	Ring-shaped trophozoites within red blood cells Classic X-shaped tetrad of merozoites also known as the Maltese cross (see Fig. 33-9)
What is the treatment for B. microti infection?	Quinine and clindamycin

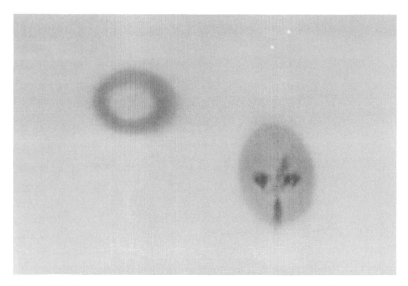

Figure 33-9. *Babesia microti* merozoites demonstrating a "Maltese cross." (See also color photo 23)

TOXOPLASMA GONDII

What disease does *T. gondii* cause?	Toxoplasmosis
What organism is the definitive host for *T. gondii*?	Cat
How is *T. gondii* transmitted?	1. Fecal–oral transmission by ingestions of oocysts in cat feces or eating undercooked contaminated meat 2. Transplacental transmission from an infected mother 3. Blood transfusion *T. gondii* is the "T" in "TORCHES" mnemonic for transplacental infections; the other organisms include rubella, cytomegalovirus, herpes simplex virus, human immunodeficiency virus (HIV), and syphilis
What are the two types of *Toxoplasma* trophozoites?	1. <u>Tachy</u>zoites are fast growing 2. <u>Brady</u>zoites are slow growing

What is the pathogenesis of both types?

Tachyzoites destroy cells, especially parenchymal and reticuloendothelial cells, e.g., macrophages
Bradyzoites are contained in cysts in the brain, muscle, and eye, and cause local inflammation and necrosis when they rupture from the cysts

What are the clinical manifestations of . . .
Acquired infection?

Generalized lymphadenopathy with a mononucleosis-like illness

Reactivation disease?

Fever, lymphadenopathy, hepatosplenomegaly, pneumonia, chorioretinitis, myocarditis, brain abscess, and encephalitis may occur in immunocompromised patients

Congenital infection?

Chorioretinitis, cataracts, seizures, mental retardation, microcephaly, encephalitis, and stillbirth

How common is *T. gondii* infection?

Ubiquitous; up to 80% of cats in the United States are infected and 30% of humans are infected, but most are usually asymptomatic

What two populations have a higher risk of symptomatic infection?

1. Neonates
2. Immunocompromised

How is *T. gondii* infection diagnosed?

1. Computed tomography (CT) demonstrates contrast-enhanced mass (reactivation)
2. Fundoscopy reveals retinal inflammation (congenital)
3. Serology indicates prior exposure or acute infection
4. Muscle biopsy demonstrates cysts
5. Polymerase chain reaction (PCR) of deoxyribonucleic acid (DNA)

How is acute *T. gondii* infection treated in immunocompetent patients?

Usually not treated unless disease is unusually severe

How is acute *T. gondii* infection treated in immunocompromised patients?

Sulfadiazine and pyrimethamine plus folinic acid

Section V

Immunology

34

Introduction to Immunology

INNATE AND ACQUIRED IMMUNITY

What is the function of the immune system?

To prevent or eliminate unwanted growth of microorganisms (such as bacteria, viruses, parasites, and fungi) and dysregulation of cells

What are the two major types of immunity?

1. Innate immunity (natural)
2. Acquired immunity (adaptive)

What are the advantages of innate immunity?

Components are preformed and are able to function immediately after a microorganism has entered the body

What are the disadvantages of innate immunity?

Components are less specific for the invading pathogen and do not develop memory for future infections

What are the two major categories of the acquired immune system?

1. Humoral (antibody-mediated) immunity
2. Cell-mediated immunity

What are the five components of acquired humoral (antibody-mediated) immunity?

1. B cells
2. Plasma cells
3. Helper T cells
4. Macrophages
5. Antibodies

What are the three components of acquired cell-mediated immunity?

1. Antigen presenting cells
2. Helper T cells
3. Cytotoxic T cells

What are the three main antigen-presenting cells?

1. Macrophages
2. Dendritic cells
3. B cells

What are the targets of humoral immunity?

Free microorganisms and toxins

What are the targets of cell-mediated immunity?	Intracellular microorganisms, parasites, and altered host cells
What are the advantages of the acquired immune system?	1. Responds to millions of different antigens 2. Provides specific immunity against the invading pathogen 3. Develops long-term memory against the specific antigen in the future Acquired immunity provides diversity, specificity, and long-term memory
What are the disadvantages of the acquired immune system?	Does not provide immediate immunity to novel pathogens because of the lag time for functionality and is responsible for autoimmune phenomenon

ACTIVE AND PASSIVE IMMUNITY

What are two ways that immunity is acquired?	1. Active 2. Passive
What is active immunity?	Immunity that is induced upon exposure to a microorganism, either in the form of infection or with preventative vaccination
What is an advantage of active immunity?	Long-term immunity
What is a disadvantage of active immunity?	Response is usually slow, requiring days for immunity to develop
What is passive immunity?	Immunity that is conferred by transferring preformed antibodies against bacteria, toxins, and/or viruses from another host
What is an advantage of passive immunity?	Large amounts of antibody can be administered quickly, generating a rapid response to the antigen
What are the disadvantages of passive immunity?	Antibodies have a short life span, may induce hypersensitivity reactions, and do not provide memory against future infections

What are three modes of acquiring passive immunity?	1. Transplacental transmission of IgG 2. IgA transmitted via breast milk 3. Injection of preformed antibodies
When is passive immunity used clinically?	For postexposure prophylaxis of diphtheria, tetanus, botulism, rabies, hepatitis A, and hepatitis B For preexposure prophylaxis of respiratory syncytial virus (RSV) in infants

ANTIGENS

What is an antigen?	Any molecule, or part thereof, that reacts with antibodies
What is an immunogen?	Any molecule, or part thereof, that induces an immune response
Are all antigens also immunogens?	No
What is a hapten?	Molecule that is not immunogenic by itself, but elicits an immune response when bound to a specific carrier protein
Give two examples of haptens.	1. Penicillin 2. Catechol
Why are haptens unable to stimulate an immune response?	They are unable to bind to major histocompatibility complex (MHC) proteins or activate B cells without a carrier protein
What is an adjuvant?	Chemical that is unrelated to an immunogen but enhances the immune response to an antigen
Give an example of an adjuvant.	Aluminum hydroxide

35

Cells & Histology of the Immune Response

CELLS OF THE INNATE IMMUNE RESPONSE

What is the innate immune response?

The initial response by the body to tissue damage or against a foreign body

What cells are involved with this response?

1. Granulocytes
2. Agranulocytes
3. Natural killer cells

What are granulocytes?

Cells derived from the bone marrow that contain cytoplasmic granules

What process is ubiquitous for normally functioning granulocytes?

Degranulation of cytoplasmic granules releasing various immune mediators

What are four types of granulocytes?

1. Neutrophils, or polymorphonuclear cells (PMNs)
2. Eosinophils
3. Basophils
4. Mast cells

What is the precursor cell to granulocytes?

Myeloid progenitor

What is the role of neutrophils in the innate immune response?

Phagocytosis of microorganisms and cellular debris

What is often found at the site of an infection?

Pus, composed of dead neutrophils and organisms
Think of neutrophils as the Marines because they are the first on the scene, ingest (destroy) the bad guy, and take a lot of casualties

What is the morphology of neutrophils?

Neutrophils have large, azurophilic granules (lysosomes) at the periphery with a multilobed nuclei (see Fig. 35-1)

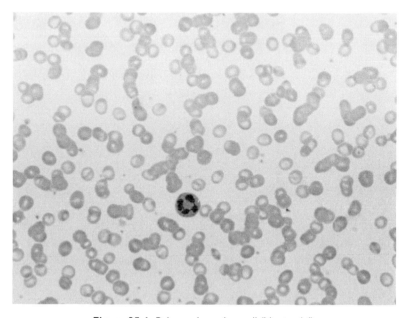

Figure 35-1. Polymorphonuclear cell (Neutrophil)

What is the role of eosinophils in the innate immune response?

1. Phagocytosis of antibody-bound microorganisms and cellular debris
2. To release histamine

What infections are associated with high concentrations of eosinophils?

Helminthic and protozoal infections

What is the morphology of eosinophils?

Eosinophils have large eosinophilic granules and a bilobed nucleus (see Fig. 35-2)

What is the role of basophils in the innate immune response?

1. Anticoagulation (heparin release)
2. Vasodilation (histamine release)

What reaction is associated with basophils?

Allergic reactions

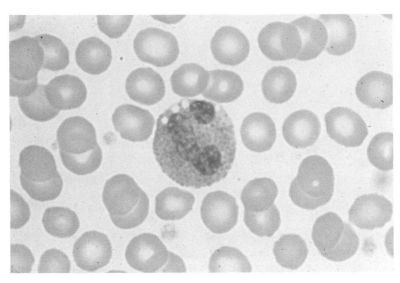

Figure 35-2. Eosinophil

What is the morphology of basophils?

Basophils have dark-blue-staining granules with a bilobed nucleus (see Fig. 35-3)

What is the role of mast cells in the innate immune response?

1. Vasodilation (histamine release)
2. Anticoagulation (heparin release)
3. Release chemotactic factors and prostaglandins

What reactions are associated with mast cells?

Allergic and anaphylactic reactions

What is the morphology of mast cells?

Mast cells have large cytoplasmic granules and a spherical nucleus

What are agranulocytes?

Cells derived from the bone marrow that lack cytoplasmic granules

What is one type of agranulocyte?

Macrophage

What is their role in the innate immune response?

1. Phagocytosis of microorganisms and cellular debris (see Fig. 35-4)
2. Antigen presentation to lymphocytes

What is the morphology of macrophages?

Macrophages are irregularly shaped cells with projections

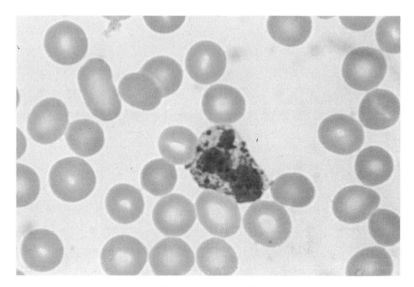

Figure 35-3. Basophil

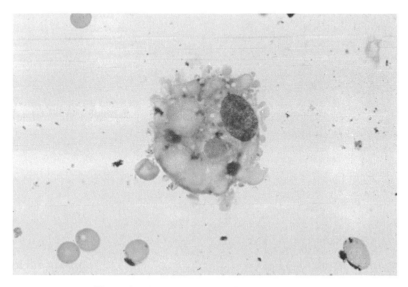

Figure 35-4. Macrophage engulfing red blood cells

What is the precursor for macrophages?	Monocytes
What other cells are produced from this precursor?	1. Kupffer cells (liver) 2. Langerhans cells (skin) 3. Alveolar macrophages (lung) 4. Osteoclasts (bone) 5. Microglia (central nervous system [CNS]) (see Fig. 35-5)
What is the morphology of the monocyte nucleus?	A kidney-shaped nucleus (see Fig. 35-6)
What are natural killer cells?	Nonphagocytic killer cells related to lymphocytes
What is the role of natural killer cells in the innate immune response?	1. Interferon release 2. Recognition of decreased major histocompatibility complex (MHC) class I surface expression
What infections are associated with natural killer cells?	Viral and intracellular bacteria

CELLS OF THE ADAPTIVE IMMUNE RESPONSE

What is the adaptive immune response?	An immune response based on specific recognition of unique foreign antigens
What are the two types of the adaptive immune response?	1. Cell-mediated response 2. Humoral response
What three cells present antigens to cells of the adaptive immune response?	Antigen presenting cells: 1. Macrophages 2. Monocytes 3. Dendritic cells
What is the progenitor cell for the adaptive immune response?	Common lymphoid progenitor
Which cells of the innate immune response share this progenitor cell?	Natural killer cells

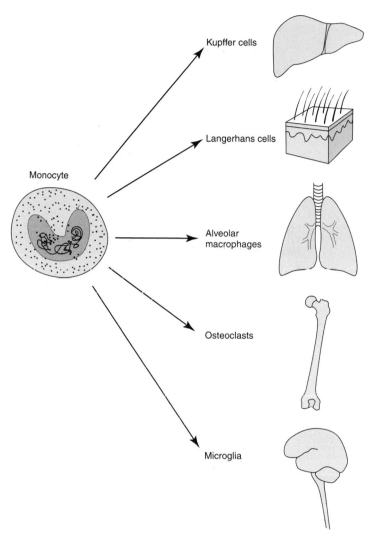

Figure 35-5. Monocyte lineage

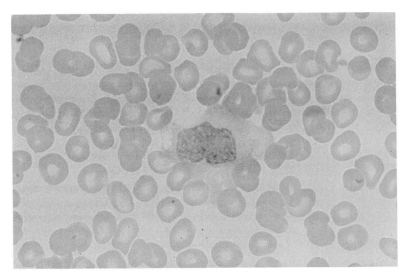

Figure 35-6. Monocyte

What specific types of differentiated common lymphoid progenitor cells are associated with each type of adaptive immune response?

Cell-mediated immune response is associated with T cells and antigen-presenting cells
Humoral immune response is associated with B cells

What is the function of T cells? What are two examples?

To develop into effector T cells that either "help" or "kill"
1. CD4+ T cells
2. CD8+ T cells or cytotoxic T cells

What is the function of B cells?

To produce antibodies and differentiate into memory cells (plasma cells)

36

The Innate Immune System

What is the first line of defense against infection?	Skin and mucous membranes
Identify the components of the innate immune system: **Cells?**	1. Neutrophils 2. Natural killer cells 3. Macrophages
Proteins?	1. Complement cascade 2. Interferons 3. Acute phase proteins
Processes?	1. Phagocytosis 2. Inflammation (acute phase response)
What are three characteristics of innate immunity?	1. Resistance is not acquired 2. Response does not improve after exposure to antigen 3. There is no "memory" for antigen-specific response
What is the initial defense of the innate immune system?	Noninflammatory, which depends on the body's static defenses (i.e., skin, gastric pH, lysozymes)
What is the subsequent response of the innate immune system?	Acute-phase response produces local inflammation and promotes migration of phagocytes and plasma proteins into the infected tissues
What are two examples of acute-phase plasma proteins?	1. C-reactive proteins 2. Mannose-binding proteins (collectins)
Where are these proteins synthesized?	In the liver

What induces acute phase protein synthesis?

Interleukin-6 (IL-6) and tumor necrosis factor-α (TNF-α)

What lab test measures the amount of acute phase proteins in the blood?

Erythrocyte sedimentation rate (ESR)

What is the clinical significance of the ESR?

Elevated ESR indicates an increase in acute-phase proteins in the blood, which may be a nonspecific indicator of infection, inflammation, autoimmune disease, or malignancy

How does the innate immune system recognize foreign microorganisms?

By detecting nonmammalian epitopes on the surface of microorganisms that differ from those on human cells

What are four examples of foreign substances?

1. Lipopolysaccharide (LPS)
2. Peptidoglycans
3. Lipoteichoic acids
4. Mannans

What is the first line of cellular defense against bacterial pathogens?

Neutrophils

What roles do the following cells play in acute inflammation:
  Neutrophils?

Phagocytosis with oxygen-dependent or independent bacterial killing mechanisms

  Macrophages?

Phagocytose and trap foreign substances, followed closely by antigen presentation

  Eosinophils?

Key inflammatory cells involved in response to helminth infections and allergens

  Basophils and mast cells?

Possess IgE receptors which bind allergens

  Natural killer cells?

Destroy abnormal host cells (virally infected or transformed) via osmotic lysis or by triggering apoptosis

How is phagocytosis enhanced?	By opsonization
What is this?	Process by which host proteins bind to antigens to make them more easily detected by phagocytic cells
What is respiratory burst?	A transient increase in oxygen uptake by phagocytic cells during bacterial killing

What are the mechanisms of oxygen-dependent killing seen in neutrophils?

1. Superoxide radical production (via nicotinamide adenine dinucleotide phosphate [NADPH] oxidase)
2. Hypochlorite ion production (via myeloperoxidase [MPO])
3. Hydroxyl radical production (formed spontaneously)

What disease is associated with NADPH oxidase deficiency?

Chronic granulomatous disease of childhood

What are patients with this disease more susceptible to?

Opportunistic infections including *Staphylococcus aureus*, gram-negative enteric rods, and *Aspergillus fumigatus*

Which disease is associated with a defect of neutrophil lysosomes?

Chediak-Higashi syndrome

What are patients with this disease more susceptible to?

Recurrent pyogenic infections by staphylococci and streptococci

What are three unique characteristics of macrophages?

1. Display receptors for molecules not normally displayed on human cells (mannose, LPS, LAM)
2. Enter connective tissue spaces forming reticuloendothelial system
3. Increased expression of class II MHC after phagocytosis

What is the difference between monocytes and macrophages?

Macrophages are mature bloodstream monocytes that have migrated into tissues

What are tissue-specific examples of macrophages?

1. Alveolar macrophages in lung
2. Kupffer cells in liver

3. Microglial cells in central nervous system (CNS)
4. Peritoneal macrophages in peritoneal fluid
5. Splenic macrophages
6. Macrophages in Peyer patches along the gut

What type of cells do natural killer cells target?

Cells that lack MHC class I molecules (viruses can induce loss of MHC class I molecules in infected cells as a way to hide from the immune system)

37

T Cells & Cell-Mediated Immunity

OVERVIEW

What is acquired immunity?

Immunity resulting from previous exposure to a pathogen

What are the two types of acquired immunity?

1. Humoral immunity
2. Cell-mediated immunity

What are five main processes of acquired immunity?

1. Maturation of lymphocytes
2. Uptake and processing foreign antigens
3. Recognizing antigenic epitopes
4. Cloning effector cells
5. Removing microorganisms by reactivity with foreign antigens

What cells are important in the acquired immune system?

1. Antigen-presenting cells
2. Lymphocytes—B cells and T cells

What are the advantages of acquired immunity over innate immunity?

1. Targets specific pathogens
2. Provides memory, which allows for a faster immune response
3. Enhanced response with repeated exposure

T CELLS

What is the origin of T cells?

Lymphoid progenitor cells

For what two types of immunity are T cells a key component?

1. Cell-mediated immunity (cytotoxic T cells)
2. Humoral immunity (helper T cells)

What are the two types of T cells?

1. Helper T cells (CD4)
2. Killer T cells (cytotoxic, CD8)

What do helper T cells do?

1. Recognize peptides presented by major histocompatibility complex (MHC) molecules
2. Assist in activation of killer T cells by elaboration of leukin-2 (IL-2)
3. Signal B cells to secrete antibodies by secreting IL-4 and IL-5
4. Help macrophages stimulate delayed-type hypersensitivity

What activates helper T cells?

Antigen-specific peptides associated with class II MHC molecules and costimulatory molecules

What do killer T cells do?

Identify and kill cells harboring viruses and other intracellular microorganisms, cancerous cells, and allografts

What activates killer T cells?

Antigen-specific peptides associated with class I MHC molecules along with costimulatory molecules

What percentage of peripheral T cells are helper T cells?

Approximately 67%

What percentage of peripheral T cells are killer T cells?

Approximately 33%

What infection causes marked lymphopenia with a reduction in the ratio of helper T cells to killer T cells?

Human immunodeficiency virus (HIV) decreases the normal CD4:CD8 ratio from 2:1 to 1:10 or worse

Where do T cells originate?

Bone marrow

Where do T cells mature?

Thymus
T cells mature in the Thymus

What do T cells acquire when they develop in the thymus?

T-cell receptors (TCRs)

What is the TCR?

A 5-chain complex of proteins forming a unique receptor for each antigen

What process occurs in the thymus after cells develop T-cell receptors?	Selection for T cells that recognize self–MHC complexes, but do not recognize self antigens (see Fig. 37-1)
What happens to immature T cells that fail to recognize self–MHC complexes?	Cell death by apoptosis
What happens to immature T cells that recognize self antigens?	Cell death by apoptosis
How many antigens does a specific T cell recognize after maturation?	Only 1 antigen bound to 1 specific MHC molecule
When does the conversion of thymocytes into mature lymphocytes predominantly occur?	From the fetal period through adolescence
How many T cells survive thymic selection?	2%
Where do T cells go after the thymus?	Into the circulation and secondary lymphoid organs

T-CELL RECEPTOR COMPLEX

What comprises the TCR complex?	Heteromeric polypeptide chains
What types of polypeptide chains form a TCR complex?	Either α/β or γ/δ along with three proteins from CD3 (zeta, ζ; eta, $\acute{\eta}$; epsilon ϵ)
How are the two chains connected?	Disulfide bonds (see Fig. 37-2)
What percentage of T cells express the α/β TCR?	95%
Why are TCRs referred to as members of the immunoglobulin supergene family?	The TCR protein structure is similar to that of antibodies

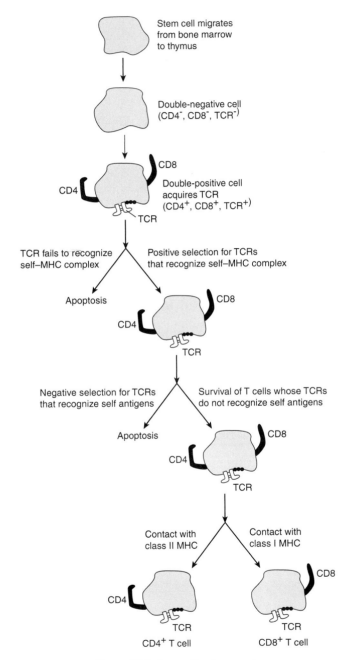

Figure 37-1. Steps in T-cell maturation

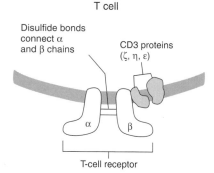

Figure 37-2. T-cell receptor

What complex transfers the signal across the cell membrane that the TCR has engaged its specific peptide?	CD3 complex
What is the result of this signal?	Activation of intracellular kinases, resulting in signal cascade and T-cell activation

MAJOR HISTOCOMPATIBILITY COMPLEX

What is the role of the MHC?	To present antigenic peptide fragments to T cells
What is the specific name for the MHC in humans?	Human leukocyte antigen (HLA)
What is the structure of an MHC molecule?	Two-chained cell-surface complex with a variable extracellular peptide binding site (see Fig. 37-3)
What is a unique characteristic of the MHC gene that allows for variability in the binding site?	Genetic polymorphism
What is genetic polymorphism?	The presence of many different rearrangements in the coding sequences for the MHC peptide binding site
How does this affect MHC molecules?	Allows for great variability of peptide binding sites for many diverse antigens

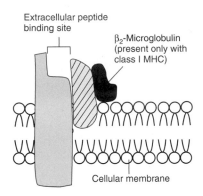

Figure 37-3. Diagram of MHC molecule

CLASS I MAJOR HISTOCOMPATIBILITY COMPLEX

Where are the peptides presented on class I MHC complexes derived from?

Proteins endogenously made inside the cell, such as viral proteins, intracellular pathogens, cross-presented tumor antigens, and normal cellular proteins

T cells that react too strongly with the normal cellular proteins that are a part of the class I MHC complex must be deselected during maturation in the thymus to prevent autoimmune disease

What are four genes that encode different types of class I MHC molecules?

1. HLA-A
2. HLA-B
3. HLA-C
4. HLA-D

What is the second chain of the class I MHC complex?

β_2-Microglobulin, a member of the immunoglobulin supergene family

What chromosome codes for the HLA gene?

Chromosome 6

What cells express class I MHC molecules?

All nucleated cells

What type of T-cell recognizes class I MHC molecules?

CD8 T cells

What occurs when the activated CD8 T cell binds to the class I MHC?	1. Clonal expansion of the T cell 2. Killing of infected cell

CLASS II MAJOR HISTOCOMPATIBILITY COMPLEX

Where are the peptides presented on class II MHC complexes derived from?	Extracellular or phagocytosed proteins
What are three gene pairs that encode different types of class II MHCs?	1. HLA-DP 2. HLA-DQ 3. HLA-DR
What do these genes encode?	Cell-surface glycoproteins made of two polypeptide chains
What are the two polypeptide chains called?	α and β
What cells express class II MHC molecules?	Mainly antigen-presenting cells
What are three antigen-presenting cells?	1. Macrophages 2. Dendritic cells 3. B cells
What type of T cell binds to class II MHCs?	CD4 T cells
	The MHC class number × T cell CD number equals 8 Class I MHC × CD8 = 8 Class II MHC × CD4 = 8
What occurs when activated CD4 T cells bind to class II MHCs?	1. Clonal expansion of the T cell 2. Secretion of cytokines to stimulate either a humor or cell-mediated response
What is the hallmark of MHC?	Diversity at the antigen-binding site
Why is diversity necessary?	To allow the immune system to identify and eliminate a wide range of pathogens

CD4 T CELLS

How is a CD4 T-cell activated?	Antigen-presenting cell (APC) presents a peptide associated with a class II MHC to a naïve T cell
What costimulatory signal is required for activation of a CD4 T cell?	B7 on antigen-presenting cell interacts with CD28 on CD4 T cell (see Fig. 37-4)

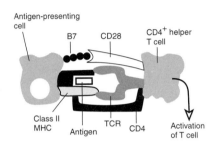

Figure 37-4. T-cell interaction with antigen-presenting cell

Where does antigen-presentation to CD4 T cells occur?	Secondary lymph tissues (e.g., spleen, lymph nodes)
What are two types of CD4 cells?	Type 1 (Th-1) and type 2 (Th-2)
What determines if a CD4 cell becomes a type 1 or a type 2?	Cytokines present in the paracortical space of lymph nodes
What cytokines lead to the development of type 1 cells?	Interferon (IFN)-γ from natural killer cells and IL-12 from macrophages
What are the actions of type 1 (Th-1) cells?	1. Produces IL-2, which stimulates CD4 T cells to divide, and activates CD8 T cells 2. Produces interferon-γ, which increases expression of class II MHC and B7 proteins on APC, enhancing the delayed-type hypersensitivity response 3. Creates a memory cell population
What type of reaction involves Th-1 cells?	Delayed-type hypersensitivity

What type of immunity do Th-1 cells primarily activate?

Cell-mediated immunity

What cytokine leads to the development of type 2 cells?

IL-4 produced by CD4 T cells

What are the actions of type 2 (Th-2) cells?

1. Expresses CD40 ligand
2. Secretes IL-4, IL-5, and IL-6, which activate B cells and facilitate antibody production (see Fig. 37-5)

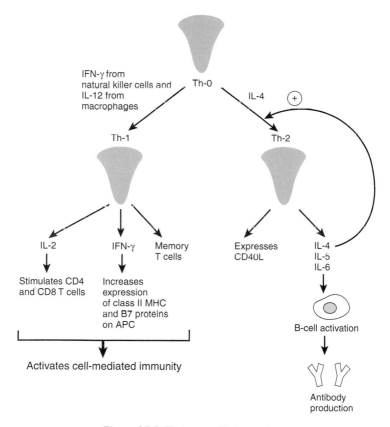

Figure 37-5. Th-1 versus Th-2 stimulation

Th-2 cells primarily activate which type of immunity?

Humoral immunity

CD8 T CELLS

How are CD8 T cells activated?	Nucleated cells present a peptide (but not the whole protein) associated with a class I MHC to a naïve T cell
What costimulatory signals are required for full activation of a CD8 cell?	IL-2 secreted from type 1 helper T cells (Th-1) or the interaction between B7 of the antigen-presenting cell with CD28 of the T cell (see Fig. 37-6)

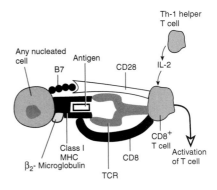

Figure 37-6. CD8+ T-cell interaction with antigen-presenting cell

What are the actions of activated CD8 T cells?	1. Stimulates CD8 T cell to divide 2. Produces and secretes interferons, tumor necrosis factor, and other cytokines 3. Kills infected cells 4. Creates a memory cell population
How does a CD8 T-cell kill its target?	1. Osmotic lysis 2. Inducing apoptosis
How does a CD8 T-cell kill target cells via osmotic lysis?	By formation and exocytosis of perforins, cytotoxic substances that form channels through the target cell's plasma membrane
How do CD8 T-cells induce apoptosis?	1. Release limited number of perforins that form pores 2. Release proteases from granules that pass through pores and degrade target cell deoxyribonucleic acid (DNA)

3. Degraded DNA stimulates apoptosis of target cell

Why don't killed viral vaccines stimulate a CD8 T-cell response?

CD8 T cells only attack cells that contain antigens displayed on class I MHC molecules; killed pathogens are not processed and displayed with class I MHC molecules

Killed viral vaccines stimulate a CD4 T-cell and antibody response, but not a CD8 T-cell response

SUPERANTIGENS

What are superantigens?

Molecules that are not processed by antigen-presenting cells, but bind class II MHC molecules and TCR-β chains outside the antigen-binding site of the MHC receptor (see Fig. 37-7)

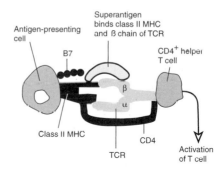

Figure 37-7. T-cell activation by a superantigen

What is the result of this interaction?

Nonspecific activation of T cells with various antigen-binding sites and massive cytokine release

What can this cause clinically?

Disseminated intravascular coagulation (DIC), hypotension, and shock

How?

Cytokines activate platelets and cause vasodilatation

What are four examples of superantigens?

1. Staphylococcal toxic shock syndrome toxin-1 (TSST-1)
2. Streptococcal pyrogenic exotoxin (Spe)

> 3. Staphylococcal enterotoxins (SE)
> 4. Exfoliative dermatitis toxin

IMMUNODEFICIENCY DISORDERS

What are three disorders characterized by immunodeficiency of T cells?

1. DiGeorge syndrome
2. Chronic mucocutaneous candidiasis
3. HIV

What is DiGeorge syndrome?

Congenital thymic aplasia or hypoplasia resulting from a defect in the embryonic development of the third and fourth pharyngeal pouches
"CATCH 22"
Congenital heart disease
Abnormal facies
Thymic aplasia
Cleft palate
Hypocalcemia
22q gene deletion

What is the result of this disorder?

Increased rate of infection because of a lack of T-cell maturation

What is chronic mucocutaneous candidiasis?

Infection of skin and mucous membranes with *Candida albicans* because of a defect in T-cell response to *Candida*

What is the T-cell response to other organisms?

Normal

What molecule does HIV bind to?

CD4

Which cells does this affect?

CD4 T cells and CD4 monocytes/ macrophages including central nervous system (CNS) microglia

38

B Cells & Humoral Immunity

B CELLS

What type of cells are B cells?

Lymphocytes

What type of immunity are B cells a key component for?

Humoral immunity

What type of pathogens do B cells mainly target with this type of immunity?

Extracellular pathogens

What are three roles of B cells?

1. Antigen-presenting cells
2. Differentiation into plasma cells that produce antibodies
3. Forming memory cells for future infections

What transmembrane proteins function as antigen receptors on B cells?

IgM and IgD antibodies expressed on the cell surface

What distinguishes the binding of B cells to antigens from the binding of T cells to antigens?

B cells bind protein, carbohydrate, lipid, or nucleic acid (not just peptides)
T cells only bind to peptides presented by major histocompatibility complex (MHC) complexes

What is the difference between a "traditional" antigen-presenting cell (e.g., a macrophage or dendritic cell) and a B cell?

In B-cell antigen presentation, repeated epitopes present in bacteria and fungi cross-link many B-cell receptors (IgM and IgD on the surface of B cells) to form aggregates, promoting endocytosis; the antigens are processed and presented in the context of class II MHC molecules to activate helper T cells

Is this process efficient for activating T cells?

Not for naïve T cells because B cells do not synthesize IL-1, but it is efficient for activating memory T cells because IL-1 is unnecessary

What is a plasma cell?

A terminally differentiated B cell that produces antibodies with the same specificity as the B-cell receptor

What stimulates B cells to become plasma cells?

Activation of B cells with antigens and helper T cells

What are three phases of B cell maturation?

1. Gene rearrangement in the bone marrow
2. Antigen-independent phase in the bone marrow
3. Antigen-dependent phase in the lymph node

What are three steps of gene rearrangement?

1. Heavy (H)-chain rearrangement
2. Kappa (κ) light-chain rearrangement
3. Lambda (λ) light-chain rearrangement

What do these chains correspond to?

The chains that make up an antibody

What occurs during each of the following?
Heavy (H)-chain rearrangement?

1. A diversity (D) segment and a joining (J) segment rearrange to form a productive DJ segment; the remaining J segment is still present
2. The DJ segment joins with a variable gene segment (V_H) to form a VDJ segment
3. Transcription of DNA with subsequent splicing of RNA to remove the remaining J segment and intervening sequences and join the VDJ segment to the constant gene
4. Translation to form a heavy chain polypeptide (see Fig. 38-1)

Kappa (κ) light-chain rearrangement?

A Vκ segment is joined with a Jκ segment to form a contiguous domain that can be transcribed, with the resultant RNA translated to form a kappa light chain

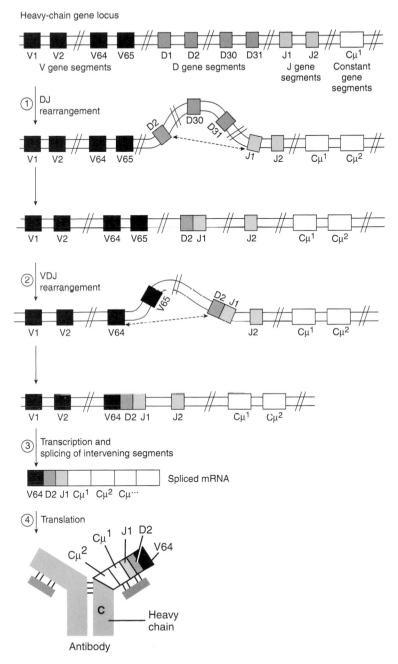

Figure 38-1. Heavy chain rearrangement.

Lambda (λ) light-chain rearrangement?

A V_λ segment is joined with a J_λ segment to form a contiguous domain that can be transcribed, with the resultant RNA translated to form a lambda light chain

H-chain rearrangement occurs in every B cell, however, only one type of light chain undergoes gene rearrangement in that cell, i.e., either κ or λ light-chain rearrangement (see Fig. 38-2)

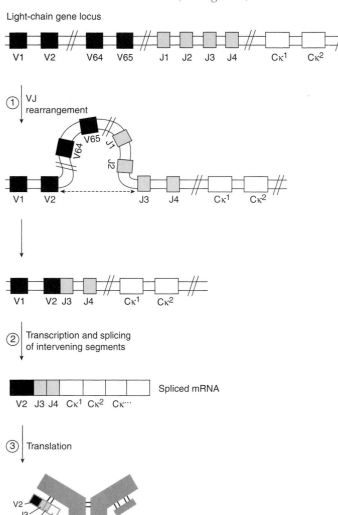

Light-chain gene locus

Figure 38-2. Light chain rearrangement.

What two enzymes are involved in gene rearrangement?

1. Recombinase
2. Exonucleases
Rearrangement is an error-prone process that is imprecise and yields unproductive products in addition to successful, highly variable gene products

What is antigen-independent maturation of B cells?

Maturation of stem cells into naïve, mature B cells without exposure to antigens

What are the different stages of B cells in antigen-independent maturation?

1. Stem cell
2. Pro-B cell
3. Pre-B cell
4. Naïve, immature B cell
5. Naïve, mature B cell (see Fig. 38-3)

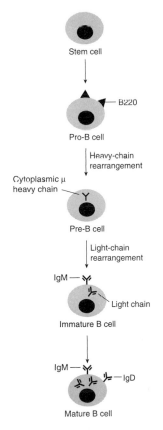

Figure 38-3. Stages of antigen-independent B-cell maturation.

Define the following:

Pro-B cell?

Cell that expresses B220 and is actively rearranging immunoglobulin genes

Pre-B cell?

Cell that synthesizes cytoplasmic μ heavy chains

Naïve, immature B cell?

Cell that expresses surface IgM after successfully synthesizing μ heavy chains and either κ or λ light chains

Naïve, mature B cell?

Cell that expresses both surface IgM and IgD after successfully synthesizing light chains, μ heavy chains, and δ heavy chains

What is antigen-dependent maturation?

Maturation of B cells that is dependent on exposure to antigen resulting in B-cell proliferation and differentiation into antibody-producing plasma cells

What are two ways that B cells become activated to differentiate into plasma cells?

1. T-helper cell activation
2. T-cell independent activation

What is T-helper cell activation?

Th-2 (and Th-1) helper T cells bind to the antigen/class II MHC complex on the surface of B cells and activate proliferation and differentiation of B cells into plasma cells by 3 methods:
1. Costimulation between CD28 on T cells and B7 on B cells induces IL-2 production by T cells
2. Costimulation between CD40L on T cells and CD40 on B cells induces class switching
3. Secretion of IL-4 and IL-5

What is T-cell–independent activation?

Activation by a large, repeating epitope that cross-links many B-cell receptors, resulting in activation of the cell without a helper T-cell signal

What is an example of a T-independent antigen?

Lipopolysaccharides (LPS) found in gram-negative bacterial cell walls

ANTIBODIES

What are antibodies?

Soluble, globular proteins that are important components of the acquired immune response

What is another name for antibodies?

Immunoglobulins

How many epitopes can an antibody recognize?

Only 1

Which cells produce antibodies?

Plasma cells

What are five functions of antibodies?

1. Opsonize bacteria
2. Neutralize toxins
3. Activate complement
4. Prevent microorganism adherence
5. Mediate lysis of microorganisms by binding

What type of antibody is made during a human response to antigen?

Polyclonal

   What does this mean?

Antibody response to antigen is heterogeneous because many different plasma cells are producing antibodies

What type of antibody can be made in the lab?

Monoclonal

   What does this mean?

The antibodies produced are identical

What are the components of an antibody?

2 heavy chains and 2 light chains

What links these chains?

Disulfide bonds (see Fig. 38-4)

What are two types of light chains?

κ and λ, corresponding to the gene used during rearrangement
Every person has both κ and λ light chains, however each antibody contains only one type

Antibody structure

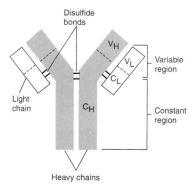

Figure 38-4. Heavy and light chains of an antibody.

What regions are found in both heavy and light chains?

Variable and constant

What fragments are created in the lab by digestion of an antibody with papain?

Two identical Fab fragments and a Fc fragment (see Fig. 38-5)

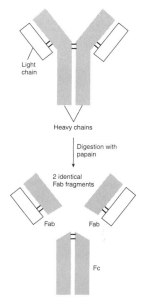

Figure 38-5. Digestion of antibody with papain to create Fab and Fc fragments

What is the role of the Fab fragment?	Bind to antigen
What is the role of the Fc fragment?	Binds complement and Fc receptors on cells
What are isotypes?	Different antibody classes based on the heavy-chain gene used during class switching
What are five examples of isotypes?	1. IgM (μ heavy chain) 2. IgD (δ heavy chain) 3. IgG (γ heavy chain) 4. IgA (α heavy chain) 5. IgE (ϵ heavy chain)
What is immunoglobulin class switching? How does this occur?	Isotype switching from IgM initially to IgD, IgG, IgA, or IgE IgM switches to IgD by alternate RNA splicing that incorporates messenger ribonucleic acid (mRNA) from a different constant gene (Cδ) IgM switches to IgG, IgA, and IgE by a second DNA rearrangement involving the constant region (see Fig. 38-6)
What triggers class switching?	Cytokines released by helper (CD4) T cells
Which isotype is . . . **Produced first in a primary immune response?**	IgM
Predominant in the secondary immune response?	IgG
Predominant in the blood?	IgG
What are allotypes?	Allelic polymorphisms within portions of the antibody genes that vary among individuals

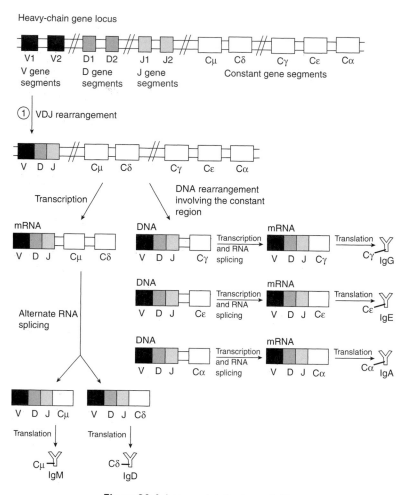

Figure 38-6. Immunoglobulin class switching

What are idiotypes?	Differing amino acid sequences in the hypervariable region that are unique for the immunoglobulin produced by a specific clone of antibody-producing cells
What is somatic hypermutation?	Process causing mutations in the hypervariable region of antibodies, resulting in generation of greater diversity, allowing selection for increased affinity for the antigen in future

IgM

What are two forms of IgM?	1. Pentameric IgM, which is found in the circulation 2. Monomeric IgM, which is found on the surface of B cells I<u>g</u>M forms <u>M</u>acromolecules
What links the pentameric IgM molecules together?	Polypeptide J chain and disulfide bonds (see Fig. 38-7)

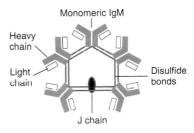

Figure 38-7. Schematic of pentameric IgM.

What other isotype is found on the surface of B cells?	IgD
What is the main action of pentameric IgM?	Activation of complement
Can IgM cross the placenta?	No
What are natural isohemagglutinins?	A subset of IgM antibodies that react against antigens resembling the ABO blood group types Natural isohemagglutinins are the reason why people with type A blood produce antibodies against type B blood and vice-versa
What is their clinical significance?	They can cause hemolytic transfusion reactions if people receive blood with an A or B type that they do not have

What type of antibodies against ABO blood types do people with . . .

    Type AB blood make? None

    Type O blood make? Antibodies against type A and type B blood

IgG

Where is IgG found? Predominant isotype found in blood, lymph, cerebrospinal fluid (CSF), and peritoneal fluid

How many subclasses of IgG exist? 5: IgG_1, IgG_{2a}, IgG_{2b}, IgG_3, IgG_4

What is the half-life of IgG? Roughly 20 days, which is the longest of all isotypes

    What is the clinical significance of this? Because of its long half-life, IgG is used for passive immunization

What is unique about the transmission of IgG? It is the only immunoglobulin that can cross the placenta

    What disease can this cause? Erythroblastosis fetalis

    Define this condition. Disease that occurs when IgG from a Rh(–) mother crosses the placenta and is directed against Rh(+) fetal red blood cell antigens, causing hemolysis in the fetus

    When can it occur? Only with the second or subsequent pregnancy because the first child generates the first Rh exposure to the Rh(–) mother

    How is it prevented? By administering RhoGAM, an Rh immune globulin that binds to and covers the Rh antigen, to prevent a maternal antibody response

How does IgG aid in cell-mediated immunity? IgG binds to antigens and enhances uptake by phagocytes through opsonization

What is ADCC?

Antibody-dependent, cell-mediated cytotoxicity, a process that occurs when IgG binds to antigen and stimulates natural killer cells to destroy the invading pathogen

Can IgG activate complement?

Yes, but not as efficiently as IgM because it is not pentavalent

IgA

Where is IgA found?

In secretions including mucus, tears, saliva, gastric fluid, sweat, and breast milk

How does IgA exist in secretions?

As dimers

What links the molecules together?

Polypeptide J chain (see Fig. 38-8)

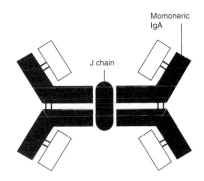

Figure 38-8. Schematic of dimeric IgA.

Where is IgA formed?

In plasma cells within the blood

How does IgA get into secretions?

It must cross epithelial cells

How does IgA achieve this?

Dimeric IgA binds to poly-Ig receptors on the basal membrane of epithelial cells and is taken into the cell by endocytosis

How is IgA released from cells?

Endocytic vesicle fuses with the luminal membrane of the epithelial cell and the poly-Ig receptor is cleaved (see Fig. 38-9)

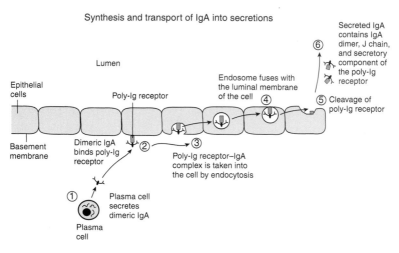

Figure 38-9. Transport of IgA into secretions.

What does secretory IgA consist of?	1. IgA dimer
	2. Polypeptide J chain
	3. Portion of the poly-Ig receptor called the secretory component

What is the main role of IgA?	Prevent adherence and penetration of microorganisms

Can IgA activate complement?	No

IgE

Where is IgE found?	At low concentrations in the serum

What is the main role of IgE?	Triggers degranulation of mast cells and basophils

How does it perform this role?	1. First exposure to an antigen causes "sensitization" whereby plasma cells synthesize IgE
	2. The Fc portion of IgE binds to mast cells and basophils
	3. In subsequent exposures, antigen binds to the F_{ab} portion of IgE, causing the IgE to cross-link and stimulate

degranulation of previously bound
mast cells/basophils (see Fig. 38-10)

**What compounds are
released by degranulation?**

Histamine, leukotrienes, prostaglandins,
heparin, and other chemicals

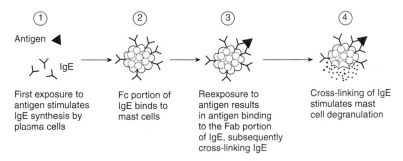

First exposure to
antigen stimulates
IgE synthesis by
plasma cells

Fc portion of
IgE binds to
mast cells

Reexposure to
antigen results
in antigen binding
to the Fab portion
of IgE, subsequently
cross-linking IgE

Cross-linking of IgE
stimulates mast
cell degranulation

Figure 38-10. Mast cell sensitization and degranulation mediated by IgE.

**What do these compounds
cause?**

Vascular permeability and increased
blood flow

**What type of allergic
reaction does IgE mediate?**

Type I hypersensitivity response

**How does this present
clinically?**

Anaphylaxis, asthma, or local wheal

**What type of infection
results in elevated IgE
levels?**

Helminth infections

IMMUNODEFICIENCY DISORDERS

**What are three disorders
characterized by
immunodeficiency of B
cells or antibodies?**

1. Bruton's agammaglobulinemia
2. Selective IgA deficiency
3. Common variable immunodeficiency (CVID)

**What are patients with
these disorders at higher
risk for?**

Recurrent infections with encapsulated
bacteria, including *Streptococcus
pneumoniae* and *Haemophilus influenzae*

**What is Bruton's
agammaglobulinemia?**

X-linked recessive disorder characterized
by a defective gene for tyrosine kinase
resulting in low levels of B cells and
immunoglobulins

What is IgA deficiency?   The most common immune deficiency resulting in a lack of IgA; most patients, however, are asymptomatic

What is common variable immunodeficiency?   An acquired immunodeficiency characterized by normal levels of B cells, but low levels of IgG and other immunoglobulins

39

Complement

What is complement?

A division of the innate immune system comprised of approximately 20 serum proteins that form a cascade to mediate direct attack, lysis, and clearance of microorganisms at the point of entry

Where are complement proteins synthesized?

Mainly in hepatocytes, but also in blood monocytes, tissue macrophages, and epithelial cells of the gastrointestinal (GI) tract

What are the two different pathways of the complement system?

1. Classic complement pathway
2. Alternative complement pathway

Why is it called the classic rather than alternative complement pathway?

No clinical reason; the classical pathway was discovered first

Which pathway is activated upon first exposure to a microorganism?
   Why?

Alternative complement pathway

An antibody response (which stimulates the classic complement pathway) does not mount until several weeks after exposure

What is common to both pathways?

Ultimately, formation of C3b, which can either generate C5 convertase or act alone as an opsonin

What is C5 convertase?

Enzyme that ultimately forms the membrane attack complex (MAC), which lyses pathogens

COMMON COMPLEMENT PATHWAY

What are four main effects of complement, regardless of the pathway by which it was activated?

1. Opsonization (enhancement of phagocytosis)
2. Generation of inflammatory mediators and chemotaxins
3. Lysis of cells such as bacteria and tumor cells
4. Immune complex clearance

What is opsonization?

Enhancement of phagocytosis by certain immunoglobulins and complement components that bind to receptors on phagocytes

What component of the complement system is most involved in opsonization?

C3b

What are the complement anaphylatoxins?

C3a, C4a, and C5a cause degranulation of mast cells and release of mediators, including histamine, leading to local inflammation

Of the three (C3a, C4a, C5a), which is the most powerful anaphylatoxin?

C5a

What parts of the complement cascade are involved in forming the membrane attack complex?

C5b, 6, 7, 8, 9, along with C5 convertase (see Fig. 39-1)

What is the mechanism of cell death via the membrane attack complex?

Osmotic cytolysis, i.e., the cell bursts as a result of an influx of ions and water

What are four endogenous methods of regulating the complement system?

1. Inhibitors of the C1 protease
2. Binding of factor H to C3b and subsequent cleavage of C3b by factor I
3. Presence of decay-accelerating factor on the surface of human cells, which degrades C3 and C5 convertases
4. Regulating the availability of IgG and IgM

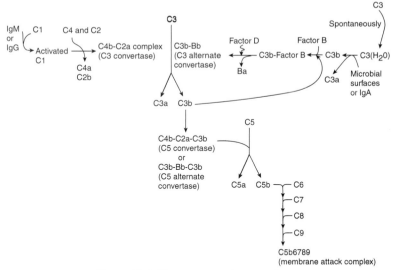

Figure 39-1. The entire complement pathway.

| The complement system is involved in which hypersensitivity reactions? | Types II and III |

CLASSIC COMPLEMENT PATHWAY

What activates the classic complement pathway?	IgM and IgG
When?	When they are bound to antigen and form antigen–antibody complexes
	IgG and IgM are known as the "complement-fixing" antibodies

| How do these antibodies initiate the classic complement pathway? | The Fc region of IgM and IgG binds to and activates C1 |

| What components of the classic complement pathway combine to form C3 convertase? | C4b and C2a, formed when the C1 protease cleaves C2 and C4 |

| What components of the classic complement pathway combine to form C5 convertase? | C4b, C2a, and C3b (see Fig. 39-2) |

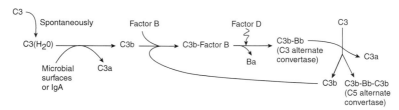

Figure 39-2. The classic complement pathway.

ALTERNATIVE COMPLEMENT PATHWAY

What activates the alternative complement pathway?

Microbial surfaces (including endotoxin) and aggregated IgA

What components of the alternative complement pathway combine to form C3 convertase?

C3b and Factor Bb

What components of the alternative complement pathway combine to form C5 convertase?

2 components of C3b with 1 component of Factor Bb (see Fig. 39-3)

Figure 39-3. The alternative complement pathway.

IMMUNODEFICIENCY DISORDERS

What condition is at increased risk if a patient has . . .

    A deficiency of C1 esterase inhibitor?

Angioedema

            Why?

Unrestrained production of anaphylatoxins from the complement cascade results in increased capillary permeability

A deficiency of C2 and C4?

Symptoms that resemble systemic lupus erythematosus and other related autoimmune diseases

Patients with systemic lupus erythematosus often have low levels of C2 and C4

What other condition is associated with low levels of C2 and C4?

Pregnancy

A deficiency of C3?

Severe, recurrent pyogenic sinus and respiratory tract infections

A deficiency of C5–C8?

Neisseria bacteremia

A deficiency of decay-accelerating factor?

Paroxysmal nocturnal hemoglobinuria, a disorder characterized by increased complement-mediated hemolysis

40

Immunodeficiency

OVERVIEW

What are four types of immunodeficiency?

1. Humoral immunity (B cell) dysfunction
2. Cellular immunity (T cell) dysfunction
3. Combined humoral and cellular immunity (B and T cell) dysfunction
4. Innate immunity (neutrophil) dysfunction

What are two examples of B-cell immunodeficiencies?

1. Bruton agammaglobulinemia (X-linked agammaglobulinemia)
2. Selective immunoglobulin deficiencies, e.g., Ig A deficiency, common variable hypogammaglobinemia

What types of pathogens generally infect patients with such immunodeficiencies?

Extracellular pathogens (mostly bacteria)

What are four examples of T-cell immunodeficiencies?

1. DiGeorge syndrome (thymic aplasia)
2. Chronic mucocutaneous candidiasis
3. Hyper IgM syndrome
4. Interleukin-12 (IL-12) receptor deficiency

What types of pathogens generally infect patients with such immuno-deficiencies?

Intracellular pathogens and opportunistic pathogens (viral and fungal)

What are three examples of combined B- and T-cell immunodeficiencies?

1. Severe combined immunodeficiency (SCID)
2. Wiskott-Aldrich syndrome
3. Ataxia-telangiectasia

What are two examples of innate immune system dysfunction?

1. Specific complement deficiency
2. Neutrophil dysfunction

What are four examples of neutrophil immuno-deficiencies?	1. Chédiak-Higashi disease 2. Chronic granulomatous disease 3. Jobs syndrome 4. Leukocyte adhesion deficiency
What types of pathogens generally infect patients with such immuno-deficiencies?	Staphylococcal infections

B-CELL DEFICIENCIES

BRUTON AGAMMAGLOBULINEMIA

What enzyme is altered in Bruton agammaglo-bulinemia?	Tyrosine kinase
What gene defect is responsible for this?	The Btx gene (X-linked recessive)
Who is commonly affected by Bruton agammaglo-bulinemia?	Males because it's X-linked
What immunoglobulins are deficient in these patients?	Almost all immunoglobins of any type
What are the common clinical manifestations of Bruton agammaglo-bulinemia?	Recurrent sinus and lung infections, including those caused by *Streptococcus pneumonia, Haemophilus influenzae, Streptococcus pyogenes,* and *Staphylococcus aureus*
When do they present?	Around 6 months of age
Why?	At around 4–6 months of age infants lose the protection of maternal antibodies

IgA DEFICIENCY

How common is IgA deficiency?	Most common cause of immunodeficiency; it is present in up to 1 in 800 people
What is the probable cause of IgA deficiency?	Failure of heavy-chain switching as a consequence of missing IgA-specific factors

What types of infections do these patients frequently contract?	Recurrent sinus and lung infections

COMMON VARIABLE HYPOGAMMAGLOBINEMIA

What characterizes common variable hypogammaglobinemia?	Recurrent pyogenic infection from reduced ability to produce IgG, IgA, and IgM

T-CELL DEFICIENCIES

DiGEORGE SYNDROME (THYMIC APLASIA)

Which two structures fail to form properly in DiGeorge syndrome?	1. Thymus 2. Parathyroid glands
What is the embryologic origin for this anomaly?	Failure of the third and fourth pharyngeal pouches to develop normally
What chromosome is involved?	Chromosome 22 Remember DiGeorge by "Catch 22" Congenital heart disease Abnormal facies Thymic aplasia Cleft palate Hypocalcemia 22q gene deletion
What is the most common clinical presentation of DiGeorge syndrome?	Tetany secondary to hypocalcemia/hypoparathyroidism
What infections are common in DiGeorge syndrome?	Severe viral, fungal, and protozoal infections, including *Pneumocystis carinii* (p. jiroveci) pneumonia and thrush

CHRONIC MUCOCUTANEOUS CANDIDIASIS

What do patients with chronic mucocutaneous candidiasis lack?	Specific T cells for *Candida albicans*

HYPER-IgM SYNDROME

Which gene is mutated in Hyper-IgM syndrome?	CD40 ligand on CD4 T cells
Which immunoglobulins are deficient?	IgG, IgA, and IgE

INTERLEUKIN-12 RECEPTOR DEFICIENCY

What infections occur in patients with IL-12 receptor deficiency?	Disseminated mycobacterial infections

COMBINED B- AND T-CELL DEFICIENCIES

SEVERE COMBINED IMMUNODEFICIENCY DISEASE

What is SCID?	A severe humoral and cell-mediated immunity dysfunction characterized by an inability to effectively fight off bacterial, fungal, viral, and protozoal infections
What are the two causes of SCID?	1. X-linked defect resulting in a defective IL-2 or ZAP-70 receptors 2. Autosomal defect resulting in recombinase enzymes mutations from defective RAG-1 or RAG-2 genes
How is the defect inherited?	1. X-linked form (75%) 2. Autosomal recessive form (25%)
What are the clinical manifestations of SCID?	Early infancy infections from bacteria, fungi, viruses, and protozoa
What are two possible treatments?	1. Bone marrow transplantation 2. Gene therapy
What is the prognosis?	Without treatment, death commonly occurs before 1 year of life

WISKOTT-ALDRICH SYNDROME

How is Wiskott-Aldrich syndrome inherited?	X-linked

What are three clinical manifestations of Wiskott-Aldrich syndrome?	1. Eczema 2. Thrombocytopenia 3. Repeated infections caused by variable cell-mediated immunity
How are immunoglobulin titers affected in this disease?	Low IgM Normal IgG and IgA Elevated IgE

ATAXIA-TELANGIECTASIA

How is ataxia-telangiectasia inherited?	Autosomally recessive
What type of gene product is defective in ataxia-telangiectasia?	Deoxyribonucleic acid (DNA) repair enzymes
What are three clinical manifestations of ataxia-telangiectasia?	1. Difficulty walking, i.e., ataxia 2. Dilated superficial capillaries seen on the face, i.e., telangiectasias 3. Recurrent infections
When do the symptoms of ataxia-telangiectasia manifest?	By age 2 years
What are the immunologic manifestations of ataxia-telangiectasia caused by?	Maldevelopment of the thymus

INNATE IMMUNE SYSTEM DYSFUNCTION

COMPLEMENT DEFICIENCIES

What are three components of the complement pathway?	1. Classic pathway 2. Alternative pathway 3. Common final pathway, i.e., membrane attack complex
What two acquired conditions cause complement deficiencies?	1. Liver failure resulting in reduced synthesis of complement proteins 2. Malnutrition resulting in reduced amino acid precursors

What is associated with C1, C2, and C4 deficiency?	Autoimmune disorders secondary to immune complexes, e.g., lupus
What is associated with C3 deficiency?	Severe pyogenic infections
What is associated with C6, C7, and C8 deficiency?	Neisseria infections

NEUTROPHIL DYSFUNCTION

CHÉDIAK-HIGASHI SYNDROME

What is Chédiak-Higashi syndrome?	Autosomal recessive defect in neutrophil lysosomes
What are two defects seen in neutrophils with this disease?	1. Cytoplasmic granule fusion 2. Defective degranulation
What pathogen are these patients commonly susceptible to?	Staphylococcal infections

CHRONIC GRANULOMATOUS DISEASE

What is chronic granulomatous disease?	Rare disease characterized by defective oxidative burst in neutrophils secondary to a lack of nicotinamide adenine dinucleotide phosphate (NADPH) oxidase
What test is used to detect it?	Nitroblue tetrazolium dye reduction test
How does the test work?	Presence of disease results in absence of clear to blue color change
How is chronic granulo-matous disease inherited?	60–80% X-linked recessive; the remainder are inherited autosomal recessively
What pathogen are these patients commonly susceptible to?	Staphylococcal infections

JOB SYNDROME

What are three characteristics of Job syndrome?	1. Frequent staphylococcal abscesses 2. Eczema 3. Elevated IgE
What is defective in this syndrome?	Helper T cells do not produce interferon-γ
What is the result of this defect?	An increased helper T-cell 2 (Th-2) response resulting in a high IgE and histamine release

LEUKOCYTE ADHESION DEFICIENCY SYNDROME

What proteins are defective in leukocyte adhesion deficiency syndrome?	Surface adhesion (leukocyte factor antigen-1 [LFA-1]) proteins on phagocytic cells
How does this defect affect neutrophils?	Impaired phagocytosis, chemotaxis, and spreading, i.e., diapedesis
What are the clinical manifestations of leukocyte adhesion deficiency syndrome?	Recurrent skin and mucosal infections

41

Hypersensitivity

OVERVIEW

What is a . . .

Type I hypersensitivity reaction?

An anaphylactic and atopic response mediated by Ig E cross-linking antigens to host cells

Type II hypersensitivity reaction?

A cytotoxic response mediated by antigen binding with IgG and IgM on host cells

Type III hypersensitivity reaction?

An immune response mediated by antibodies binding to host tissue with ensuing inflammation

Type IV hypersensitivity reaction?

A delayed, cell-mediated response mediated by T lymphocytes that encounter antigens and release inflammatory components

TYPE I HYPERSENSITIVITY REACTION

What is a type I hypersensitivity reaction?

An anaphylactic and atopic response mediated by IgE cross-linking antigens to host cells (see Fig. 41-1)

What are two examples?

1. Systemic anaphylactic reaction
2. Atopic reaction

What is systemic anaphylaxis?

A life-threatening IgE-mediated hypersensitivity, characterized by severe hypotension, bronchoconstriction, and massive release of mast cell and basophil mediators

What are three common causes of systemic anaphylaxis?

1. Drugs
2. Insect venom
3. Food

What is an atopic reaction?

A non–life-threatening IgE-mediated hypersensitivity, characterized by a localized inflammatory process

Type I hypersensitivity

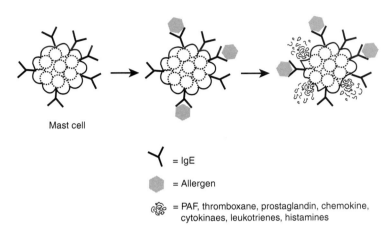

Mast cell

Y = IgE

⬡ = Allergen

🦠 = PAF, thromboxane, prostaglandin, chemokine, cytokinaes, leukotrienes, histamines

Figure 41-1. Type I hypersensitivity. PAF = platelet-activating factor.

What is a common example of an atopic reaction?	Atopic dermatitis seen in asthmatics, i.e., eczema
What host cell receptors does IgE target?	Fc receptors of mast cells and basophils
What common factor do mast cells and basophils release?	Histamine
What are five other substances released by mast cells?	1. Platelet-activating factor (PAF) 2. Thromboxanes 3. Prostaglandins 4. Chemotactic factors for eosinophils and neutrophils 5. Slow-reacting substance of anaphylaxis (SRS-A)
What is the difference between anaphylaxis and anaphylactoid reactions?	Anaphylactoid reactions do not involve IgE

TYPE II HYPERSENSITIVITY REACTION

What is a type II hypersensitivity reaction?	A cytotoxic response mediated by antigens binding with IgG and IgM on host cells (see Fig. 41-2)

Type II hypersensitivity

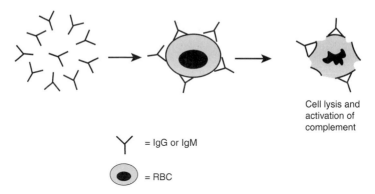

Cell lysis and
activation of
complement

Y = IgG or IgM

● = RBC

Figure 41-2. Type II hypersensitivity. RBC = red blood cell.

What are two mechanisms for Type II hypersensitivity reactions?

1. Lysis of cells because of either complement activation (direct) or opsonization (indirect)
2. Antibody-dependent cell-mediated toxicity (ADCC) predominately by natural killer (NK) cells

What are three common targets of cytotoxic hypersensitivity?

1. Erythrocyte membrane, e.g., transfusion reactions
2. Antigens of basement membranes, e.g., Goodpasture disease
3. Acetylcholine (ACh) receptors

What are three clinical manifestations of type II hypersensitivity against the erythrocyte membrane?

1. ABO incompatibility, i.e., transfusion reactions
2. Rh incompatibility, i.e., erythroblastosis fetalis
3. Drug-induced hemolytic anemia

What class of antibody is associated with ABO incompatibility?

IgM
IgM is primarily found in the serum

What class of antibody is associated with erythroblastosis fetalis?
  What is the mechanism?

IgG
IgG is the only immunoglobulin that can cross the placenta
Maternal antibody that is formed to previous exposure to Rh antigen, which subsequently crosses the placenta in a pregnancy

What two conditions predispose the mother to develop this particular IgG?	1. Second, or subsequent, Rh+ fetus born to an Rh– mother 2. Exposure to the Rh antigen, e.g., in a blood transfusion
How does penicillin cause a type II hypersensitivity drug-induced hemolytic anemia?	Covalent linkage of penicillin to erythrocyte membrane proteins
What is another mechanism by which penicillin can cause a hypersensitivity reaction?	By a type III hypersensitivity
What are two autoimmune clinical manifestations of type II hypersensitivity?	1. Goodpasture disease 2. Myasthenia gravis
What is Goodpasture disease?	Disease characterized by an immune response against the lung and kidney parenchyma basement membranes
What is myasthenia gravis?	Disease causing fatigable skeletal muscular weakness because of autoantibodies to ACh receptor
Which muscles are most seriously affected in myasthenia gravis?	Diaphragm and muscles innervated by cranial nerves

TYPE III HYPERSENSITIVITY REACTION

What is a type III hypersensitivity reaction?	An immune response mediated by antibodies binding to host tissue with ensuing inflammation
What initiates a type III hypersensitivity reaction?	Insoluble antigen-antibody complexes (see Fig. 41-3)
What are two mechanisms of type III hypersensitivity?	1. Complement activation with neutrophil diapedesis 2. Factor XII (Hageman factor) activation
What three coagulation cascade factors are activated in type III hypersensitivity via Hageman factor?	1. Kinin 2. Fibrin 3. Plasmin

Type III hypersensitivity

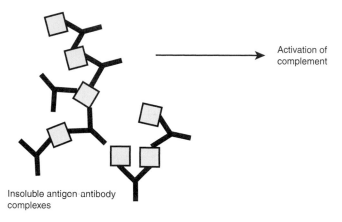

Figure 41-3. Type III hypersensitivity

What are general common presentations of immune complex-mediated reactions?	Rash, fever, lymphadenopathy, and arthralgia
What are six clinical manifestations associated with type III hypersensitivity?	1. Serum sickness 2. Arthus reaction 3. Polyarteritis nodosa (PAN) 4. Poststreptococcal glomerular nephritis 5. Systemic lupus erythematosus (SLE) 6. Rheumatoid arthritis
What is serum sickness?	Immune complex vasculitis 7–10 days following drug or allergen exposure
What symptoms are seen in serum sickness?	Fever, arthralgia/arthritis, acute glomerular nephritis, vasculitis, urticaria, purpura, and lymphadenopathy
Is the severity of serum sickness dose-dependent?	Yes
What are two common causes of serum sickness?	1. Drugs, e.g., penicillin and streptokinase 2. Antibody therapy, i.e., monoclonal or polyclonal

What is another mechanism by which penicillin can cause a hypersensitivity reaction?	By a type II hypersensitivity
What is the Arthus reaction?	Preformed antibodies activate complement to subcutaneously injected antigen causing inflammatory cell attraction and increased vascular permeability resulting in edema
What is an example of an Arthus reaction?	Immune complex hypersensitivity reaction to tetanus toxoid in an individual previously immunized with the tetanus vaccine

TYPE IV HYPERSENSITIVITY REACTION

What is a type IV hypersensitivity reaction?	A delayed, cell-mediated response mediated by T lymphocytes that encounter antigens and release inflammatory components (see Fig. 41-4)
What type of cell initiates the host response?	CD 4+ T-helper cells
What are three steps of a type IV reaction response?	1. Antigen processing in macrophage 2. T-helper cells stimulated by macrophage antigen-major histocompatibility complex class II (MHC_{II}) complex and interleukin (IL)-1 3. Activation of other T-helper cells and macrophages
What are three examples of type IV hypersensitivity reactions?	1. Tuberculin skin test, i.e., purified protein derivative (PPD) 2. Contact dermatitis, e.g., poison ivy 3. Transplant reaction
How is the PPD response evaluated?	Diameter of induration, i.e., swelling PPD is read by the diameter of induration, not the surrounding reddened area
When is the PPD response evaluated?	48–72 hours after injection

Type IV hypersensitivity

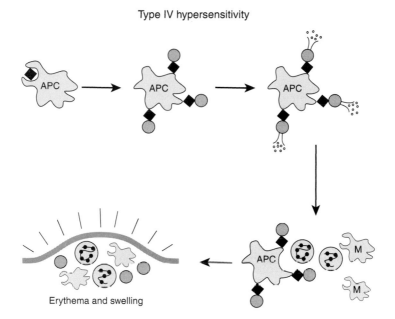

= Antigen

APC = Antigen presenting cell

= T cell

= Cytokines

= PMNs

M = Macrophages

Figure 41-4. Type IV hypersensitivity. PMNs = polymorphonuclear neutrophils.

Is a positive PPD diagnostic   No
of active disease?
  What does it indicate?   PPD tests only indicates that an infection
                                     has occurred at some point or that the
                                     person has received bacillus
                                     Calmette-Guérin (BCG) vaccine

42

Autoimmune Disease

What is an autoimmune disease?

A disease caused by an immune reaction against the body's own antigens and tissues

What are four possible mechanisms of autoimmunity?

1. Molecular mimicry
2. Alteration of normal proteins (i.e., via drugs)
3. Superantigens
4. Release of antigens from previously "privileged" sites (i.e., central nervous system [CNS], eye, testes) by trauma

What is molecular mimicry?

Phenomenon where an environmental trigger (e.g., microorganism) resembles a component of the body resulting in an immune response directed against the environmental trigger that cross-reacts with that body component

Which neoplasm are autoimmune diseases most commonly associated with?

Thymomas

What are the organ-specific autoimmune diseases that affect each of the following:
Thyroid gland?

1. Graves disease
2. Hashimoto thyroiditis

Skin?

1. Pemphigus vulgaris
2. Dermatitis herpetiformis
3. Autoimmune alopecia
4. Vitiligo

Neurons?

1. Multiple sclerosis
2. Guillain-Barré syndrome

Heart?

Rheumatic fever

Kidney?

Goodpasture syndrome

Stomach?	Pernicious anemia
Pancreas?	Type 1 diabetes mellitus
Adrenal gland?	Autoimmune Addison disease
Red blood cells?	Autoimmune hemolytic anemia
Platelets?	Idiopathic thrombocytopenic purpura
Muscle?	Myasthenia gravis

What are six systemic autoimmune diseases?
1. Systemic lupus erythematosus
2. Rheumatoid arthritis
3. Systemic necrotizing vasculitis
4. Wegener granulomatosis
5. Antiphospholipid syndrome
6. Sjögren syndrome

Rheumatoid arthritis is associated with which human leukocyte antigen (HLA) type?
HLA-DR4

Systemic lupus erythematosus is associated with which HLA types?
HLA-DR2 or HLA-DR3

Ankylosing spondylitis is associated with which HLA type?
HLA-B27

What autoimmune conditions are associated with HLA-B27?
1. Psoriasis
2. Ankylosing spondylitis
3. Inflammatory bowel disease
4. Reiter syndrome
"PAIR" is an acronym for the autoimmune conditions associated with HLA-B27

What disease is associated with each of the following: Antimicrosomal antibodies?
Hashimoto's thyroiditis

Antinuclear antibodies?
Systemic lupus erythematosus

Anti–double-stranded deoxyribonucleic acid (dsDNA) antibodies?	Systemic lupus erythematosus
Anti-Smith antibodies?	Systemic lupus erythematosus
Antihistone antibodies?	Systemic lupus erythematosus (drug-induced form)
Anti–SS-B antibodies?	Sjögren syndrome
Antiimmunoglobulin (Ig) G antibodies?	Rheumatoid arthritis
Anticentromere antibodies?	Scleroderma (limited; calcinosis cutis, Raynaud phenomenon, esophageal motility disorder, sclerodactyly, and telangiectasia [CREST] syndrome)
Antineutrophil antibodies?	Vasculitis
Anti–Scl-70 antibodies?	Scleroderma (diffuse)
Antiepithelial cell antibodies?	Pemphigus vulgaris
Antigliadin antibodies?	Celiac disease
Antimitochondrial antibodies?	Primary biliary cirrhosis
Antibasement membrane antibodies?	Goodpasture disease

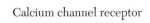

What is the target of the immune response in each of the following: Lambert-Eaton syndrome?	Calcium channel receptor
Myasthenia gravis?	Acetylcholine receptor
Graves disease?	Thyroid-stimulating hormone (TSH) receptor
Hashimoto thyroiditis?	Thyroid peroxidase and thyroglobulin

Idiopathic thrombocyto-penic purpura?	Platelet glycoproteins IIb/IIIa
Pernicious anemia?	Intrinsic factor and parietal cells
Insulin-dependent diabetes mellitus?	Pancreatic islet β cells
Addison disease?	Adrenal cortex
Polyarteritis nodosa?	Small and medium-size arteries
Guillain-Barré syndrome?	Myelin protein

Section VI

Organ Systems

43

Respiratory System

OVERVIEW

What infection-prone structures are found in each of the following:

Upper respiratory tract?
1. Oral cavity
2. Nasal cavity
3. Sinuses
4. Pharynx
5. Tonsils

Middle respiratory tract?
1. Larynx
2. Epiglottis
3. Trachea

Lower respiratory tract?
1. Bronchi
2. Bronchiole
3. Alveoli
4. Extra-alveolar lung tissue, i.e., pulmonary parenchyma

What four latent pathogens can be found in the respiratory tract?
1. *Pneumocystis carinii*, (*P. jiroveci*) in the lung
2. *Mycobacterium tuberculosis* in a dormant primary tubercle
3. Cytomegalovirus in the lymph nodes
4. Herpes simplex in neurons
5. Epstein-Barr virus in the mucosa

UPPER RESPIRATORY TRACT INFECTIONS

What is the most common pathogen that causes upper respiratory infections?

Viruses

What type of infection commonly complicates viral infections?

Bacterial infections

ORAL CAVITY

What pathogen is implicated in each of the following:

Dental carries? *Streptococcus mutans*

Oral thrush? *Candida albicans*

Periodontal disease? Anaerobic bacteria, e.g., bacteroides, actinomycetes or *Prevotella*

NASAL CAVITY AND SINUSES

What pathogens commonly cause infections of the nasal cavity (rhinitis) or sinuses (sinusitis)?
Viruses are the most common cause of rhinitis, e.g., rhinovirus, coxsackievirus A, echovirus, coronavirus, influenza virus, respiratory syncytial virus (RSV), adenovirus
Bacterial pathogens commonly infect the nasal cavity following damage caused by a viral infection

What are the common pathogens associated with each of the following:

Acute sinusitis? *Streptococcus pneumoniae*
Haemophilus influenzae

Chronic sinusitis? Mixed aerobic and anaerobic bacteria in addition to the same organisms that cause acute sinusitis
Opportunistic fungal pathogens may also infect immunocompromised persons, such as *Aspergillus*

PHARYNX

What is pharyngitis? Inflammation of the pharynx, occasionally involving the tonsils

What is the most common cause of pharyngitis? Viruses are the most common cause of pharyngitis (~60%), i.e., rhinoviruses, adenovirus, and coronavirus

What are less-common causes of pharyngitis? *Corynebacterium diphtheriae, Chlamydia pneumoniae, Neisseria gonorrhoeae,* influenza, herpes simplex virus,

Epstein-Barr virus (EBV), *Mycoplasma* and *Bordetella pertussis*

What is the most common bacterial cause of pharyngitis?

Streptococcus pyogenes

What is this condition commonly called?

Strep throat

What are the clinical manifestations?

Sore erythematous throat, temperature >39.5°C (103.1°F), general malaise, lack of cough, grayish-yellow exudates on tonsils, headache, cervical lymphadenopathy, and leukocytosis

What is a pertinent negative that helps confirm the diagnosis of strep throat?

Lack of cough

What are three possible complications of strep throat?

1. Rheumatic fever
2. Acute glomerulonephritis
3. Scarlet fever

How is pharyngitis diagnosed?

1. History and physical
2. Properly administered rapid strep test (*S. pyogenes*)
3. Monospot test (EBV)
4. Culture

What are three clinical manifestations of *Corynebacterium diphtheriae*?

1. Pseudomembrane formation
2. "Bull neck" cervical adenopathy
3. Mild pharyngitis

Pseudomembrane formation is a classic manifestation of *C. diphtheriae*

What causes pseudo-membrane formation?

An exotoxin

What are the components of the exotoxin?

The A component is a adenosine diphosphate (ADP) ribosyl transferase that ribosylates elongation factor 2 (EF-2), shutting down protein synthesis in eukaryotic cells

The B component is a trigger that induces uptake of the A component by specific cells in the host

What other organism forms pseudomembranes? **Where?**	*Clostridium difficile* In the intestine
Which two cell types other than upper respiratory tract epithelium are susceptible to *C. diphtheriae*?	1. Cardiac myocytes 2. Neurons
Are they exposed to *C. diphtheriae*?	No, only to the *C. diphtheriae* exotoxin
What are three complications of these infections?	1. Myocarditis of variable severity 2. Potential arrhythmias secondary to conduction abnormalities 3. Soft-palate paralysis and other forms of neuritis may occur later in the illness, including cranial nerve palsies
How is *C. diphtheriae* infection diagnosed?	1. History and physical 2. Culture on tellurite plate or Löffler agar 3. "Chinese characters" seen with microscopy after Gram stain
How is *C. diphtheriae* infection treated?	Airway support, diphtheria antitoxin, corticosteroids, and erythromycin/penicillin G
How is *C. diphtheriae* infection prevented?	Vaccination with DTaP, a combination of formalin-inactivated diphtheria toxoid, tetanus toxoids, and acellular *B. pertussis*
What are the clinical manifestations of *B. pertussis*?	Whooping cough, commonly seen in children too young to be vaccinated, in nonimmunized children, and in adults whose immunity has waned
Describe the course of *B. pertussis*: **Incubation period?**	Asymptomatic stage lasting 1–3 weeks
Catarrhal stage?	Runny nose (rhinorrhea) and bloodshot eyes (hyperemia) progressing to a dry cough
Paroxysmal stage?	Worsening of the cough where the patient will often cough 5–20 times violently and

Convalescent stage?

then inhale rapidly against a swollen upper airway and glottis, producing a characteristic "whoop"

Less-severe cough that may persist for weeks or even months

How is *B. pertussis* diagnosed in the laboratory?

Polymerase chain reaction (PCR)

How can a comprehensive blood count (CBC) be helpful in diagnosis?

Leukocytosis (i.e., an increase in white blood cells) and specifically lymphocytosis (i.e., increase in lymphocytes)

How is *B. pertussis* treated?

Erythromycin, which decreases toxin production, but has no affect on existing toxin
Erythromycin is also given prophylactically to sick contacts

What two vaccines exist for *B. pertussis*?

1. Purified *B. pertussis* proteins (acellular)
2. Killed whole cells

Which of these is used in the United States?

Acellular type

MIDDLE RESPIRATORY TRACT INFECTIONS

LARYNX

What is laryngitis?

Inflammation of the larynx most commonly caused by viruses, e.g., influenza, parainfluenza, and adenovirus

What are the clinical manifestations of laryngitis?

Acute onset of hoarseness or voice changes; usually self-limited

EPIGLOTTITIS

What is epiglottitis?

Cellulitis of the epiglottis and surrounding structures; it affects children more frequently than adults

What are the two most common cause of epiglottitis?

1. *S. aureus*
2. *H. influenzae*
Since the implementation of "H. flu" vaccination programs, it is not as commonly associated with epiglottitis as it has in the past

What types of strains exist?

Both encapsulated and nonencapsulated strains exist

Where do they normally exist?

They can be normal components of the upper respiratory flora in humans

How is the organism spread?

1. Respiratory droplets from colonized or diseased hosts
2. Humans are the only reservoir

Which serotype causes the most potent disease?

Of the encapsulated strains, type B is the most potent at causing local disease and disseminated spread

What are the clinical manifestations of encapsulated strains?

1. Life-threatening epiglottitis
2. Acute bacterial meningitis

What are the clinical manifestations of nonencapsulated strains?

Pharyngitis, otitis media, and sinusitis from colonized oropharynx
Bronchitis and pneumonia is possible in the elderly, immunocompromised, or chronic obstructive pulmonary disease (COPD) patients

What does the *H. influenzae* vaccine contain?

Only the *H. influenzae* type b polysaccharide capsule complexed to a protein conjugate, i.e., diphtheria toxoid, or to *Neisseria meningitidis* outer membrane coat

What is the purpose of the protein conjugate?

To induce a strong T-cell antibody response

Are vaccinated individuals still susceptible to infection?
Why?

Yes

The vaccine only covers type b *H. influenzae* and does not protect against unencapsulated or the other capsule strains

TRACHEA

What is tracheitis?	A rare inflammation of the trachea caused by *S. aureus* or *S. pyogenes* that can cause life-threatening abscesses

LOWER RESPIRATORY TRACT INFECTIONS

BRONCHITIS AND BRONCHIOLITIS

What is bronchitis?	Inflammation of the tracheobronchial tree, commonly caused by viruses; frequently presents with a cough
How is it diagnosed?	History and physical
How is it treated?	With supportive care
What is bronchiolitis?	A common acute viral infection of the lower respiratory tract affecting children less than 2 years old
What are the two most common causes of bronchiolitis?	1. RSV, a negative-sense, enveloped RNA virus of the *Paramyxoviridae* family 2. Parainfluenza virus, a negative sense, enveloped RNA virus of the *Paramyxoviridae* family
Why are children particularly prone to bronchiolitis?	Children have inherently smaller bronchioles which are more easily occluded from inflammation and swelling
How is RSV infection diagnosed?	1. History and physical 2. RSV antigen detection/culture from respiratory secretions
How is RSV infection treated?	1. Supportively 2. Bronchodilators, e.g., albuterol 3. Palivizumab (Synagis) "Ribavirin" may appear as the treatment of choice for RSV on tests, but since the mid-1990s, this antiviral has not been used by many institutions to treat RSV; still, some use it if the infection occurred within the past 1–2 days

PNEUMONIA

What is pneumonia?	A lower respiratory tract infection that can be caused by bacteria, viruses, fungi, mycobacteria, or parasites
What is atypical pneumonia?	A usually milder lower respiratory tract infection most commonly caused by *Mycoplasma pneumoniae, Chlamydiae pneumoniae,* or *Legionella pneumophila* Also known as "walking pneumonia" because the patient often remains ambulatory throughout the entire illness
What are three ways in which pneumonia is classified?	1. Where/how the illness was acquired 2. Patient's age 3. Patient's state of health
What are three ways that pneumonias can be classified based on where/how the illness was acquired?	1. Community acquired 2. Nosocomial acquired 3. Aspiration acquired
What are the most common causes of each of the following:	
Community-acquired pneumonia?	1. *S. pneumoniae* 2. *H. influenzae* 3. *M. pneumoniae*
Nosocomial-acquired pneumonia?	1. *S. aureus* 2. Gram-negative bacteria, e.g., *Klebsiella, Escherichia coli, Enterobacter*
Aspiration-acquired pneumonia?	Mixed anaerobic flora
What are four ways in which pneumonias can be classified based on the patient's age?	1. Children and adolescents, i.e., birth to 18 years of age 2. Younger adults, i.e., 18–40 years of age 3. Older adults, i.e., 40–65 years of age 4. Elderly, i.e., older than 65 years of age

What are the most common causes of pneumonia each of the following:

Children and adolescents, i.e., birth to 18 years of age?

1. Respiratory syncytial virus
2. *M. pneumoniae*
3. *C. pneumoniae*
4. *S. pneumoniae*

Younger adults, i.e., 18–40 years of age?

1. *Mycoplasma*
2. *C. pneumoniae*
3. *S. pneumoniae*

Older adults, i.e., 40–65 years of age?

1. *S. pneumoniae*
2. *H. influenzae*
3. Anaerobic organisms
4. Viruses, i.e., *Orthomyxoviridae, Rhinoviridae, Coronaviridae, Arenaviridae,* etc.
5. Mycoplasma

Elderly, i.e., older than 65 years of age?

1. *S. pneumoniae*
2. Viral
3. Anaerobes
4. *H. influenzae*
5. Gram rods
6. *M. tuberculosis*, i.e., reactivation tuberculosis

What are two viral causes of pneumonia?

1. Coronavirus, e.g., severe acute respiratory syndrome (SARS)
2. Influenza, especially in the elderly

What are five common etiologies of pneumonia in the immunocompromised host?

P. carinii (P. jiroveci), cytomegalovirus (CMV), *Cryptococcus, Aspergillus,* and tuberculosis

What are the clinical manifestations of pneumonia?

Depends on underlying etiology, but common symptoms include mucopurulent sputum production which may be blood streaked, cough, fever, chills, chest pain, and shortness of breath, i.e., dyspnea

What are three methods for diagnosing pneumonia?

1. History and physical
2. Sputum cultures
3. Chest x-ray

How is pneumonia treated?   Antimicrobial for the responsible organism

How is pneumococcal pneumonia prevented?   In adults, a pneumococcal polysaccharide vaccine (PPV) exists that contains 23 of the most common capsular serotypes (Pneumovax)
In infants, a heptavalent vaccine exists that is linked to a conjugate to aid in immunogenicity and protects against 7 capsular serotypes (Prevnar)

44

Cardiovascular System

OVERVIEW

What are five infection-prone components of the cardiovascular system?	1. Blood 2. Endocardium 3. Myocardium 4. Pericardium 5. Blood vessels

BLOOD INFECTIONS

What is bacteremia?

Viable bacteria in circulating blood

What are four common portals of entry and associated pathogens that cause bacteremia?

1. Urinary tract, e.g., *Escherichia coli*
2. Respiratory tract, e.g., *Streptococcus pneumoniae, Haemophilus influenzae, Streptococcus pyogenes*
3. Skin, e.g., *S. aureus*
4. Gastrointestinal (GI) tract, e.g., *Salmonella typhi, Enterobacter*

What pathogen is a common cause of bacteremia in neonates?

Streptococcus agalactiae, a group B streptococci (GBS)

What are three types of bacteremia?

1. Transient
2. Intermittent
3. Continuous

What is transient bacteremia?

Short periods of viable bacteria in the blood, i.e., 15–20 minutes

What are two common causes of transient bacteremia?

1. Tooth brushing
2. Menstruation

What makes it transient?

Bacteria are cleared by reticuloendothelial system, e.g., macrophages

What is intermittent bacteremia?

Recurrent episodes of viable bacteria in the blood

What is a common cause of intermittent bacteremia? Abscesses, especially in the liver or kidney

What are the signs and symptoms of intermittent bacteremia? Recurrent episodes of bacteremia often accompanied by malaise, fever, and/or chills

What is continuous bacteremia? Constant presence of bacteria in the blood

What are common causes of continuous bacteremia? Multisystem disease, typhoid, leprosy, pericarditis, endocarditis, thrombophlebitis

How is the diagnosis of bacteremia made? Multiple, sterilely drawn blood cultures from different percutaneous sites over time

What is viremia? Presences of virus in the blood

What are four examples of viruses that can be found in the blood?
1. Human immunodeficiency virus (HIV)
2. Hepatitis B, C, and D
3. Coxsackievirus
4. Poliovirus

What virus is the most commonly associated with myocarditis and pericarditis? Coxsackie B
With the increased prevalence of acquired immune deficiency syndrome (AIDS), HIV is also a major contributor to the etiology of myocarditis

What is fungemia? Presence of fungus in the blood

What should be considered in a patient with fungemia? Immunocompromised status

What fungal infection is associated with intravenous (IV) drug use and endocarditis? *Candida albicans*

What parasite affects the cardiovascular system? *Trypanosoma cruzi*
    What condition does it cause? Chagas disease

    Where is it most common? Central and South America

How is it transmitted?	Reduviid bug
What are the cardiovascular clinical manifestations?	Myocarditis, cardiomyopathy, arrhythmias, death after latent period of more than 10 years
How is it diagnosed?	Blood smear, as well as bone marrow aspirate and culture

ENDOCARDITIS

What is endocarditis?	Inflammation of the valves or lining of the heart
What is the most common age of affected patients?	Middle-age individuals with a median age of 50 years
Which valve is most commonly affected?	Mitral
What is the second most common valve affected?	Aortic
What valve is most commonly affected by endocarditis in patients with a history of IV drug use?	Tricuspid
Why?	IV drug users inject into veins and the tricuspid valve is the first valve to come in contact with venous blood return
What are the causes of endocarditis?	Bacteremia with seeding of a modified endocardial surface
What are predisposing factors for endocarditis?	Acute rheumatic fever, congenital valve problems, prosthetic heart valves, IV drug use, presence of immune complexes, congenital heart defects, direct trauma
What deposits on this modified endocardial surface predispose patients to endocarditis?	Platelets and fibrin
What do they create?	A biofilm
What does it do?	Protects the bacteria from phagocytic and humoral defenses

What are some clinical manifestations of endocarditis?	New murmur, anemia, fever, emboli, fever, chills, anorexia, splinter hemorrhages, Osler's nodes, Janeway lesions, Roth's spots
Define each of the following: **Osler's nodes?**	Tender, raised lesions on fingers and toes from septic embolization
Janeway lesions?	Non-tender lesions on palms and soles of feet
Roth's spots?	Round white spots surrounded by hemorrhage on the retina
Where are splinter hemorrhages commonly found?	Nail beds
What are the two main types of endocarditis?	Acute and subacute
What are four methods of diagnosing endocarditis?	1. History and physical 2. Clinical signs and symptoms 3. Echocardiogram of the heart showing vegetations 4. Blood cultures
What are the complications of endocarditis?	Valvular insufficiency, arrhythmias, chordae tendineae rupture, glomerulonephritis, suppurative pericarditis, emboli, microinvasion of brain or coronary arteries
What are the microemboli of endocarditis composed of?	Immune complexes
What known bacteria are associated with endocarditis?	1. S. aureus 2. Viridans streptococcus 3. HACEK bacteria
What does HACEK stand for?	*Haemophilus aphrophilus* or *paraphrophilus* *Actinobacillus actinomycetem-comitans Cardiobacterium hominis*

Eikenella corrodens
Kingella kingae

Where are the normal flora for these organisms?

Mouth

What is the treatment against these pathogens?

Ceftriaxone

What pathogen is the most common cause of acute endocarditis?

S. aureus

What is its virulence?

Highly virulent, locally destructive, and devastating

What predisposes one to acute endocarditis?

IV drug use

What is the appearance of vegetations in acute endocarditis?

Large conglomerate masses on normal valves that are prone to dislodge and cause emboli

What is the treatment for acute endocarditis?

IV antibiotics depending on blood culture sensitivities, e.g., penicillinase-resistant penicillins: nafcillin and gentamicin

What is the onset of subacute endocarditis?

Insidious onset characterized with vague flu-like symptoms lasting from weeks to months

What pathogens are the most common cause of subacute endocarditis?

Viridans streptococcus, e.g., *Streptococcus sanguinis*, *Streptococcus salivarius*, *Streptococcus mutans*, *Streptococcus bovis*
Enterococci, e.g., *Enterococcus faecalis*

What is their virulence?

Less virulent and less aggressive than *S. aureus*

What pathogen most commonly colonizes prosthetic heart valves leading to endocarditis?

Staphylococcus epidermidis

What organism most commonly infects native valves?

Viridans streptococcus

What predisposes susceptible individuals to be colonized with this pathogen?	Dental work or periodontal disease
How is this prevented?	Prophylactic antibiotics, i.e., penicillin, prior to dental procedures in patients with preexisting valvular damage
What is the appearance of vegetations in subacute endocarditis?	Small vegetations on abnormal valves
Do these vegetations usually produce emboli?	No
What is the treatment for subacute endocarditis?	Antibiotics, depending on blood culture sensitivities

MYOCARDITIS

What is myocarditis?	Inflammation of the heart muscle
What are the clinical manifestations of myocarditis?	Chest pain, congestive heart failure, fatigue, cardiac enlargement often with ventricular dilatation, arrhythmias, and valvular insufficiency
What are five viral pathogens that cause myocarditis?	1. Coxsackievirus B 2. Echoviruses 3. HIV 4. Influenza 5. Poliovirus
What are common bacterial pathogens that cause myocarditis?	Staphylococci, *Neisseria gonorrhoeae*, *S. pneumoniae*, *Neisseria meningitidis*, *Rickettsia rickettsii*, *Coxiella burnetii*, *Corynebacterium diphtheriae*, *Treponema pallidum*, *Mycobacterium tuberculosis*, *Mycobacterium leprae*
What parasite causes myocarditis?	*Trichinella* sp.
What are two protozoal pathogens that cause myocarditis?	*Toxoplasma* sp., *Trypanosoma cruzi*

What is the most common overall organism that causes myocarditis?	Coxsackievirus B With the increased prevalence of AIDS, HIV is also a major contributor to the etiology of myocarditis
How is myocarditis treated?	Supportively and with antibiotics if a bacterial or parasitic/protozoal organism is identified

PERICARDITIS

What is pericarditis?	Inflammation of the sac enclosing the heart, i.e., the pericardium
What are two sources of infection for bacterial pericarditis? **What are the most common bacterial causes?**	1. Direct spread from lung or mediastinal lymph nodes after trauma or surgery 2. Bloodstream *Mycobacterium tuberculosis, Staphylococcus, Neisseria, S. pneumoniae, Borrelia burgdorferi*
What is a source for viral pericarditis? **What are the most common viral causes?**	Upper respiratory infection Coxsackievirus B, echovirus, poliovirus, influenza
What type of pericardial effusion is associated with coxsackievirus?	Serous, or clear transudative-like effusion
What type of pericardial effusion is associated with M. tuberculosis?	Caseous, or "cottage cheese-like" effusion
What are complications of pericarditis?	Pericardial effusions, constrictive pericarditis, cardiac tamponade, congestive heart failure, and death
What is the treatment for pericarditis?	Supportive measures, antibiotics if a bacterial etiology exists, and pericardectomy if constrictive enough to cause heart failure

THROMBOPHLEBITIS

What is thrombophlebitis?	Venous inflammation of blood vessel walls with thrombus formation that can involve superficial to deep veins

What are common causes of superficial thrombophlebitis?

Skin ulcers or trauma from abrasion, laceration, IV site, and surgical sites

What are the most common bacterial causes?

S. aureus, anaerobic streptococci, *Rickettsia, Brucella,* and *T. pallidum*

What are the most common fungal causes?

Candida, Mucor, and *Rhizopus*

Which blood vessel does *T. pallidum* commonly affect?

Ascending aorta

What is the pathogenesis of *T. pallidum*?

Following primary and secondary syphilis, tertiary syphilis can result in the disruption of the vas vasorum of the aorta at which point viable *Treponema* is rarely seen

What is the classic appearance of the aorta?

Tree-bark appearance

What are the complications?

Dilation/aneurysm of the ascending aorta and aortic valvular insufficiency from a "stretched" annulus

Genitourinary System

OVERVIEW

What are six female genitourinary structures prone to infections?	1. Urethra, (urethritis) 2. Bladder (cystitis) 3. Kidneys (pyelonephritis) 4. Vulva and vagina (vulvovaginitis) 5. Cervix (cervicitis) 6. Female reproductive organs (pelvic inflammatory disease [PID])
What are six male genitourinary structures prone to infections?	1. Urethra (urethritis) 2. Bladder (cystitis) 3. Kidneys (pyelonephritis) 4. Prostate (prostatitis) 5. Epididymis (epididymitis) 6. Testicles (orchitis)

URINARY TRACT INFECTIONS: URETHRITIS, CYSTITIS, AND PYELONEPHRITIS

What are the clinical manifestations of urinary tract infections (UTIs)?	Painful urination, i.e., dysuria, and sometimes urethral discharge
What is pyelonephritis?	Infection of the kidneys following an ascending UTI
What are three clinical manifestations of pyelonephritis?	1. Fever 2. Costovertebral tenderness, i.e., flank pain 3. Dysuria
Why are UTIs more common in women than in men?	1. Shorter urethra 2. Proximity of urethral meatus to anal area/feces
What are risk factors for developing UTIs?	Obstructions, sexual intercourse, catheters, diaphragms, and voiding impairment

What is the most common cause of UTIs?

Uropathogenic *Escherichia coli*

What are nine other causes?

1. *Staphylococcus saprophyticus*
2. *Streptococcus agalactiae* (GBS)
3. *Enterococcus faecalis*
4. *Proteus mirabilis*
5. *Neisseria gonorrhoeae*
6. *Chlamydia trachomatis*
7. *Ureaplasma urealyticum*
8. *Mycoplasma hominis*
9. Noninfectious causes, e.g., allergic reaction or chronic irritation

How does *E. coli* damage the genitourinary tract?

1. Adheres to the mucosa via pili
2. Induces inflammation with endotoxin (lipopolysaccharide [LPS])

What gram-positive bacteria are associated with UTIs?

1. *S. saprophyticus*
2. *S. agalactiae*, i.e., group B streptococci (GBS)
3. *E. faecalis*

Which bacterium causes a mild genital tract infection and can result in fulminant neonatal meningitis?

Group B streptococci (GBS)

How do you prevent this?

Prophylactic maternal antibiotic treatment

Which bacterium causes UTIs in sexually active young females?

S. saprophyticus

What makes *E. faecalis* UTIs difficult to manage?

Antibiotic resistance

What distinguishes *P. mirabilis* from other pathogens?

Urease production that hydrolyzes urea into ammonia and CO_2
Proteus and *Helicobacter pylori* both produce urease

What is the result of this?

Increased rate of kidney struvite stone formation because of magnesium precipitation

What two bacteria can cause urethritis, pelvic inflammatory disease, and newborn conjunctivitis?

N. gonorrhoeae and *C. trachomatis* (serotypes D–K)

What is gonococcal urethritis?	Urinary tract infection caused by *N. gonorrhoeae*
What age group has the highest incidence of *N. gonorrhoeae*?	15–25-year-olds because they are the most sexually active age group
What percentage of women and men infected with *N. gonorrhoeae* are asymptomatic?	30% of women, 10% of men
Should you treat partners of patients infected with *N. gonorrhoeae*?	Yes, they should visit their physician, be counseled, cultured, treated, and encouraged to use condoms
What are five other types of mucous membrane infections caused by *N. gonorrhoeae*?	1. Ophthalmia neonatorum 2. Endocervicitis 3. Rectal infections 4. Pharyngitis 5. Disseminated infection
What is ophthalmia neonatorum? **How is it acquired?**	Neonatal conjunctivitis secondary to *N. gonorrhoeae* During passage through the birth canal
How is neonatal conjunctivitis treated?	Tetracycline or topical silver nitrate
What are two long-term consequences of repeated *N. gonorrhoeae* infections?	1. Sterility 2. Increased risk of ectopic pregnancy
What pathogen frequently coinfects patients with gonorrhea and also requires treatment?	*Chlamydia*, which can be treated with azithromycin or doxycycline
What are clinical manifestations of *C. trachomatis* subtypes D–K?	Nongonococcal urethritis, pelvic inflammatory disease in adult women Inclusion conjunctivitis and pneumonia in neonates
What are clinical manifestations of *C. trachomatis* subtypes L1–L3? **What is this?**	Lymphogranuloma venereum Suppurative, inguinal adenitis

VULVOVAGINITIS AND PELVIC INFLAMMATORY DISEASE

What are three causes of vulvovaginitis?

What is the pathogenesis of each?

1. *Gardnerella vaginalis*, i.e., bacterial vaginosis
2. *Candida albicans*, i.e., yeast infection
3. *Trichomonas vaginalis*, i.e., trichomoniasis or "trich"
G. vaginalis overproliferates, replacing normal flora, i.e., *Lactobacillus*
C. albicans overgrowth is seen with too much estrogen, antibiotics suppressing normal flora, or immunosuppression, e.g., from human immunodeficiency virus (HIV) or diabetes
Trichomoniasis is commonly acquired sexually and results in mucosal inflammation, vaginal discharge and irritation

What is PID?

Colonization of the endometrium, fallopian tubes, adnexa, and/or peritoneum

What five organisms commonly cause PID?

1. *C. trachomatis*, serotypes D–K
2. *N. gonorrhoeae*
3. *Mycoplasma hominis*
4. *U. urealyticum*
5. *Fusobacterium*

What are some specific clinical manifestations of PID?

1. Endometritis
2. Salpingitis
3. Pelvic peritonitis
4. Tuboovarian abscess
5. Adhesion formation
6. Ectopic pregnancy
7. Sterility

What risk factors are associated with PID?

Young women who are sexually active and have a history of multiple sexual partners

PROSTATITIS, EPIDIDYMITIS, AND ORCHITIS

What are two classifications of prostate infections?
What causes each?

1. Acute bacterial prostatitis
2. Chronic bacterial prostatitis
Acute bacterial prostatitis is usually caused by gram-positive bacteria, e.g., *E. faecalis* and *S. saprophyticus*

Chronic bacterial prostatitis is usually caused by gram-negative bacteria, e.g., *Enterobacteriaceae* spp. and *Pseudomonas* spp.

What is important in treating these infections?

Longer courses of antibiotics because of poor antimicrobial penetration of the prostate

What three pathogens are associated with epididymitis?

1. *Pseudomonas* spp.
2. *C. trachomatis*
3. *N. gonorrhoeae*

What is orchitis?
What pathogens are associated with this?

Infection of the testicles
Gram-negative bacteria, e.g., *E. coli*, *Klebsiella pneumoniae*, *Pseudomonas* spp.

GENITAL LESIONS

What type of lesion is associated with each of the following:
Syphilis?

Painless, raised ulcers

What is the pathogen?

Treponema pallidum
T. pallidum is visualized with darkfield microscopy (see color photo 18)

Chancroid?

Painful, ragged, soft chancre

What is the pathogen?

Haemophilus ducreyi

Herpes?

Painful vesicles

What is the pathogen?

Herpes simplex virus types I and II

46

Infections of the Skin, Eye, & Ear

SKIN INFECTIONS

OVERVIEW

Define each of the following:

Maculopapular rash?
Generalized erythematous rash which can have a combination of flat and raised areas

Papule?
Raised palpable lesion less than one centimeter in diameter

What are two forms of papules?
1. Smooth papule
2. Verrucous papule, i.e., rough and wart-like papule

Wheal?
Papule characterized by erythema, edema, and normal overlying skin

Annular plaque?
Ring-like lesion with central clearing greater than 1 cm

Nodule?
Round, deep lesion in the dermis or subcutaneous tissue that is less than 1.5 cm

Bullae?
Skin blisters greater than 1 cm in diameter

Vesicle?
Skin blisters less than 1 cm in diameter

Pustule?
Pus-filled vesicle

Ulcer?
Area of skin denuded of overlying epidermis

Necrotic tissue?
Dead tissue, also known as gangrenous tissue

MACULOPAPULAR RASHES

What are three types of maculopapular rashes?	1. Scarlet fever 2. Toxic shock syndrome 3. Morbilliform eruptions
What is scarlet fever?	A less-severe maculopapular rash that is similar to staphylococcal scalded skin syndrome and is characterized by a "sandpaper-like rash," erythematous eruption, and desquamation after 4 days, which is caused by a superantigen, i.e., erythrogenic toxin
What pathogen causes it?	Group A streptococcus, i.e., *Streptococcus pyogenes*
How is it treated?	Penicillinase-resistant penicillins
What is toxic shock syndrome?	Generalized eruption of a "sunburn-like rash" accompanied with desquamation and systemic dysfunction, i.e., hypotension and organ failure
What pathogen causes it?	*Staphylococcus aureus*
How is it treated?	Penicillinase-resistant penicillins
What is a morbilliform rash?	A measles-like rash with a "webbed" appearance
What pathogens cause it?	1. Rubella, i.e., German measles 2. Rubeola (measles)
How is it treated?	Supportive therapy

SMOOTH PAPULAR LESIONS

What are two types of smooth papular lesions? **What pathogens cause these clinical manifestations?**	1. Molluscum contagiosim 2. Condyloma latum Molluscum contagiosum is caused by pox virus Condyloma latum is caused by *Treponema pallidum* during the secondary stage of syphilis

VERRUCOUS PAPULAR LESIONS

What are four types of verrucous papular lesions?	1. Condyloma acuminatum, i.e., genital warts

2. Common warts
3. Cutaneous tuberculosis
4. Fungi, e.g., blastomycosis and coccidioidomycosis

What pathogen causes condyloma acuminatum and the common wart?

Human papillomavirus (HPV)

How is it treated?

Although prone to recur, lesions are excised, e.g., by freezing them off

ANNULAR PLAQUE LESIONS

What two infectious diseases manifest themselves with annular plaques?

1. Lyme disease
2. Erythema multiforme

What is the etiology of each?

Lyme disease is caused by *Borrelia burgdorferi*

Erythema multiforme is caused by a variety of viruses, bacteria, and drugs

ERYTHEMATOUS PATCHES AND NODULES

What are two causes of erythematous plaques?

1. Streptococcal cellulitis
2. Necrotizing cellulitis (gas gangrene)

What are two clinical manifestations of streptococcal cellulitis?

1. Cellulitis
2. Erysipelas

What is the difference between them?

Cellulitis is a diffuse spreading infection of the skin accompanied by a confined exudative lesion frequently affecting the leg usually caused by *Staphylococcus* spp.

Erysipelas is an edematous, spreading, circumscribed, hot erythematous area frequently affecting the face usually caused by *S. pyogenes* (GAS)

What is necrotizing cellulitis, i.e., gas gangrene?

Infection that results in the irreversible destruction (necrosis) of soft tissue by anaerobic organisms, commonly associated with *Clostridial* spp.

How does gas gangrene commonly present?	Destruction of infected tissue surrounding the healthy tissue after a severe traumatic wound
What is the treatment for gas gangrene?	1. Penicillin 2. Debridement 3. Hyperbaric oxygen 4. Amputation
What toxin makes clostridia pathogenic? **Why?**	Alpha toxin, i.e., lecithinase Damages cellular membranes
What clinical manifestation is associated with erythematous nodules?	Erythema nodosum
What are the clinical features of this condition?	Tender, inflamed nodules on the extensor surfaces, e.g., shin
What is the pathogenesis?	Hypersensitivity reaction to a variety of factors, including *Mycobacterium tuberculosis*, fungi, bacteria, viruses, and ulcerative colitis

ERYTHEMATOUS AND HYPOPIGMENTED PLAQUES

What condition is associated with each of the following symptoms? **Erythematous plaques?**	Cutaneous candidiasis
Hypopigmented plaques?	Tinea
Erythematous plaques and hypopigmented plaques?	Pityriasis versicolor
What characterizes cutaneous candidiasis?	Erythematous, well-defined plaques found in body folds
What are six types of tinea infections?	1. Tinea pedis 2. Tinea corporis 3. Tinea capitis 4. Tinea cruris 5. Tinea unguium 6. Tinea barbae

What is the clinical manifestation and responsible pathogen in each of the following:

Tinea pedis?

Infected tissues between toes which can spread to nails (*Trichophyton rubrum*)

Tinea corporis?

"Ring worm"—advancing annular rings with scaly centers (*Epidermophyton floccosum*)

Tinea capitis?

Scaling patches on head with extensive hair loss (*Microsporum*)

How can tinea capitis be diagnosed?

Hair appears green when exposed to ultraviolet (UV) light fluorescence, e.g., from a Wood lamp, secondary to hyphae

Tinea cruris?

"Jock itch"—advancing annular rings with scaly centers in moist groin areas (*E. floccosum*)

Tinea unguium?

Thick, brittle, and discolored nails. (*T. rubrum*)

Tinea barbae?

Infection localized in bearded areas (*T. rubrum*)

What is a general term for these fungal infections? Why?

Dermatophytoses

These fungal infections use keratin as a nutritional source and affect the hair, skin, or nails

How are they treated?

Topical antifungals, e.g. Miconazole or systemic antifungals, e.g. ketoconazole

What pathogen is associated with pityriasis versicolor?

Malassezia furfur

What is the clinical manifestation of this?

Slightly raised plaques, which can be red, pink, tan, brown, or white, that appear like "spaghetti and meatballs" under microscopy when scrape-biopsied

How is it treated?

Topical antifungals, e.g., miconazole or selenium sulfide

VESICULAR, BULLOUS, AND ULCERATIVE LESIONS

What are eight forms of vesicular and/or bullous lesions?	1. Staphylococcal scalded skin syndrome 2. Impetigo 3. Chickenpox 4. Herpes simplex 5. Herpes zoster 6. Hand-foot-and-mouth disease 7. Sporotrichosis 8. Smallpox
What is staphylococcal scalded skin syndrome?	Bullae and desquamated skin usually seen in children This is the most severe manifestation of S. *aureus*
What is responsible for the pathogenesis of this disease?	Exfoliative toxin (ET)
What is the characteristic skin finding?	Splitting of dermal layers by proteolysis of intercellular junctions
How is it treated?	Penicillinase-resistant penicillins
What are the two types of impetigo? **How are they different?**	1. Impetigo 2. Bullous impetigo Impetigo is a superficial skin infection that begins as a vesicular lesion progressing to a yellow, crusted lesion Bullous impetigo is different from impetigo because bullae quickly erupt, rupture, and leave a light brown crust
What causes impetigo and bullous impetigo?	Impetigo is usually caused by S. *pyogenes* (GAS) Bullous impetigo is usually caused by S. *aureus*
Who usually gets impetigo?	Children
How are impetigo and bullous impetigo treated?	Impetigo is treated with penicillin Bullous impetigo is treated with a penicillinase-resistant penicillin
What herpesviruses commonly cause skin manifestations?	1. Herpes virus 2. Varicella zoster virus, i.e., chicken pox

What are the characteristic skin findings of each?	Herpes causes shallow, ulcerated painful vesicles that group to form larger vesicles Chicken pox causes vesicles resembling "dew drops on rose petals" that become pustular and crust
What diagnostic test is used to identify these viruses?	Tzanck test
What is the implication of harboring herpesviruses after an initial infection?	Reactivation
What precipitates this?	Stress, trauma, fever, and hormones
What drugs decrease the intensity of reactivation?	Acyclovir or valacyclovir
What is hand-foot-and-mouth disease? **What pathogen is responsible for this?**	Small, fragile vesicles found in the mouth and on the hands and feet Enteroviruses (*Picornaviridae*), particularly coxsackievirus A and enterovirus 71
What is sporotrichosis? **What pathogen causes it?**	Mycoses which invades subcutaneous tissue, dermis, and bone *Sporothrix schenckii*
How is it acquired?	Traumatic lacerations or puncture wound, e.g., puncture with a rose thorn Sporotrichosis is also called "rose gardener's disease"
What are the clinical manifestations?	Granulomatous ulcer at the puncture wound, producing secondary lesions tracking along lymphatics

PUSTULES AND ABSCESSES

What are four conditions that may present with pustules?	1. Acne 2. Folliculitis 3. Furuncles 4. Kerion
What pathogen is associated with acne?	*Propionibacterium acnes*

What is folliculitis?	Infection of the follicular orifices
Where does folliculitis commonly present?	Bearded regions and burn or surgical wounds
What pathogens are associated with this?	1. *S. aureus* 2. *Pseudomonas aeruginosa* from hot tubs or swimming pools
What is a furuncle?	A subcutaneous abscess formed around an imbedded body or inoculation by a foreign body
What pathogen is associated with this?	*S. aureus*, e.g., from inoculation by a splinter
What is a kerion?	Painful, boggy, erythematous growth, commonly seen on the scalp, which is caused by a fungal infection
What is a mycetoma?	Localized abscess, usually of the feet, that drains pus, serum, and blood through sinus tracts
What causes it?	*Madurella grisea*
How is it diagnosed?	Presence of colored grains (red, black, yellow, white) in exudates
How is it treated?	With excision

PETECHIA, PURPURA, AND ECCHYMOSES

What are five infectious causes of petechia, purpura, or ecchymoses?	1. Meningococcemia 2. Infective endocarditis 3. Disseminated gonococcal infection 4. Rocky Mountain spotted fever 5. Dengue fever

EYE INFECTIONS

BACTERIAL EYE INFECTIONS

What are the two most common resident flora of the eye?	*Staphylococcus epidermidis* and then *S. aureus*.
What are two eye infections that can cause blindness in neonates?	1. *C. trachomatis* 2. *N. gonorrhoeae*

What is the cause of trachoma?	*C. trachomatis* subtypes A–C
What is trachoma?	A chronic infection that causes the eyelashes to scar the cornea leading to blindness
How is trachoma spread?	Personal contact (i.e., eye to eye droplets)
What is the cause of inclusion conjunctivitis?	*C. trachomatis* subtypes D–K
How does inclusion conjunctivitis infection begin?	Inoculation of eye with genital secretions during birth
How is *C. trachomatis* infection treated?	Doxycycline
In whom is gonococcal ophthalmia usually seen?	Neonates born at home without receiving prophylactic medicine
When does gonococcal ophthalmia usually affect neonates?	First 5 days of life
What does gonococcal ophthalmia cause?	A rapidly destructive hyperpurulent conjunctivitis
What can untreated gonococcal ophthalmia ultimately result in?	Blindness
What disease is caused by *Haemophilus influenza*, biotype *aegyptius*?	Bacterial "pinkeye"
How does this present?	Epidemic purulent conjunctivitis
Who is usually affected by this infection?	School-aged children
What is the leading cause of chronic bacterial conjunctivitis following a break in the corneal epithelium?	*S. aureus*

What is the cause of a hordeolum, i.e., sty, in the eye?	An infected meibomian gland in the eyelid
What bacterium usually causes a sty?	*S. aureus*

VIRAL EYE INFECTIONS

How does herpes simplex virus (HSV) keratitis present?	Corneal ulcers, red eye, moderate pain, and photophobia
What virus is worrisome in acquired immune deficiency syndrome (AIDS) patients with eye pain?	Varicella-zoster virus (VZV)
What does this virus cause in AIDS patients?	Acute retinal necrosis
What is the most common cause of acute conjunctivitis in children?	Adenovirus
With is adenoviral conjunctivitis associated with?	Acute febrile pharyngitis
What is the course of adenoviral conjunctivitis?	Usually resolves on its own, after 7–10 days
What is the treatment for adenoviral conjunctivitis?	No treatment is available
What virus can cause congenital cataracts?	Rubella

PARASITIC EYE INFECTIONS

What nematode causes river blindness?	*Onchocerca volvulus*
How is onchocerciasis transmitted?	The female blackfly
How is onchocerciasis diagnosed?	Microfilariae in the skin on biopsy

How is onchocerciasis treated?	Ivermectin and/or surgery
What nematode may be seen crawling in the subconjunctival space?	*Loa loa*
How is loiasis transmitted?	Deer flies
What is the most common cause of infectious keratitis?	Herpes simplex virus types 1 and 2

EAR INFECTIONS

What is the lay term for otitis externa?	Swimmer's ear
What is otitis externa?	An inflammation of the external ear canal that can also involve the pinna
What population is generally affected?	Diabetic patients
What is the most common bacterial infection of children?	Otitis media
What is this?	Infection of the internal ear canal
What are the three most common causes of otitis media in infants older than age 2 months?	1. *S. pneumoniae* 2. *H. influenzae* 3. *Moraxella catarrhalis*
How is otitis media treated?	Although the majority resolve spontaneously, β-lactam antibiotics are sometimes prescribed

47

Nervous System: Peripheral & Central

MENINGITIS

What are the two main categories of meningitis?

1. Bacterial meningitis
2. Aseptic meningitis

What is aseptic meningitis?

Inflammation of the meninges not caused by a bacterial pathogen
Viral meningitis is a type of aseptic meningitis, but aseptic meningitis does not exclusively infer a viral etiology (fungal infection or inflammatory reactions can cause aseptic meningitis)

What are the cardinal signs of bacterial meningitis?

Nuchal rigidity, headache, fever, photophobia, nausea, and vomiting

What diagnostic tests are used for evaluation of meningitis?

Lumbar puncture with Gram stain, cell count, lab chemistries, and culture of the cerebrospinal fluid (CSF)

What are the characteristic CSF findings seen in bacterial meningitis?

1. Increased neutrophils secondary to the immune response mounted against bacteria
2. Decreased glucose
3. Increased protein
4. Increased opening pressure
5. Frank pus in severe cases

What are three differences between bacterial and viral meningitis?

1. Bacterial disease is more severe and aggressive
2. CSF neutrophils are elevated in bacterial meningitis, whereas CSF lymphocytes are elevated in viral meningitis
3. CSF glucose is significantly lower in bacterial meningitis but is usually normal in viral meningitis

What are two ways that microorganisms reach the meninges?

1. Hematogenous spread—organisms infect the blood or cells in the blood and cross the blood–brain barrier to the meninges
2. Neural spread—organisms infect neurons and spread retrograde to the meninges

What are the two most common causes of bacterial meningitis in adults?

1. *Neisseria meningitides* (meningococcal meningitis)
2. *Streptococcus pneumoniae*

What are the three most common causes of meningitis in neonates?

1. Group B streptococci, i.e., *Streptococcus agalactiae*
2. *Escherichia coli*
3. *Listeria monocytogenes*

What vaccine has dramatically lowered the incidence of bacterial meningitis in newborns?

Conjugated *Haemophilus influenzae* vaccine against capsular polysaccharide b has been very successful in reducing the incidence of bacterial meningitis caused by *H. influenzae*

How does *N. meningitidis* infect the meninges?

N. meningitidis penetrates the epithelial lining of the nasopharynx and enters the bloodstream
Once in the blood, it can cross the blood–brain barrier and infect the meninges

What additional sign may be detected by physical exam in meningococcal meningitis?

Petechial rash

What is acute fulminating meningococcal septicemia in young children called?

Waterhouse-Friedrich syndrome

What are the clinical manifestations of Waterhouse Friedrich syndrome?

Adrenal necrosis, large skin hemorrhages, circulatory collapse, disseminated intravascular coagulation (DIC), and death within 10–12 hours

What are the first-line drugs used to treat meningococcal meningitis?

Intravenous antibiotics, e.g., ceftriaxone and ampicillin

What drug is used to treat close contacts of individuals infected with N. *meningitides* or H. *influenzae* meningitis?

Rifampin

What vaccine is available for meningitis prophylaxis in older children and adults?

A capsular vaccine effective against serogroups A, C, W, and Y of N. *meningitidis*

Why is serogroup B not included in the meningitis vaccine?

Serogroup B does not elicit an immune response

How is L. *monocytogenes* meningitis usually acquired?

Foodborne acquisition through the gastrointestinal tract

What populations are at higher risk for L. *monocytogenes* causing meningitis?

Pregnant women, the elderly, neonates, and the immunocompromised

What opportunistic organisms may cause meningitis in patients infected with human immunodeficiency virus (HIV)?

1. *Mycobacterium tuberculosis*
2. *Cryptococcus neoformans*
3. *Toxoplasma gondii*
4. Cytomegalovirus
5. JC virus

How can pseudomonas infect the meninges and possibly cause meningitis?

Secondary to trauma, surgery, or tumors of the head or neck

In what stage of syphilis can syphilitic meningitis be seen?

Tertiary syphilis

In what seasons does viral meningitis mainly occur?

Summer and fall

What organisms are the major recognizable causes of aseptic meningitis?

Enteroviruses of the *Picornaviridae* family (poliovirus, coxsackievirus, echovirus, enterovirus)
All enteroviruses can cause central nervous system (CNS) disease

What is significant about enterovirus 70 and enterovirus 71?

Associated with particularly virulent CNS disease

What *Arenaviridae* family virus is a common cause of viral meningitis?

Lymphocytic choriomeningitis virus (LCMV)

What sexually transmitted virus can cause meningitis?

Herpes simplex virus (HSV)

What is the cardinal finding with this infection?

Retrograde infection of the temporal lobe with hemorrhage

What mycotic organism causes meningitis and yields a positive India ink stain?

Cryptococcus neoformans

In what patient population is *C. neoformans* a common cause of meningitis?

Acquired immune deficiency syndrome (AIDS) patients

What drug is used for prophylaxis against *C. neoformans* meningitis in this population?

Fluconazole

ENCEPHALITIS

What category of viruses is a common cause of encephalitis?

Arboviruses

What are they?

Viruses transmitted by arthropods, e.g., mosquitoes and ticks
Arbovirus is an acronym for
A̲rthropod-b̲orne virus

What arboviruses cause encephalitis that are part of each of the following:
Togaviridae family?

1. Eastern equine encephalitis virus
2. Western equine encephalitis virus
3. Venezuelan equine encephalitis virus

***Flaviviridae* family?**

1. St. Louis encephalitis virus
2. Japanese encephalitis virus
3. West Nile virus

***Bunyaviridae* family?**	1. California encephalitis virus 2. La Crosse encephalitis virus
How are all the previously mentioned viruses spread?	By infected mosquitoes
What *Rhabdoviridae* can cause encephalitis?	Rabies virus
What *Paramyxoviridae* can cause encephalitis?	Measles virus can rarely cause postmeasles encephalitis

"SLOW DISEASES" CAUSED BY VIRUSES

What are "slow diseases"?	A fatal set of diseases that affect the central nervous system that are caused by agents with long incubation periods, characterized by a gradual onset of symptoms, with a progressively deteriorating course
What are three "slow diseases" caused by viruses?	1. Progressive multifocal leukoencephalopathy (PML) 2. Subacute sclerosing panencephalitis (SSPE) 3. AIDS
What is PML?	A fatal disease of white matter that affects oligodendrocytes, leading to demyelination of neurons
What causes PML?	JC virus
What are the clinical manifestations of PML?	Impaired speech, vision, and mental capacity that rapidly progresses to paralysis, blindness, dementia, and coma
Which patient population is at increased risk for this disease?	Patients with impaired cell-mediated immunity; especially AIDS patients
What is SSPE?	Disease characterized by regions of inflammation diffusely throughout the brain

What causes SSPE?

Measles virus

What is the typical time course of SSPE after infection?

Usually does not present until several years after measles virus infection

What virus causes AIDS?

HIV

What are the central nervous system manifestations of AIDS?

AIDS encephalopathy resulting in severe dementia. (See Chapter 30, "Human Immunodeficiency Virus," for a more detailed review of AIDS)

PRIONS

What are prions?

Highly resistant agents composed of protein but no nucleic acid

What type of diseases do prions cause?
What are five examples?

Spongiform encephalopathies

1. Creutzfeldt-Jakob disease (CJD)
2. Kuru
3. Gerstmann-Straussler-Schinker (GSS) syndrome
4. Fatal familial insomnia
5. Bovine spongiform encephalopathy (mad cow disease)

What is seen on pathologic examination of prion-infected brains?

Spongiform (sponge-like) appearance secondary to neuronal vacuolation and degeneration

What are three forms of spongiform encephalopathies?

1. Infectious
2. Hereditary
3. Sporadic

48

Gastrointestinal System

DEFENSE MECHANISMS OF THE GASTROINTESTINAL TRACT

What are three types of barriers of the gastrointestinal tract?	1. Anatomical 2. Physiological 3. Biochemical
What are the special defenses of each of the following: **The mouth?**	1. Secretory IgA 2. Flow of liquids 3. Lysozymes 4. Normal flora, i.e., predominantly anaerobes
The esophagus?	1. Flow of liquids 2. Peristalsis
The stomach?	1. Low pH 2. Peristalsis 3. Mucus
The small intestine?	1. Flow of liquids 2. Peristalsis 3. Shedding of epithelium 4. Peyer patches 5. IgA 6. Mucus
The large intestine?	1. Normal flora, e.g., predominantly anaerobes including *Bacteroides fragilis* 2. Peristalsis 3. Shedding of epithelium
How does normal bacterial flora act as a defense mechanism?	1. Stimulates mucosal defenses 2. Competes with pathogens for nutrients 3. Directly inhibits growth or attachment

Are most gastrointestinal infections caused by bacterial, viral, or protozoal infections?	Viral infections

BACTERIAL PATHOGENS OF THE GASTROINTESTINAL TRACT

What are four ways that infectious agents overcome natural defenses?	1. Adherence to mucosal epithelium 2. Intracellular growth 3. Invasion of intestinal epithelium 4. Toxin production (endotoxin and exotoxin)
Where in the gastrointestinal tract does invasion of epithelium usually occur?	Through M cells of Peyer patches
What are three types of exotoxins that cause pathogenesis?	1. Enterotoxins 2. Cytotoxins 3. Neurotoxins
What is the pathogenesis of enterotoxins?	Alteration of metabolic activity resulting in an outpouring of electrolytes and fluid into the lumen
What are two types of enterotoxins?	Heat-labile toxin and heat-stable toxin
What is the mechanism of heat-labile enterotoxin?	Subunit B: extracellularly binds G_{M1} ganglioside at the brush border of the small intestine and facilitates the entry of Subunit A Subunit A: intracellularly activates adenylate cyclase, increases cyclic adenosine monophosphate (cAMP), increases secretion of water and Cl^- and inhibits Na^+ reabsorption leading to electrolyte imbalance, hypermotility and diarrhea
What is the mechanism of heat-stable enterotoxin?	Activates guanylate cyclase in epithelial cells of the small intestine, increases cyclic guanosine monophosphate (cGMP) and leads to fluid secretion

Heat-stable toxins can be ingested, but heat-labile toxins are produced by bacteria after ingestion

What makes exotoxins different from endotoxins?

Exotoxins are released from bacteria while endotoxins are found in the lipopolysaccharide (LPS) complex in gram-negative bacteria

What is a common component found in most endotoxins?

Toxic lipid A core

What is the pathogenesis of cytotoxins?

Cause alterations in cell function resulting in cell death, e.g., exotoxin B produced by *Clostridium difficile*

What is the pathogenesis of neurotoxins?

Cause alterations in neurological function, e.g., botulinum toxin

What percentage of the inpatient hospital population is affected by nosocomial enteric infections?

5–10%

What are the most common complications of nosocomial enteric infections?

Bacteremia and shock

Are nosocomial enteric infections or community-acquired enteric infections more resistant to bacteria?

Nosocomial enteric infections are more likely to be resistant to antibiotics as a result of antibiotic use

What is the general incubation period for enteric bacteria?

1–2 days

What is the leading cause of foodborne gastrointestinal illness in the United States?

Campylobacter causes 15% of foodborne illness

What is the most common cause of enteric fever?

Salmonella

Which bacteria cause inflammatory, bloody diarrhea?	1. *Campylobacter jejuni* 2. *Shigella* 3. Enteroinvasive *Escherichia coli* (EIEC) 4. Enterohemorrhagic *E. coli* (EHEC) 5. *Salmonella*
What protozoa causes inflammatory, bloody diarrhea?	*Entamoeba histolytica*
Which bacteria cause emesis secondary to ingestion of preformed toxins?	1. *Bacillus cereus* 2. *Staphylococcus aureus* 3. *Clostridium botulinum*
Which bacteria cause diarrhea secondary to ingestion of preformed toxins?	1. *B. cereus* 2. *Clostridium perfringens* 3. Enterotoxigenic *E. coli* (ETEC) 4. *Vibrio cholerae*
Which bacteria cause diarrhea secondary to colonization and multiplication?	1. *C. jejuni* 2. *Salmonella* species 3. *E. coli* species, i.e., EPEC, EHEC, EIEC 4. *Yersinia* species 5. *Vibrio* species 6. *Listeria monocytogenes*

BACTERIA CAUSING EMESIS SECONDARY TO INGESTION OF PREFORMED TOXIN

BACILLUS CEREUS

What food is associated with *B. cereus* infection causing emesis?	Fried rice
How does *B. cereus* cause disease?	Gram-positive, spore-forming rod produces both heat-stable and heat-labile toxins
What is the pathogenesis of *B. cereus*?	Heat-stabile toxin is released from spores when the food cools Heat-stabile toxin causes emesis, whereas heat-labile toxin causes diarrhea

What are the symptoms of B. cereus infection?	Rapid onset nausea (1–6 hours)
What is the duration of the vomiting disease?	8–10 hours

STAPHYLOCOCCUS AUREUS

What foods are associated with S. aureus infection?	Foods high in salt (ham), sugar (custard), and cream sauces
How does S. aureus cause disease?	Gram-positive cocci produce heat-stable emetic toxin
What is the pathogenesis of S. aureus?	Ingestion of only a small amount of heat-stable emetic toxin binds to neural receptors of upper gastrointestinal tract and stimulates emesis
What are the clinical manifestations of S. aureus infection?	Rapid onset nausea (1–6 hours), abdominal pain, vomiting, and diarrhea
What is the duration of the disease?	24–48 hours

CLOSTRIDIUM BOTULINUM

What foods are associated with C. botulinum infection?	Improperly canned vegetables, smoked fish, and honey
How does C. botulinum cause disease?	Gram-positive, spore-forming rod produces botulinum toxin
What is the pathogenesis of C. botulinum?	Botulinum exotoxin causes paralysis of cholinergic nerve fibers at the myoneural junction and suppresses the release of acetylcholine (ACh)
What disease does C. botulinum cause?	Botulism
What are the symptoms?	Nausea, dizziness, cranial palsy, double vision, swallowing and speech problems, muscle weakness, respiratory paralysis, and death in 20% of cases

Infant botulism: constipation, weakness, loss of head and limb control, i.e., "floppy baby syndrome"

BACTERIA CAUSING DIARRHEA SECONDARY TO INGESTION OF PREFORMED TOXIN

BACILLUS CEREUS

What foods are associated with B. cereus infection causing diarrhea?	Cream sauces, pudding, beef, sausage, chicken soup, and fried rice
How does B. cereus cause disease?	Gram-positive, spore-forming rod produces both heat-stable and heat-labile toxins
What is the pathogenesis of B. cereus?	Heat-labile enterotoxin causes increased cAMP levels and fluid secretion, resulting in diarrhea Heat-stabile toxin causes emesis, whereas heat-labile toxin causes diarrhea **USMLE**
What are the symptoms of B. cereus infection?	Watery diarrhea 10–12 hours after ingestion
What is the duration of the diarrheal disease?	20–36 hours

CLOSTRIDIUM PERFRINGENS

What foods are associated with C. perfringens infection?	Beef, poultry, gravy, fish, and stew that have been cooked and reheated
Which seasons are associated with higher incidence of C. perfringens infection?	Fall and winter
How does C. perfringens cause disease?	Gram-positive spore-forming rod produces heat-labile toxin during sporulation
What is the pathogenesis of C. perfringens?	Heat-labile enterotoxin inhibits glucose transport and damages intestinal epithelium via alpha toxin and lecithinase

How many organisms are required for symptoms to occur?	Large inoculum needed ($>10^8$)
What are the symptoms of *C. perfringens* infection?	Watery diarrhea, crampy abdominal pain, vomiting, fever, chills, and headache occurring 8–24 hours after ingestion
What is the duration of the disease?	Less than 24 hours

ENTEROTOXIGENIC *ESCHERICHIA COLI*

What foods are associated with ETEC infection?	Salads, fruits, vegetables
How does ETEC cause disease?	Gram-negative rod produces heat-stable and heat-labile toxins
What is the pathogenesis of ETEC?	Heat-stable and heat-labile enterotoxins cause hypersecretion of chloride ions and water from intestinal mucosal cells while inhibiting reabsorption of sodium Heat-labile enterotoxin acts much like cholera toxin
What are the symptoms of ETEC infection?	"Traveler's diarrhea" secretory diarrhea within 16–72 hours of ingestion

VIBRIO CHOLERA

What foods are associated with *V. cholera* infection?	Shellfish and other uncooked foods with contaminated water
How does *V. cholera* cause disease?	Gram-negative rod produces heat-labile enterotoxin, i.e., cholera toxin
What is the pathogenesis of *V. cholera*?	Cholera toxin adenosine diphosphate (ADP) ribosylates G_s causing constitutive activation of adenylate cyclase resulting in increased cAMP and opening the cystic fibrosis transmembrane conductance regulator (CFTR) chloride channel
What are the symptoms of *V. cholera* infection?	Watery diarrhea referred to as "rice water stools" within 48–72 hours of ingestion
Do symptoms occur with a small inoculum?	No, a large dose is needed to cause disease

What is a complication of *V. cholera* infection? **What is the mortality rate of this complication?**	Hypovolemic shock 60% if unmanaged
What is the treatment for cholera?	Replacement of fluids and electrolytes can reduce death rates from 50% to less than 1% Tetracycline can shorten symptoms

BACTERIA CAUSING DIARRHEA SECONDARY TO COLONIZATION AND MULTIPLICATION

CAMPYLOBACTER JEJUNI

What is the reservoir for *C. jejuni*?	Large animal reservoir, especially poultry
What foods are associated with *C. jejuni* infection?	Chicken, other poultry, milk, and contaminated water
What is the pathogenesis of *C. jejuni*?	Gram-negative rod colonizes the intestinal mucosa and invades epithelium, causing ulceration and bleeding
Does *C. jejuni* cause bacteremia?	Rarely enters the bloodstream, but more likely to do so in the immuno-compromised
What are the symptoms of *C. jejuni* infection? **What is the duration of these symptoms?**	Acute enteritis with bloody diarrhea following a 2- to 10-day incubation period 1 week
What are uncommon symptoms of *C. jejuni* infection?	Traveler's diarrhea and pseudoappendicitis
What are three complications of *C. jejuni* infection?	1. Bacteremia 2. Reactive arthritis 3. Guillain-Barré syndrome

SALMONELLA SPECIES

Which strains of *Salmonella* cause gastrointestinal disease?	1. *S. enterica* serotype *enteritidis* 2. *S. enterica* serotype *typhimurium* 3. *S. typhi* 4. *S. paratyphi*

What is the mode of transmission used by _S. enterica_ serotypes _enteritidis_ and _typhimurium_?

Contact with pet turtles and consumption of chicken eggs, poultry, and dairy products

What is the pathogenesis of these serotypes?

Invasion of epithelial cells of the small intestine resulting in the release of prostaglandins and cytokines

What are the symptoms of infection with either _S. enterica_ serotype _enteritidis_ or _typhimurium_?

16–48 hours after ingestion, nausea and vomiting ensue, followed by abdominal cramping and nonbloody diarrhea

What is the duration of disease?

3–4 days

What is the mode of transmission used by _S. typhi_ and _S. paratyphi_?

Person-person transmission; _S. typhi_ is only a human pathogen

What is the pathogenesis of _S. typhi_ and _S. paratyphi_?

Bacterial invasion of M cells and replication in macrophages of Peyer patches enables the bacteria to enter the reticuloendothelial system and disseminate into the bloodstream

What disease is caused _S. typhi_ and _S. paratyphi_?

Enteric typhoid fever

What are the symptoms of this disease?

After an incubation period of 5–21 days, fever, abdominal pain, and rose spots develop; diarrhea occurs late in the infection

S. paratyphi infection causes a milder form of this disease

What are the complications of this disease?

Intestinal hemorrhage and endocarditis

ESCHERICHIA COLI

Which strains of _E. coli_ cause gastrointestinal disease through colonization and multiplication?

1. Enteropathogenic _E. coli_ (EPEC)
2. Enterohemorrhagic _E. coli_ (EHEC)
3. Enteroinvasive _E. coli_ (EIEC)

What is the mode of transmission used by EPEC?

Newborn infected during birth or _in utero_

What is the pathogenesis of EPEC?

Tissue destruction and effacing lesions secondary to colonization resulting in a malabsorptive surface

What are the symptoms of EPEC?

Chronic, watery diarrhea in infants
EPEC is a significant cause of infant diarrhea in developing countries

What foods are associated with EHEC infection?

Beef, apple juice, and radish roots

What is the pathogenesis of EHEC?

Similar to EPEC, but at very low bacterial inoculums (< 100 organisms), bacteria produce Shiga-like toxins which remove a base from 28s ribosomal ribonucleic acid (rRNA), disrupting protein synthesis; the attaching/effacing lesions destroy microvilli resulting in severe bloody diarrhea

What are the symptoms of EHEC?

What is a major complication of this disease?

Ranges from mild watery diarrhea to hemorrhagic colitis with abdominal cramps and bloody diarrhea
Hemolytic uremic syndrome (HUS), which consists of microangiopathic hemolytic anemia, thrombocytopenia, and acute renal failure caused by thrombosis of glomerular capillaries
HUS is a major cause of renal failure in children when treated with antibiotics

What serotype of EHEC causes most infections?

E. coli 0157:H7

What is the mode of transmission used by EIEC?

Foodborne, most similar to *Shigella*

What is the pathogenesis of EIEC?

Invades and destroys colonic epithelium

What are the symptoms of EIEC?

Which patient population is most likely to present with these symptoms?

Initially watery diarrhea which progresses to dysentery-like syndrome with fever and bloody stools
Children younger than 5 years old in developing countries; EIEC is rare in the United States

YERSINIA SPECIES

What species of Yersinia cause gastrointestinal disease?

Y. enterocolitica and *Y. pseudotuberculosis*

How are Y. enterocolitica and Y. pseudotuberculosis transmitted?

Ingestion of food (especially pork and milk) contaminated by colonized domestic animals or raw meat

What is unique about Yersinia?

Can grow at 4°C (39.2°F), although it prefers to grow at 22°C (71.6°F) to 25°C (77°F)

What is the pathogenesis of Y. enterocolitica and Y. pseudotuberculosis?

Produces a toxin that causes increased cGMP and bacterial invasion of M cells; replication in mesenteric lymph nodes causes inflammation and ulcerative lesions in the terminal ileum

What are the symptoms of Y. enterocolitica and Y. pseudotuberculosis infection?

Symptoms appear 4–6 days after ingestion and include fever, pain, and bloody diarrhea, mimicking appendicitis

   What are the complications?

Septicemia, arthritis, intraabdominal abscess, hepatitis, and osteomyelitis

   Who is at risk for infection?

Infants and children; however, infection is rare in the United States

   Does infection require a high or low dose of organisms?

High dose of bacteria is required for symptoms to appear

VIBRIO SPECIES

Which species of Vibrio cause gastrointestinal disease through colonization and multiplication?

V. parahaemolyticus

What foods are associated with Vibrio infection?

Contaminated raw seafood

   What is the pathogenesis of infection?

Bacteria invade intestinal cells, but usually do not cause bacteremia or systemic spread

What are the symptoms of Vibrio infection?	Explosive watery diarrhea and fever 16–72 hours after ingestion
Does infection require a high or low dose to cause symptoms?	High dose is required for symptoms to appear

LISTERIA MONOCYTOGENES

What foods are associated with L. monocytogenes infection?	Contaminated milk, soft cheeses, vegetables, and coleslaw
How else is L. monocytogenes transmitted?	Crosses the placenta
What is unusual about L. monocytogenes?	Can grow at 4°C (39.2°F)
What are the symptoms of L. monocytogenes?	Meningitis in neonates and immunocompromised; mild intestinal distress in healthy adults

GASTROINTESTINAL INFECTIONS NOT ASSOCIATED WITH FOOD

SHIGELLA SPECIES

Which species of Shigella cause gastrointestinal disease?	S. sonnei, S. boydii, S. flexneri, and S. dysenteriae
What is the natural reservoir for Shigella?	Human-only pathogen
How is Shigella transmitted?	Person to person transmission usually by poor hygiene or by contact with contaminated stools
What is a common setting for Shigella transmission?	Child day care centers
What type of gastrointestinal disease is caused by Shigella?	Shigellosis
What is another name for this disease?	Bacillary dysentery

What are the symptoms?	Frequent, scant diarrhea with blood, mucus, and painful abdominal cramping
How does *Shigella* cause disease?	Colonizes and destroys large intestinal mucosa; *S. dysenteriae* serotype 1 elaborates Shiga-toxin
What is the pathogenesis of this toxin?	Inhibits protein synthesis by removing one base from 28S rRNA
What other toxin has a similar mechanism of action?	"Shiga-like" toxin elaborated by enterohemorrhagic *E. coli* (EHEC)
Is this toxin necessary for the organism to cause disease?	No, but presence of the toxin increases the severity of disease
Does infection require a high or low dose of organisms?	Low dose of organisms is required because the bacteria is highly infectious
What is a serious complication of infection?	HUS

CLOSTRIDIUM DIFFICILE

Is *C. difficile* part of the normal flora?	Yes, it is carried in 3% of healthy adults
What group of patients is at higher risk of symptomatic *C. difficile* infection? Why?	Patients on antibiotics Antibiotics reduce normal flora while allowing overgrowth of other pathogenic species
Which antibiotics predispose patients to symptomatic *C. difficile* infection?	Clindamycin and β-lactams
How does *C. difficile* cause disease?	Gram-positive, spore-forming rod that produces toxins
What is the pathogenesis of *C. difficile*?	Enterotoxin (toxin A) and cytotoxin (toxin B) kill mucosal cells, causing gastrointestinal distress

What gastrointestinal diseases are caused by C. difficile?	1. Pseudomembranous colitis 2. Antibiotic-associated diarrhea
What is the treatment for C. difficile infection?	Removal of offending antibiotics and possibly starting metronidazole; reconstituting flora by eating yogurt also improves symptoms

HELICOBACTER PYLORI

What is the main reservoir for H. pylori?	Humans
How is H. pylori transmitted?	Only person to person (fecal–oral)
What is an important virulence factor of H. pylori? **Why?**	Urease Produces ammonia that neutralizes stomach acid, facilitating bacterial colonization of the stomach; stimulates monocytes and neutrophils and increases inflammation
What is the pathogenesis of H. pylori?	Mobile, gram-negative, flagellated rod colonizes gastric mucosa in the stomach, and metaplastic epithelium in the esophagus and duodenum, leading to chronic inflammation
What gastrointestinal diseases are caused by H. pylori?	1. Duodenal and gastric ulcers 2. Acute gastritis, sometimes with diarrhea
What disease does H. pylori infection increase the risk for?	Gastric adenocarcinoma and gastric mucosa-associated lymphoid tissue (MALT) lymphoma

BACTEROIDES FRAGILIS

What type of gastrointestinal disease is caused by B. fragilis?	Abdominal pain secondary to gastrointestinal abscesses that form after damage to mucosal barriers
How is B. fragilis transmitted?	Part of the normal flora of the colon which causes disease only when it gains

access to the blood or peritoneum usually following surgery or trauma; there is no human transmission

What are the pathogenic mechanisms used by B. fragilis?

Weak endotoxin and polysaccharide capsule

VIRAL PATHOGENS OF THE GASTROINTESTINAL TRACT

How are most gastrointestinal viruses transmitted?

Fecal–oral transmission

What are the general characteristics of gastrointestinal viruses?
  What are three exceptions?

Usually they are nonenveloped positive single-stranded RNA viruses

1. Rotavirus has a segmented double-stranded RNA genome
2. Adenovirus has a double-stranded DNA genome
3. Enteric coronaviruses have an envelope

What population is at a higher risk for severe diarrheal disease?

Children
Diarrheal disease accounts for 25% of all deaths in children younger than 5 years of age in developing countries

What is endemic diarrhea?

Diarrhea caused by viruses or offending agents restricted to a certain geographical area

  What is a common etiology?

Group A rotavirus

What is epidemic diarrhea?

Diarrhea caused by viruses or offending agents that cross geographical areas

  What are three common etiologies?

1. Norwalk virus
2. Group B rotavirus
3. Group C rotavirus

What is the typical incubation period for gastrointestinal viruses?

12–36 hours

What does a faster incubation period suggest?	Bacterial infection with symptoms caused by preformed bacterial toxins
How does gastrointestinal viral infection typically cause diarrhea?	Virus causes a breakdown in the lumen of the small intestine, resulting in an area of malabsorption, osmotic diarrhea, and fluid loss
How are gastrointestinal viral infections detected?	Symptomatic individuals can be diagnosed by viral cultures or by a fourfold (or greater) increase in antibody titer
Are gastrointestinal viruses usually detectable in the feces?	Yes, most viruses achieve high titers in feces

ROTAVIRUS

What disease does rotavirus cause?	Acute gastroenteritis
What are the symptoms?	Low-grade fever, diarrhea, and vomiting for 5–8 days
Whom does this disease typically affect?	Infants and children
What is the incubation period for rotavirus?	1–3 days
How many serotypes of rotavirus exist?	Several serotypes have been identified, at least six of which have been isolated from humans
What type of nucleic acid does the rotavirus genome contain?	Segmented, dsRNA
How does rotavirus cause diarrhea?	Replicates in mucosal cells of small intestine, damaging transport mechanisms resulting in a loss of water, glucose, and salt into the lumen
Does rotavirus cause inflammatory diarrhea?	No, the diarrhea is watery and nonbloody
Does a vaccine for rotavirus exist?	Yes, Rotashield vaccine contains a live-attenuated virus

Why is the vaccine no longer used in the United States?	Vaccine was linked to higher rates of intussusception

NORWALK VIRUS

What disease does Norwalk virus cause?	Acute gastroenteritis
Who is typically affected by this disease?	School-aged children and adults
Where do outbreaks of this disease usually occur?	In confined populations, e.g., schools and cruise ships
How long do symptoms typically last?	12–24 hours

ENTERIC PICORNAVIRUSES

What are four enteric picornaviruses?	1. Poliovirus 2. Echoviruses 3. Coxsackievirus 4. Hepatitis A (see Chapter 29, "Viral Hepatitis")
What disease does poliovirus cause?	Poliomyelitis
What are the three types of this disease?	1. Abortive poliomyelitis 2. Nonparalytic poliomyelitis 3. Paralytic poliomyelitis
What symptoms can occur with each type?	Abortive poliomyelitis symptoms include nonspecific symptoms such as headache, nausea, and vomiting Nonparalytic poliomyelitis symptoms include fever, headache, stiff neck Paralytic poliomyelitis symptoms include asymmetric muscle weakness followed by muscle paralysis
How often are patients with poliovirus infection symptomatic?	1% of infections are symptomatic
Which cells are initially infected by poliovirus?	Poliovirus infects and replicates within cells of the oropharynx and intestinal lymphoid tissue

What is the treatment for symptomatic treatment?

Only supportive treatment

Is there a vaccine for poliovirus?

Yes, a live-attenuated vaccine (Sabin) and a killed vaccine (Salk) have effectively eradicated poliovirus from the western hemisphere

What diseases do echoviruses cause?

1. Aseptic meningitis
2. Upper respiratory infections
3. Infantile diarrhea
Coxsackieviruses and echoviruses are two of the leading causes of aseptic meningitis

What diseases do coxsackieviruses cause?

1. Herpangina (group A)
2. Hand-foot-and-mouth disease (group A)
3. Aseptic meningitis (groups A and B)
4. Epidemic pleurodynia (group B)
5. Myocarditis (group B)
6. Pericarditis (group B)

What is herpangina?

Disease with symptoms including fever, sore throat, and vesicles in the oropharynx

What is hand-foot-and-mouth disease?

Disease characterized by vesicular rash of hands and feet and ulcerations in the oropharynx

ADENOVIRUSES

What gastrointestinal disease do adenoviruses cause?

Infantile gastroenteritis

What serotypes of adenovirus are associated with this disease?

Types 40 and 41

How do the symptoms of this disease compare to that caused by rotavirus?

Milder form of gastroenteritis, but symptoms last longer (about 11 days)

MINOR VIRAL PATHOGENS

What are two minor enteric viral pathogens?

1. Coronavirus
2. Astrovirus

What gastrointestinal disease has been linked to coronavirus?	Necrotizing enterocolitis
Who is at risk for this disease?	Neonates
What disease does astrovirus cause?	Acute gastroenteritis
What are the symptoms?	Watery diarrhea in children, similar to symptomatic rotavirus infection

PARASITES OF THE GASTROINTESTINAL SYSTEM

PROTOZOA

What three protozoa are major intestinal pathogens?	1. *Giardia lamblia* 2. *Cryptosporidium parvum* 3. *Entamoeba histolytica*

Giardia Lamblia

How is *Giardia* transmitted?	Ingestion of cysts in fecally contaminated food and water
How does *Giardia* cause disease?	Trophozoite attaches to gut, causing inflammation of duodenal mucosa and malabsorption of protein and fat *Giardia* does not invade epithelial cells
What disease does *Giardia* cause?	Giardiasis
What are the symptoms?	Nonbloody, foul-smelling, watery diarrhea associated with nausea and abdominal cramps
How long do symptoms persist?	Left untreated, generally spontaneous recovery can occur after 10–14 days, although multiple relapses may occur
What is the treatment of choice?	Metronidazole

Cryptosporidium Parvum

How is *Cryptosporidium* transmitted?	Ingestion of oocysts in fecally contaminated food and water

How does *Cryptosporidium* cause disease?	Trophozoite attaches to surface of intestinal epithelium, matures by schizogony, and then fertilization *Cryptosporidium* invades just within brush-border epithelium, but does not penetrate the basal layer
What disease does *Cryptosporidium* cause?	Cryptosporidiosis
What are the symptoms?	Nonbloody, watery diarrhea lasting approximately 10 days
In which population are the symptoms most severe?	Immunocompromised

Entamoeba Histolytica

How is *E. histolytica* transmitted?	Ingestion of cysts in fecally contaminated food and water
How does *E. histolytica* cause disease?	Trophozoite invades colonic epithelium and secretes enzymes, causing extensive local necrosis; trophozoite invades portal circulation and forms abscesses in liver *E. histolytica* invades epithelial cells
What diseases do *E. histolytica* cause?	Amebic dysentery and liver abscess
What are the symptoms?	Bloody diarrhea containing mucous associated with right upper quadrant abdominal pain and tenesmus
What are three minor intestinal protozoal pathogens?	1. *Cyclospora cayetanensis* (cyclosporiasis) 2. *Isospora belli* (isosporosis) 3. *Balantidium coli* (dysentery)

TREMATODES

Which three trematodes are major intestinal pathogens?	1. *Schistosoma mansoni* 2. *Schistosoma japonicum* 3. *Clonorchis sinensis*

How do S. mansoni and S. japonicum affect the gastrointestinal tract?	Live in the mesenteric veins and produce eggs that that migrate to the liver, spleen, or wall of the intestine
What do these trematodes cause?	Portal hypertension Schistosomiasis is the number one cause of portal hypertension worldwide
How is C. sinensis transmitted?	Eating raw or undercooked fish
Where does C. sinensis live in the body? **What does it cause?**	Biliary tract Cholangitis or even cholangiocarcinoma

CESTODES

What four cestodes are major intestinal pathogens?	1. *Taenia solium*, i.e., pork tapeworm 2. *Taenia saginata*, i.e., beef tapeworm 3. *Diphyllobothrium latum*, i.e., fish tapeworm 4. *Echinococcus granulosus*, i.e., dog tapeworm
How is T. solium transmitted?	Eating raw or undercooked pork
Does T. solium itself cause much damage to the gastrointestinal tract?	No, most of the damage is caused by the tissue cysts that develop
What does T. solium cause?	Cysticercosis and neurocysticercosis, i.e., cysts develop in the brain
How is T. saginata transmitted?	Eating raw or undercooked beef
Does T. saginata cause cysticercosis?	No
How is D. latum transmitted?	Eating raw or undercooked fish
What does D. latum cause? How?	Megaloblastic anemia The parasite preferentially takes up vitamin B_{12}, causing vitamin B_{12} deficiency and megaloblastic anemia

What is the most important definitive host for *E. granulosus*?	Dogs (with sheep as important intermediate hosts)
What does *E. granulosus* cause?	Hydatid cyst disease
What organs does this disease typically affect?	Liver, lung, and brain
What happens if the cyst ruptures?	May cause a severe anaphylactic reaction, therefore surgical removal is carefully considered

NEMATODES

What seven nematodes are major intestinal pathogens?	1. *Enterobius vermicularis*, i.e., pinworm 2. *Trichuris trichiura*, i.e., whipworm 3. *Ascaris lumbricoides*, i.e., giant roundworm 4. *Ancylostoma duodenale*, i.e., old world hookworm 5. *Necator americanus*, i.e., new world hookworm 6. *Strongyloides stercoralis*, i.e., small roundworm 7. *Trichinella spiralis*
What is the most common symptom of *E. vermicularis* (i.e., pinworm) infection?	Perianal pruritus
How is *E. vermicularis* infection diagnosed?	Scotch tape test in the morning
What symptoms do *T. trichiura* (i.e., whipworm) cause?	Diarrhea, abdominal pain, flatulence, and possibly rectal prolapse
What can an infection with a heavy worm burden cause?	Intestinal obstruction
How do *A. duodenale* and *N. americanus* affect the gastrointestinal tract? **What does this cause?**	These hookworms attach to the small intestine and suck blood from the intestinal wall Microcytic anemia

How does *S. stercoralis* affect the gastrointestinal tract?

Larvae penetrate skin; adult female worms attach to small intestine, causing inflammation and watery diarrhea

What is unique about the transmission of *S. stercoralis*?

May cause autoinfection where larvae infect the host without leaving the host

How does *S. stercoralis* infection differ in the immunocompromised?

Can cause a hyperinfection syndrome, with larvae migrating to many organs

How is *T. spiralis* transmitted?

Eating raw or undercooked meat, including pork or homemade sausage

How does *T. spiralis* affect the gastrointestinal tract?

Larvae are released in the stomach causing gastroenteritis and diarrhea

How does *T. spiralis* spread?

Larvae travel through the blood to many organs, but encyst in striated muscle cells

What are the symptoms that occur later in infection?

Fever, myositis, myalgia, and periorbital edema

Section VII

Appendices

Appendix A

Antibacterial Drugs

OVERVIEW

What are bactericidal antibiotics?

Drugs that kill bacteria

What are bacteriostatic antibiotics?

Drugs that inhibit the growth of bacteria, but do not immediately kill them

When are bactericidal antibiotics preferable to bacteriostatic antibiotics?

1. Immunocompromised patients
2. Infections that are immediately life-threatening, e.g., meningitis or endocarditis
3. Infections that are protected from the host's immunity, e.g., abscess

What is MIC?

Minimal Inhibitory Concentration, or the lowest concentration of a drug that inhibits bacterial growth *in vitro*

What is MBC?

Minimal Bactericidal Concentration, or the lowest concentration of drug that kills bacteria *in vitro*

What is synergism?

An effect where the action of combining two or more drugs is significantly greater than the sum of the drugs acting separately

What is antagonism?

An effect where the action of combining two or more drugs is significantly lower than the sum of the drugs acting separately

What are broad-spectrum antibiotics?

Drugs that are effective against several different classes of bacteria, e.g., both gram-positive and gram-negative bacteria (imipenem is an example)

What are narrow-spectrum antibiotics?	Drugs that are effective against few types of bacteria; e.g., first-generation cephalosporins are effective against only gram-positive bacteria
What four parts of the bacterial cell are common targets for antibacterial drugs?	1. Cell walls 2. Cell membranes 3. Ribosomes (protein synthesis) 4. Nucleic acid and biosynthetic enzymes

PENICILLIN-FAMILY ANTIBIOTICS

What structure do all penicillin-family antibiotics contain?	β-Lactam ring
What enzymes do penicillin-family antibiotics inhibit?	Transpeptidases
What is the effect of inhibiting these enzymes?	Prevents the final cross-linking step in the synthesis of peptidoglycan
Are penicillin-family antibiotics bactericidal or bacteriostatic?	Bactericidal
What are some mechanisms that allow organisms to resist actions of penicillin?	1. Altered penicillin-binding proteins (PBPs), including transpeptidases, to prevent binding of the drug to cell membranes and walls 2. Contain β-lactamase enzymes that cleave the β-lactam ring, inactivating the drug
What other mechanism do gram-negative bacteria uniquely use to develop resistance against penicillins?	Alter their porins to prevent penicillin from entering the organism
What side effect can occur from administration of penicillins?	Hypersensitivity reaction characterized by anaphylactic shock, hives, and rash
What are five classes of penicillin-family antibiotics?	1. Penicillin G and V 2. Aminopenicillins 3. Penicillinase-resistant penicillins

4. Antipseudomonal penicillins
5. Cephalosporins

What is the main difference between penicillin G and V?

Penicillin G is administered intravenously
Penicillin V is administered orally
   Think "<u>GIVE</u>" pen <u>G</u> by <u>IV</u>

What is the spectrum of activity for penicillin G and V?

1. *Streptococcus pneumoniae*
2. *Streptococcus pyogenes*
3. Gram-positive rods, including *Bacillus anthracis*, *Clostridium perfringens*, and *Corynebacterium diphtheriae*
4. *Neisseria* sp.
5. *Treponema pallidum*

What are two aminopenicillins?

1. Ampicillin
2. Amoxicillin

How do the aminopenicillins differ in their spectrum of activity from penicillin G and V?

Provide better gram-negative coverage and also cover enterococci (group D streptococci)

What antibiotic is commonly added to ampicillin for broader gram-negative coverage?

Gentamicin
Amp-Gent (ampicillin-genta-
   micin) is a common combination used on the wards

What are three penicillinase-resistant penicillins?

1. Methicillin
2. Nafcillin
3. Oxacillin

What are the therapeutic uses for penicillinase-resistant penicillins?

Staphylococcus aureus infections, especially for penicillinase-producing strains

What are four antipseudomonal penicillins?

1. Carbenicillin
2. Ticarcillin
3. Piperacillin
4. Mezlocillin

What are the therapeutic uses for antipseudomonal penicillins?

1. *Pseudomonas aeruginosa*
2. Anaerobes

What are three β-lactamase inhibitors that are often given with penicillins to prevent resistance?

1. Clavulanic acid
2. Sulbactam
3. Tazobactam

Common combinations on the wards include ampicillin-sulbactam, amoxicillin-clavulanic acid, ticarcillin-clavulanic acid, and piperacillin-tazobactam

What are three organisms that produce β-lactamase?

1. *Staphylococcus aureus*
2. *Haemophilus influenzae*
3. *Bacteroides fragilis*

What are the major examples of each of the following:

First-generation cephalosporins?

1. Cephalexin
2. Cefazolin

Second-generation cephalosporins?

1. Cefuroxime
2. Cefoxitin
3. Cefotetan

Third-generation cephalosporins?

1. Ceftriaxone
2. Cefotaxime
3. Ceftazidime

Fourth-generation cephalosporins?

Cefepime

How does the spectrum of the cephalosporins change from first through third generations?

Increasing spectrum for gram-negative bacteria and decreasing spectrum for gram-positive bacteria

What is the spectrum of activity for each of the following:

First-generation cephalosporins?

Gram-positive bacteria

Second-generation cephalosporins?

Increasing activity against gram-negative bacilli and variable activity against gram-positive bacteria

Third-generation cephalosporins?

More increased activity against gram-negative bacilli and less activity against gram-positive bacteria; some types active against *P. aeruginosa*

Fourth-generation cephalosporins?	Extended activity against gram-positive and gram-negative bacteria, including *P. aeruginosa*
What is the main advantage of cephalosporins over the other penicillins?	They contain an adjacent 6-member ring, making their β-lactam ring more resistant to β lactamases
What percentage of people with a penicillin allergy are also allergic to cephalosporins?	10%

ANTIBIOTICS THAT TARGET CELL WALL SYNTHESIS AND CELL MEMBRANES

Which antibiotics target cell wall synthesis?	1. Penicillin-family antibiotics 2. Carbapenems 3. Monobactams 4. Vancomycin 5. Bacitracin 6. Cycloserine 7. Fosfomycin
Which antibiotic targets cell membranes?	Polymyxin
What are two carbapenems?	1. Imipenem 2. Meropenem
What is the spectrum of activity for carbapenems?	Gram-positive bacteria, gram-negative bacteria, and anaerobes
Why is imipenem so powerful?	1. Resistant to β-lactamases 2. Small size allows it to pass through porins
What drug is commonly given with imipenem? Why?	Cilastin Cilastin inhibits the renal enzyme that metabolizes imipenem, thereby increasing the half-life of imipenem
What is an example of a monobactam?	Aztreonam
What is the spectrum of activity for aztreonam?	Only gram-negative bacteria

What is the spectrum of activity for vancomycin?	All gram-positive bacteria, including methicillin-resistant *S. aureus* (MRSA) and most enterococci (except vancomycin-resistant *Enterococcus* [VRE])
What is the mechanism for vancomycin?	Inhibits transpeptidation of D-alanine, which is one step earlier than the penicillin-family antibiotics

DRUGS THAT TARGET THE 50S RIBOSOMAL SUBUNIT

What drugs target the 50S ribosomal subunit?

1. Chloramphenicol
2. Macrolides
3. Lincosamides
   The average age of "CML" is 50(S)

What is the spectrum of activity for chloramphenicol?

Gram-positive bacteria, gram-negative bacteria, and anaerobes

What is the toxicity of chloramphenicol?

1. Bone marrow toxicity–aplastic anemia
2. Gray baby syndrome

What are three macrolides?

1. Azithromycin
2. Clarithromycin
3. Erythromycin
   Remember "ACE" for the macrolides

What is the spectrum of activity for erythromycin?

Erythromycin is better incorporated into gram-positive bacteria
1. *Mycoplasma pneumoniae*
2. *Legionella*
3. *Streptococcus pneumoniae*
4. *Chlamydia trachomatis*
5. *Bordetella pertussis*
6. *Corynebacterium diphtheriae*

For which patient population is erythromycin an acceptable choice?

Penicillin-allergic patients

What is the toxicity of erythromycin?

Relatively benign, but can cause gastrointestinal distress and, rarely, reversible cholestatic hepatitis

What are two lincosamides?

1. Clindamycin
2. Lincomycin

Lincosamides contain the letters "lin"

What is the spectrum of activity for lincosamides?

Anaerobes, gram-positive organisms

What side-effect does clindamycin have?
How does it occur?

Pseudomembranous colitis

Kills natural gastrointestinal (GI) flora, allowing *Clostridium difficile* to grow and release an exotoxin, causing cell death, ulceration, exudative membrane formation and severe bloody diarrhea

How is this condition treated?

Oral vancomycin or metronidazole

DRUGS THAT TARGET THE 30S RIBOSOMAL SUBUNIT

Which drugs target the 30S ribosomal subunit?

1. Aminoglycosides
2. Tetracyclines

What are five aminoglycosides?

1. Streptomycin
2. Gentamicin
3. Tobramycin
4. Amikacin
5. Neomycin

Are aminoglycosides bactericidal or bacteriostatic?

Bactericidal

What is the spectrum of activity for aminoglycosides?

Aerobes including gram-negative rods, *Francisella tularensis*, *Klebsiella pneumoniae*, *Proteus mirabilis*, and *P. aeruginosa*

Why are aminoglycosides only effective against aerobes?

Require an oxygen-dependent transport system to deliver the antibiotic across cell membranes

Why are aminoglycosides often used with penicillins?

Penicillins break down cell walls, allowing aminoglycosides to enter, i.e., they have a synergistic effect

What are the side effects of aminoglycosides?	1. Ototoxicity—cranial nerve (CN) VIII toxicity 2. Nephrotoxicity 3. Neurotoxicity—neuromuscular blockade
What are two tetracyclines?	1. Tetracycline 2. Doxycycline
Are tetracyclines bactericidal or bacteriostatic?	Bacteriostatic
What is the spectrum of activity for tetracyclines?	*Rickettsia rickettsii, Chlamydia* sp., *Mycoplasma pneumoniae, Borrelia burgdorferi, Treponema pallidum, Haemophilus influenzae, Vibrio cholerae,* and *Corynebacterium acnes*
What are the side effects of tetracyclines?	1. Teratogenic effects in fetus 2. GI irritation 3. Phototoxic dermatitis 4. Superinfections—*Candida* and *C. difficile* 5. Hepatic toxicity 6. Renal toxicity 7. Fanconi syndrome 8. Bone deposition and discoloration
What foods should patients taking tetracyclines avoid?	Dairy products because the drug chelates with the calcium ions and does not absorb in the intestine
What is an absolute contraindication to treatment with tetracyclines?	Pregnancy

DRUGS THAT TARGET NUCLEIC ACID

What drugs target messenger ribonucleic acid (mRNA) synthesis?	Rifampin
How?	Inhibits DNA-dependent RNA polymerase
What is the spectrum of activity for rifampin?	*Mycobacterium tuberculosis* and leprosy; prophylaxis for patients exposed to *Neisseria meningitidis*

What are the side effects of rifampin?

Secretions become orange (including urine, sweat, and tears); asymptomatic jaundice; hepatotoxicity

What drugs target DNA synthesis by inhibition of DNA gyrase?

1. Fluoroquinolones
2. Nalidixic acid

Are fluoroquinolones bactericidal or bacteriostatic?

Bactericidal

What are five fluoroquinolones?

1. Nalidixic acid (first generation)
2. Ciprofloxacin (second generation)
3. Ofloxacin (second generation)
4. Levofloxacin (third generation)
5. Moxifloxacin (fourth generation)

What is the spectrum of activity for each generation of fluoroquinolones?

All fluoroquinolones have good gram-negative coverage

  First generation

Oral use only, narrow spectrum

  Second generation

Systemic infections, urinary tract infections, hospital-acquired infections, gram-negative intracellular organisms

  Third generation

Expanded gram-positive and atypical pneumonia coverage (*Legionella, Mycoplasma, Chlamydia*)

  Fourth generation

Anaerobic activity and enhanced gram-positive coverage

Why are fluoroquinolones good for treating urinary tract infections?

They achieve high renal and prostate drug levels

Why are fluoroquinolones used for treating diarrhea?

They have good coverage of gram-negative organisms including *E. coli, Salmonella, Shigella*, and *Campylobacter*

Why are fluoroquinolones used for treating infections in patients with cystic fibrosis?

They have good *Pseudomonas* coverage

What are the side effects of fluoroquinolones?	Gastrointestinal distress, Achilles tendon rupture (rare), central nervous system (CNS) effects in the elderly
Why should fluoroquinolones not be prescribed for children?	May damage cartilage
What drugs target tetrahydrofolate synthesis (and therefore nucleotide synthesis)?	1. Sulfonamides 2. Trimethoprim
What is a common combination of these drugs?	Trimethoprim-sulfamethoxazole (TMP-SMX)
Why are these drugs usually given together?	They have a synergistic effect Trimethoprim inhibits dihydrofolate (DHF) reductase; sulfamethoxazole inhibits *para*-aminobenzoic acid (PABA) conversion to DHF
What is the spectrum of activity for TMP-SMX?	*Pneumocystis carinii, Neisseria gonorrhoeae, Neisseria meningitides, E. coli, H. influenzae, Legionella pneumophila, P. mirabilis, S. typhi, Shigella,* and *C. difficile*
What are the side effects of TMP-SMX?	1. Gastrointestinal distress 2. Allergic reactions to sulfa drugs 3. Skin rash 4. Bone marrow suppression in acquired immune deficiency syndrome (AIDS) patients 5. Macrocytic anemia in patients with low folate 6. Hemolysis in glucose-6-phosphatase deficiency (G6PD) patients 7. Kernicterus in infants secondary to increased red blood cell (RBC) turnover and possibly other mechanisms

ANTIMYCOBACTERIAL DRUGS

What four drugs are commonly used to treat tuberculosis (TB)?	1. R̲ifampin 2. I̲soniazid 3. P̲yrazinamide

4. Ethambutol
Think "RIPE" for the treatment
of tuberculosis

**Are these drugs
bactericidal or
bacteriostatic?**

All are bactericidal except for ethambutol,
which is bacteriostatic

**What is the mechanism of
action for isoniazid?**

Inhibits mycolic acid synthesis

**What are the treatment
options for active TB?**

1. 6 months treatment: 2 months of
isoniazid, rifampin, and pyrazinamide,
followed by 4 months of isoniazid and
rifampin
2. 9 months of isoniazid and rifampin

**Why is treatment with
pyrazinamide limited to
only 2 months?**

Increased risk of hepatotoxicity

**What other drugs are
hepatotoxic?**

Isoniazid and rifampin
It is important for patients not to
consume alcohol while on
treatment for tuberculosis
because of increased risk for
hepatotoxicity

**What is an additional side
effect of isoniazid?**

Peripheral neuropathy secondary to
vitamin B_6 deficiency; extensive vitamin
B_6 deficiency causes pellagra
characterized by neuropathy, rash, and
anemia

**What is a side effect of
ethambutol?**

Dose-dependent, reversible, ocular
toxicity

**When is it acceptable to
add just one medicine to a
patient's regimen when the
patient is not clinically
improving while on "RIPE"
therapy?**

Never, because resistance spreads quickly
in tuberculosis; failure to show clinical
improvement is a sign of resistance and
adding only one drug is likely to breed
multiple-resistant strains

Appendix B

Antifungal Drugs

OVERVIEW

What are fungi?

Eukaryotic organisms that have a cell membrane composed of ergosterol and a rigid cell wall composed of chitin and polysaccharides

What are fungal infections called?

Mycoses

TREATMENT OF SYSTEMIC AND SUBCUTANEOUS MYCOSES

What are two mechanisms of action for antifungals used in treating systemic and subcutaneous mycoses?

1. Alteration of cell membranes, i.e., fungicidal
2. Inhibition of replication, i.e., fungistatic

What are four drugs that alter cell membranes?

1. Amphotericin B
2. Ketoconazole
3. Fluconazole
4. Itraconazole

What drug inhibits replication?

Flucytosine (5-FC)

What type of drug is amphotericin B?

A polyene produced by *Streptomyces nodosus* that can be either fungistatic or fungicidal, depending on the organism and dosage

What is its mode of action?

Several polyene molecules bind to fungal ergosterol forming pores that allow for the efflux of potassium, as well as other electrolytes and small molecules

What type of drugs are ketoconazole, fluconazole, and itraconazole?

Azoles that can be either fungistatic or fungicidal, depending on the dosage

What is their mode of action?	Prevent synthesis of ergosterol from lanosterol by interacting with cytochrome P450 enzymes
What is the difference between the three drugs?	Ketoconazole was the first widely used azole; the latter two are newer azoles that have fewer side effects, e.g., decreased endocrinological disruption of the sexual hormone production
What type of drug is 5-FC?	A synthetic pyrimidine antimetabolite that is fungistatic
What is its mode of action?	5-FC enters the mycotic cell through a cytosine-specific enzyme not found in mammalian cells, is converted into an active form that serves as a false nucleotide, inhibits thymidylate synthetase, and deprives the cell of thymidylic acid, an essential deoxyribonucleic acid (DNA) component

TREATMENT OF SUPERFICIAL MYCOSES

What fungi cause superficial skin infections?	Dermatophytes
What are two modes of action for antifungals used in treating dermato-phytoses?	1. Alteration of cell membranes 2. Disruption of the cytoskeleton
What drugs alter cell membranes?	1. Azoles, including miconazole, clotrimazole, and econazole 2. Polyenes, including nystatin
What drugs disrupt the cytoskeleton?	Griseofulvin
What is the mode of action of azoles?	Prevent synthesis of ergosterol from lanosterol by interacting with cytochrome P450 enzymes They can be either fungistatic or fungicidal, depending on the dosage
What is the mode of action of polyene?	Several polyene molecules bind to fungal ergosterol forming pores that allow for the efflux of potassium, as well as other electrolytes and small molecules

Polyenes can be either fungistatic or fungicidal, depending on the organism and dosage

What type of drug is griseofulvin?

A fungistatic drug that accumulates in infected, newly synthesized keratin-containing tissues

What is its mode of action?

Disruption of the mitotic spindle's microtubules inhibiting mitosis

Appendix C

Antiviral Drugs

OVERVIEW

What are viruses?

Obligate intracellular parasites that lack a cell wall and/or cell membrane; they are incapable of independently performing metabolic processes and are dependent on host cells for reproduction

When do most clinically useful drugs exert their antiviral effect?

During viral replication

What type of compound are many antiviral drugs? What are they?

Antimetabolite

Compounds that are normally used by viruses but that have been altered to be toxic to the virus when activated

What are four classes of antivirals?

1. Antiinfluenza agents
2. Antiherpetic agents
3. Anti-HIV agents
4. Antiviral agents used against viral hepatitis

ANTIINFLUENZA AGENTS

What are the subtypes of influenza?

Influenza A and B

What agents are used to treat each?

Influenza A is treated with amantadine and rimantadine
Influenza A and B are treated with oseltamivir and zanamivir

What is the mechanism of action for amantadine and rimantadine?

Inhibition of the M2 viral membrane matrix protein, preventing the orthomyxovirus from binding to the host cell

What is the role of this protein?	M2 is an ion channel protein which is required for viral membrane fusion to the host cell membrane
What is the mechanism of action for oseltamivir and zanamivir? **What is the role of this enzyme?**	Inhibition of the neuraminidase (NA) enzyme preventing released progeny virions to infect new cells NA cleaves sialic (neuraminic) acid sugars from the cell surface proteins/glycolipids, preventing virion binding back to infected cells and allowing released progeny virions to infect new cells
When are antiinfluenza agents most effective?	Within 48 hours of symptom onset
Who gets an antiinfluenza agent?	The very young, the very old, and the immunocompromised

ANTIHERPETIC AGENTS

What herpes viruses are effectively treated with antiherpetic agents?	1. Herpes simplex virus (HSV) 2. Cytomegalovirus (CMV) 3. Varicella-zoster virus (VZV)
What is the first-line agent used to treat each?	HSV is treated with acyclovir CMV is treated with ganciclovir or foscarnet VZV is treated with acyclovir
What is acyclovir? **What is its mechanism of action?**	Acyclovir is a guanosine analog Acyclovir is activated by a viral kinase specific to HSV and VZV creating a competitive substrate for deoxyribonucleic acid (DNA) polymerase leading to nucleic acid chain termination
What is it used for?	HSV and VZV
What are three antiviral agents that have similar characteristics to acyclovir?	Famciclovir, valacyclovir, and penciclovir
What is the mechanism of action of foscarnet?	Foscarnet reversibly inhibits viral DNA and ribonucleic acid (RNA) polymerases and HIV reverse transcriptase
What is it used for?	CMV retinitis

What is the mechanism of action of ganciclovir?	Ganciclovir is a guanine derivative that is phosphorylated to form a nucleotide that inhibits CMV and HSV DNA polymerases without causing chain termination
What is it used for?	CMV prophylaxis and treatment
What is the mechanism of action of cidofovir?	Cidofovir is activated by *host cell kinases* and inhibits the DNA polymerases of HSV, CMV, adenovirus, and papillomavirus
What is it used for?	CMV retinitis

ANTIHUMAN IMMUNODEFICIENCY VIRUS AGENTS

What are three categories of anti-HIV agents?	1. Nucleoside reverse transcriptase inhibitors (NRTIs) 2. Nonnucleoside reverse transcriptase inhibitors (NNRTIs) 3. Protease inhibitors
What are NRTIs?	Agents that are phosphorylated by host cell kinases that terminate and/or inhibit reverse transcriptase
What are some examples?	Lamivudine, stavudine, zalcitabine, zidovudine, didanosine, and abacavir
What are NNRTIs?	Agents that bind to a site on reverse transcriptase that is different than the NRTI's and inhibit the action of reverse transcriptase
What are some examples?	Delavirdine, efavirenz, and nevirapine
What are protease inhibitors?	Agents that inhibit HIV-1 protease preventing cleavage of viral precursors creating uncleaved, nonfunctional proteins
What are some examples?	Indinavir, nelfinavir, ritonavir, saquinavir, and amprenavir
How are anti-HIV agents administered when treating HIV?	As a "cocktail," i.e., a combination of drug classes to minimize the development of resistance and to maximize the antimetabolite action of the drugs

ANTIVIRAL AGENTS USED AGAINST VIRAL HEPATITIS

What are two agents used to treat viral hepatitis?

1. Interferon-α
2. Lamivudine

Which one is approved for use in pregnancy?

Interferon-α

What is the mechanism of action for interferon-α?

Interferon-α has multiple actions that impede viral RNA and DNA synthesis, e.g., activation of protein kinase RNA-dependent (PKR) 2-5A synthetase and inducing apoptosis

Appendix D

Antiparasitic Drugs

ANTIHELMINTIC DRUGS

What drugs paralyze helminths by each of the following mechanisms: Inhibiting microtubule synthesis?	1. Mebendazole 2. Thiabendazole 3. Albendazole
Producing persistent nicotinic (depolarizing) stimulation?	Pyrantel pamoate
Increasing calcium permeability, resulting in a loss of calcium in the helminth?	Praziquantel
What drug kills helminths by opening chloride channels, resulting in an influx of chloride ions in the helminth?	Ivermectin
What drug induces changes to the microfilarial surface, making the parasite more susceptible to the host's defenses?	Diethylcarbamazine
What adverse reaction can this drug cause?	Mazzotti reaction, characterized by pruritus, fever, hypotension, and facial edema in Onchocerca infections
What drug inhibits oxidative phosphorylation in helminths, thus preventing adenosine triphosphate (ATP) formation?	Niclosamide

CESTODES

What are five common cestodes that can infect humans?	1. *Taenia solium* 2. *Taenia saginata* 3. *Hymenolepis nana* 4. *Echinococcus* 5. *Diphyllobothrium latum*
Name the drug that corresponds to each of the following: **The first-line treatment for *T. solium*, *T. saginata*, *H. nana*, and *D. latum*?**	Praziquantel
The second-line treatment for *T. solium*, *T. saginata*, *H. nana*, and *D. latum*?	Niclosamide
Used to treat *Echinococcus*?	Albendazole (with possible surgical excision or aspiration of cysts)

NEMATODES

Intestinal Nematodes

What are six intestinal nematodes that can infect humans?	1. *Enterobius vermicularis* 2. *Trichuris trichiura* 3. *Ascaris lumbricoides* 4. *Strongyloides stercoralis* 5. *Necator americanus* 6. *Ancylostoma duodenale*
What drug is used to treat each of the following: **E. vermicularis, A. lumbricoides, N. americanus, and A. duodenale?**	Mebendazole or pyrantel pamoate
T. trichiura?	Mebendazole
S. stercoralis?	Thiabendazole

Tissue Nematodes

What are six tissue nematodes that can infect humans?	1. *Trichinella spiralis* 2. *Brugia malayi* 3. *Wuchereria bancrofti* 4. *Loa Loa* 5. *Onchocerca volvulus* 6. *Toxocara canis*
What drug is used to treat each of the following: ***T. spiralis?***	Thiabendazole (effective against adult worms in early stages of infection)
B. malayi. W. bancrofti, **and *L. loa?***	Diethylcarbamazine
O. volvulus?	Ivermectin
T. canis?	Diethylcarbamazine

TREMATODES

What are six trematodes that can infect humans?	1. *Schistosoma* species 2. *Clonorchis sinensis* 3. *Paragonimus westermani* 4. *Fasciola hepatica* 5. *Fasciolopsis buski* 6. *Heterophyes heterophyes*
What drug is used to treat these trematode infections?	Praziquantel

ANTIPROTOZOAL DRUGS

INTESTINAL PROTOZOA

What are six intestinal protozoa that can infect humans?	1. *Entamoeba histolytica* 2. *Giardia lamblia* 3. *Cryptosporidium parvum* 4. *Isospora belli* 5. *Cyclospora cayetanensis* 6. *Balantidium coli*
What drugs are used to treat *E. histolytica* infections?	Metronidazole followed by iodoquinol

How does metronidazole work?

Selectively forms cytotoxic compounds in parasites and anaerobic organisms by serving as an electron acceptor

What is the treatment for each of the following:
G. lamblia?

Metronidazole

C. parvum?

No effective drug therapy

I. belli and C. cayetanensis?

Trimethoprim-sulfamethoxazole

B. coli?

Tetracycline

How does trimethoprim-sulfamethoxazole work?

Synergy between these two drugs inhibits the formation of tetrahydrofolate (which is not found in human cells), thereby inhibiting DNA synthesis in the parasite

UROGENITAL PROTOZOA

What is the major pathogenic urogenital protozoan?

Trichomonas vaginalis

What is the treatment?

Metronidazole for all partners

BLOOD AND TISSUE PROTOZOA

What are seven blood and tissue protozoa that can infect humans?

1. *Naegleria fowleri*
2. *Acanthamoeba* species
3. *Leishmania* species
4. *Trypanosoma* species
5. *Plasmodium* species
6. *Toxoplasma gondii*
7. *Babesia microti*

What is the treatment for each of the following:
N. fowleri?

Amphotericin B

Acanthamoeba species?

Ophthalmic solution: topical 0.1% propamidine isethionate plus neomycin-polymyxin B-gramicidin

Leishmania species?	Sodium stibogluconate
Trypanosoma rhodesiense and *Trypanosoma gambiense*?	Suramin ± melarsoprol (for central nervous system [CNS] infection)
Trypanosoma cruzi?	Nifurtimox
T. gondii?	Sulfadiazine and pyrimethamine
B. microti?	Quinine and clindamycin

ANTIMALARIALS

What drug is used as prophylaxis against malaria in areas where there is no resistance?

Chloroquine

Why is it ineffective as a single treatment against *Plasmodium vivax* and *Plasmodium ovale*?

Chloroquine only kills erythrocytic forms of *Plasmodium* and will not kill the liver hypnozoites present in *P. vivax* and *P. ovale* infections

What drugs are used as prophylaxis against malaria when the strains are resistant to chloroquine?

1. Mefloquine
2. Doxycycline
3. Atovaquone-proguanil

What is the treatment for *P. ovale* and *P. vivax*?

Chloroquine and primaquine (to kill hypnozoites)

What is the treatment for *Plasmodium malariae* and nonresistant *Plasmodium falciparum*?

Chloroquine

What is the treatment for chloroquine-resistant *P. falciparum*?

1. Quinine and pyrimethamine-sulfadoxine
2. Mefloquine
3. Atovaquone-proguanil
4. Artemether

What is an adverse reaction seen with chloroquine, quinine, and primaquine?

Acute hemolytic anemia in patients with glucose-6-phosphate dehydrogenase (G6PD) deficiency

What is the name for the constellation of symptoms that can occur as a side effect with quinine treatment?

Cinchonism, which is characterized by headache, fever, nausea, vomiting, diarrhea, vertigo, tinnitus, and visual disturbances

Appendix E

Diagnostic Techniques Used in Microbiology

STAINS USED TO
IDENTIFY BACTERIA, FUNGI, AND PARASITES

What is a stain?

A dye used in histologic and bacteriologic techniques

Define each of the following:

Acid-fast Ziehl-Neelsen stain?

Staining technique that denotes bacteria that resist decolorization with hydrochloric acid while non–acid-fast bacteria are successfully counterstained with methylene blue
Used to identify *Mycobacteria* spp.

Hematoxylin and eosin stain?

Stain for tissues whereby nuclei are stained deep blue or black and the cytoplasm is stained pink
Used to identify Rickettsiae, protozoa, and helminths

India ink stain?

Staining technique, Gram crystal violet, that indirectly denotes organism capsules based on lack of stain uptake, resulting in clear-appearing capsule against a dark background
Used to identify *Cryptococcus neoformans* and *Streptococcus pneumoniae*

Gram stain?

Method for differential staining organisms by smearing on a slide, heat fixing, staining with crystal violet, treating with iodine solution, rinsing, decolorizing. and then counterstaining them with safranin O
Gram-positive organisms appear purple
Gram-negative organisms appear pink
Used to identify bacteria

Periodic-acid Schiff (PAS) stain?

Method for staining tissues rich in polysaccharides, which entails periodic acid oxidization of polysaccharide aldehyde groups, which then react with the Schiff stain resulting in red or violet coloration of glycogen, basement membranes, etc.

Potassium hydroxide?

Strongly basic liquid that breaks down cells, revealing the rigid chitin/ polysaccharide fungal cell walls
Used to identify fungi

Wright Giemsa stain?

Compound of methylene blue and eosin for demonstrating intracellular organisms
Used to identify *Chlamydia, Borrelia, Trypanosoma* spp., *Leishmaniasis* spp., *Plasmodium* spp. *Toxoplasma gondii, Babesia microti,* and *Histoplasma*

IMMUNOLOGIC (SEROLOGIC) ASSAYS

What is an immunologic (serologic) assay?

Technique whereby a substance being investigated serves as an antigen and an added substance serves as an antibody

Define each of the following:
Counterimmunoelectro-phoresis?

Immunologic (serologic) assay whereby an unknown antigen is applied to a gel near the cathode and a known antibody, e.g., antiserum, is placed opposite near the anode
With the addition of an electric field, the two substances migrate and the maximum amount of complex precipitation occurs when the concentration of the antigen and matching antibody are equivalent
Used to identify circulating antigens in those infected with *Haemophilus influenzae, Neisseria meningitidis, S. pneumoniae,* and *Streptococcus agalactiae* (GBS)

Enzyme-linked immunosorbent assay (ELISA)?

Rapid immunologic (serologic) assay whereby an enzyme covalently linked to an antigen or antibody is added to a solution

When the enzyme that is covalently linked to an antigen or antibody binds to its substrate, a reaction occurs that can be visualized, quantified, etc.

Used to identify circulating bacterial, fungal, parasitic antigens or viruses

Immunofluorescence?

Immunologic (serologic) assay whereby an antibody to the target is applied, specimen is washed, an antibody labeled with a fluorescent molecule that is specific to the antibody bound to the target is applied, and specimen is washed; target is identified if it shows fluorescence

Used to identify *Borrelia burgdorferi*, *Rickettsia* spp., *Bordetella pertussis*, *Chlamydia trachomatis*, *H. influenzae*, *N. meningitidis*, *S. pneumoniae*, *Streptococcus pyogenes* (GAS), *S. agalactiae* (GBS), *Legionella*, *Giardia*, *Cryptosporidium*, and *Entamoeba histolytica*

Latex agglutination?

Immunologic (serologic) assay whereby the antibody is bound to latex particles and the substance being investigated is suspended and exposed to the latex particles

Used to identify *H. influenzae*, *N. meningitidis*, *S. pneumoniae*, *S. pyogenes* (GAS), *S. agalactiae* (GBS), *Trichomoniasis*, *Clostridium difficile*, and *Cryptococcus*

Radioimmunoassay?

Immunologic (serologic) assay that uses the principle of competitive antibody/antigen binding between the substance being investigated (antigen) and a radioactive homologous antigen

The mixture of antibody–antigen complexes is then quantified with a scintillation counter

Used to identify *Legionella* and *Histoplasma*

Quellung reaction?

Example of an immunologic (serologic) assay whereby the bacterial capsule

"swells" when mixed with specific antibodies and is visualized with India ink (see color photo 3)
Used to identify *S. pneumoniae*, but other capsular organisms can be seen with this assay

AGARS AND CULTURE MEDIUM

What is agar?

A polysaccharide derived from seaweed used in the preparation of culture medium

Describe the type of culture medium for each of the following:
Bordet-Gengou agar?

Agar containing glycerin, potato, and blood

Chocolate agar?

Agar that contains blood that is heated until cells breakdown, becoming brown or "chocolate" in appearance

Löwenstein-Jensen agar?

Agar containing eggs

Loeffler agar?

Agar containing beef products and eggs

MacConkey agar?

Agar containing bile salts, peptone, and red and violet dyes

Sabouraud agar?

Agar containing peptones and sugar

Tellurite agar?

Agar containing elemental tellurite

Thayer-Martin (VCN) agar?

Agar containing beef products, peptones starch, sheep blood, and antibiotics

What organisms are selectively isolated with each of the following:
Bordet-Gengou agar?

B. pertussis

Chocolate agar with nicotinamide adenine dinucleotide (NAD) and hematin (factors V and X)?

H. influenzae

Löwenstein-Jensen agar?	*Mycobacterium tuberculosis*
Loeffler agar?	*C. diphtheriae*
MacConkey agar?	Distinguishes between lactose-fermenting gram-negative organisms whereby lactose fermenters, e.g., *Escherichia coli, Klebsiella*, and *Enterobacter*, have red colonies and nonfermentors, e.g. *Salmonella, Shigella*, and *Proteus* appear colorless
Sabouraud agar?	Fungi
Tellurite agar?	*C. diphtheriae*
Thayer-Martin (VCN) agar?	*N. gonorrhoeae*

DIAGNOSTIC TECHNIQUES USED TO IDENTIFY VIRUSES

What are five techniques used to identify viruses?	1. Cytology 2. Molecular biological techniques 3. Cultures 4. Detection of viral antigens 5. Immunologic (serologic) assays
What is cytology?	Technique by which cells are visualized microscopically
What is an example of a commonly used cytologic technique?	Papanicolaou smear, also known as the Pap smear
How is cytology used to identify viruses?	Cells infected by virus have characteristic inclusion bodies
What is an example of such a finding?	Negri bodies, are intracellular inclusions found with rabies infection (see color photo 21)
What are three molecular biological techniques used to identify viruses?	1. Polymerase chain reaction (PCR) 2. Blots, e.g., Western blots 3. Enzyme-linked immunosorbent assay (ELISA)

What is PCR?

Technique used to synthesize many copies of deoxyribonucleic acid (DNA) from a small amount of original DNA

How does PCR work?

1. DNA is subject to heat, resulting in the dissolution of the double helix, i.e., denatured
2. Short-chain primers, nucleotides, and heat-stable DNA polymerases are added
3. DNA is allowed to cool
4. Primers anneal to the denatured DNA with heat-stable DNA polymerases
5. Formation of a new double strand by DNA polymerase using primers as starting points and nucleotides as reagents
   This process is repeated several times, resulting in an exponential increase in DNA

What are the advantages of PCR?

Technique is highly specific and sensitive, requires no culture, and is unaffected by previous administration of antibiotics

What are four types of blotting techniques (interactions)?

1. Southern blot (DNA to DNA)
2. Northern blot (DNA to ribonucleic acid [RNA])
3. Western blot (antibody to protein)
4. Southwestern (DNA to protein)

What steps are involved with each of the following:
Southern blot?

1. DNA sample is run on a gel electrophoresis
2. Samples in gel are transferred to a filter paper
3. Filter is exposed to a radioactive single-strand deoxyribonucleic acid (ssDNA) probe, which is complementary to a sequence on the original strand, and binds to it
4. Filter is exposed to film allowing for visualization of the DNA probe/sample hybrid

Northern blot?

1. RNA sample is run on a gel electrophoresis
2. Samples in gel are transferred to a filter
3. Filter is exposed to a radioactive ssDNA probe, which binds to part of the original protein sample
4. Filter is exposed to film allowing for visualization of the RNA/DNA probe hybrid

Western blot?

1. Protein sample is run on a gel electrophoresis
2. Samples in gel are transferred to a filter
3. Filter is exposed to a radioactive antibody probe (protein), which binds to a part of the original protein
4. Filter is exposed to film allowing for visualization of the protein sample/antibody hybrid

Southwestern blot?

1. Protein sample run on a gel electrophoresis
2. Samples in gel are transferred to a filter
3. Filter is exposed to a radioactive DNA probe, which binds to part of the original protein sample
4. Filter is exposed to film allowing for visualization of the DNA probe/protein hybrid

Appendix F

Vaccines

OVERVIEW

What are the two types of immunity?

Passive and active

PASSIVE IMMUNITY

What is passive immunity?

Immunity that is conferred by receiving preformed antibodies (immuno-globulins)

When is passive immunization desired?

When exposure to the pathogen has already occurred in someone that lacks active immunity

Why?

To initiate a rapid immune response in those that would otherwise not mount a rapid response

Does passive immunization activate the immune system?

No

Does passive immunization create a memory response?

No

How quickly does passive immunity act?

Immediately

What types of antibodies are used to provide passive immunity?

IgG

What are the major risks of using equine immunoglobulins in passive immunization?

Anaphylaxis and serum sickness, especially following high doses or second exposures

What are examples of pathogens against which human immunoglobulins are available for passive immunity?	Hepatitis A, hepatitis B, rabies, varicella-zoster virus (chickenpox), *Clostridium tetani* (tetanus), *Clostridium botulinum* (botulism), *Corynebacterium diphtheriae* (diphtheria)

ACTIVE IMMUNITY

What is active immunity?	Immunity that is conferred by exposure to pathogens, modified pathogens, or their products
Does active immunization activate the immune system?	Yes
Does active immunization create a memory response?	Yes
How quickly does active immunity act?	Over days to months
What are the different formulations of vaccines that provide active immunization?	1. Live-attenuated vaccines 2. Killed vaccines 3. Microbial extracts 4. Vaccine conjugates 5. Inactivated toxins (toxoids)
What are live-attenuated vaccines?	Weakened live organisms that are used to create an effective immune response yet aim to eliminate the clinical consequences of infection with the live organism
Can the organisms contained in these vaccines multiply within the host?	Yes
What is the benefit of live-attenuated vaccines?	They induce a more robust and long-lasting immune response than does vaccination with killed organisms
What type of an immune response is elicited by live-attenuated vaccines?	Cytotoxic T-cell response
For what type of pathogen is this response effective?	Intracellular organisms, including viruses

What is the greatest risk of giving live-attenuated vaccines?

Reversion to pathogenicity

In what group of individuals should live-attenuated vaccines not be used? Why?

Immunocompromised individuals, as well as those in close contact with immunocompromised individuals

Reversion to pathogenicity occurs at in increased rate in immunocompromised individuals

What are the advantages of killed vaccines?

There is no risk of vaccine causing an infection

What are the disadvantages of killed vaccines?

They often provide only a short-term immune response

What molecules are most commonly used in creating vaccines from microbial extracts?

Surface antigens

What is the purpose of conjugating capsular polysaccharides to a protein antigen?

To enable the recipient to produce a strong T-cell–dependent antibody response
Without conjugation, the poly-saccharide only mounts a weak T-cell–independent antibody response

Which protein antigen is commonly used in conjugation?

Diphtheria toxoid

Which conjugated vaccines may be administered to children younger than age 18 months?

The vaccines for *Haemophilus influenzae*, *Streptococcus pneumoniae*, and *Neisseria meningitidis*

What type of immune response do vaccines containing killed pathogens or antigenic components of pathogens elicit?
For what type of pathogen is this response effective?

B-cell–mediated humoral response

Extracellular organisms

What are toxoid vaccines?	Vaccines using harmless or chemically altered natural exotoxins to create an immune response
What is an adjuvant?	A substance injected along with an antigen that serves to enhance the immunogenicity of the antigen
What is a commonly used adjuvant?	Aluminum hydroxide

COMMON BACTERIAL VACCINES

What does the DTaP vaccine target?

1. *C. diphtheriae*
2. *C. tetani*
3. *Bordetella pertussis*

What does the DTaP vaccine contain?

1. <u>D</u>iphtheria toxoid
2. <u>T</u>etanus toxoid
3. <u>A</u>cellular <u>P</u>ertussis vaccine containing purified proteins

What vaccines are available for *B. pertussis*?

An acellular vaccine containing purified proteins has replaced the vaccine containing killed bacteria

What is the target of the pneumococcal vaccine?

S. pneumoniae

What are the two types of pneumococcal vaccine?

1. Pneumococcal polysaccharide vaccine (which contains 23 serotypes)—Pneumovax
2. Pneumococcal polysaccharide-protein conjugate vaccine (which contains 7 serotypes conjugated to diphtheria toxoid)—Prevnar

For whom is the pneumococcal polysaccharide vaccine recommended?

Adults older than age 60 years

For whom is the pneumococcal polysaccharide-protein conjugate vaccine recommended?

Infants up to age 24 months

What vaccine must individuals receive after splenectomy?	S. *pneumoniae* vaccine
Why?	Asplenic patients have a poor ability to clear encapsulated organisms
What does the vaccine for N. *meningitidis* contain?	Capsular polysaccharides of 4 different serotypes: A, C, W135, and Y
Who should receive the N. *meningitidis* vaccine?	College students living in dormitories, military recruits, and travelers visiting endemic areas
What does the vaccine for H. *influenzae* contain?	Type b polysaccharide conjugated to diphtheria toxoid or other carrier protein

BACTERIAL VACCINES USED IN SPECIAL SITUATIONS

What type of vaccine is used for Lyme disease?	A noninfectious recombinant vaccine
What does the vaccine for Lyme disease contain?	Lipoprotein OspA, an outer surface protein of *Borrelia burgdorferi*
How does the vaccine for Lyme disease work?	When a tick bites and ingests the blood of an immunized individual, antibodies in the blood kill *B. burgdorferi* species inside the tick
What type of vaccine(s) is (are) available for each of the following:	
Typhoid fever?	1. Vaccine containing the polysaccharide capsule of *Salmonella typhi* 2. Vaccine containing live-attenuated *S. typhi* 3. Vaccine containing killed *S. typhi*
Cholera?	Vaccine containing killed *Vibrio cholerae*
Plague?	Vaccine containing killed *Yersinia pestis*
Anthrax?	Vaccine containing "protective antigen" purified from the organism
Tuberculosis?	Bacille Calmette-Guérin (BCG), a vaccine containing live-attenuated *Mycobacterium bovis*

Tularemia?	Vaccine containing live-attenuated *Francisella tularensis*
Typhus?	Vaccine containing killed *Rickettsia prowazekii*
Q fever?	Vaccine containing killed *Coxiella burnetii*

COMMON VIRAL VACCINES

What is the MMR vaccine?	A combination vaccine against measles, mumps, and rubella
What type of vaccine is the MMR?	Vaccine containing live-attenuated viruses from all three strains
Who should receive the MMR vaccine?	Young children prior to entering school
What type of vaccine is given for varicella-zoster?	A live-attenuated, temperature-sensitive vaccine
What is the traditional vaccine given for influenza?	A killed vaccine
What is a newer method for influenza vaccination?	A new live-attenuated vaccine has been developed for intranasal administration
How often must the influenza vaccine be administered to be effective?	The vaccine should be given annually
Why must the influenza vaccine be given annually? What is this?	To cover for the newer strains of influenza that have undergone antigenic drift A process whereby minor antigenic changes in outer viral proteins allow the organism to evade previously formed host antibodies
Who should receive the influenza vaccine?	Adults older than age 65 years and health care staff
Who should not receive the influenza vaccine?	Those with hypersensitivity to any components of the vaccine (egg), with active influenza infection, or who are pregnant and in their first trimester

What are the two types of vaccines for polio?	1. Killed poliovirus vaccine (Sa<u>l</u>k) 2. Live-attenuated poliovirus vaccine (Sabin) Sa<u>l</u>k is a <u>k</u>illed vaccine
What are the advantages of the Salk vaccine?	Because the vaccine contains killed virus, it cannot cause poliomyelitis, and is safer for use in the immunocompromised
What are the disadvantages of the Salk vaccine?	1. Administration is by injection only 2. It provides less gastrointestinal (GI) immunity, increasing the risk of asymptomatic GI infection, which could be spread to other people
What are the advantages of the Sabin vaccine?	1. It may be administered orally 2. Provides better GI immunity 3. 95% of people respond to a 3-dose course with life-long immunity
What are the disadvantages of the Sabin vaccine?	1. There is a small risk of infection (1 in 2.4 million doses) 2. It cannot be administered to the immunocompromised
What is the current recommendation for polio vaccination?	The Salk vaccine is exclusively used in the United States
What type of vaccine is available for hepatitis A?	Killed virus
Why is the hepatitis A vaccine not recommended for children less than 2?	Residual antihepatitis A virus (anti-HAV) (antibody) acquired from the mother may interfere with the vaccine
What type of vaccine is available for hepatitis B?	A vaccine containing recombinant hepatitis B surface antigen

VIRAL VACCINES USED IN SPECIAL SITUATIONS

What type of vaccine is available for each of the following: **Rotavirus?**	Live-attenuated virus (which is not currently used in children because of concerns with intussusception)

Rabies?	Killed virus
Yellow fever?	Live-attenuated virus
Japanese encephalitis?	Killed virus
Adenovirus?	Live-attenuated virus; each of the 3 current vaccines is effective against only one serotype
Smallpox?	Live-attenuated vaccinia virus
Why was the smallpox vaccine successful in eradicating the disease?	1. Smallpox virus has only one stable serotype 2. Humans are the only host and there is no animal reservoir 3. Antibody response is prompt 4. Disease is easily recognized clinically 5. There is no carrier state 6. Most infected people are symptomatic

Index

Page numbers in *italics* denote figures; those followed by t denote tables.